AGE ERASING SECRETS

500 Fast and Easy Ways to Look Younger and Feel Great

KEVIN IRELAND

BARNES & NOBLE BOOKS
NEW YORK

Notice

The information in this book has been carefully researched, and all efforts have been made to ensure accuracy. Rodale Inc. and Barnes & Noble, Inc. assume no responsibility for any injuries suffered or damages or losses incurred during or as a result of following this information. All information should be carefully studied and clearly understood before taking any action based on the information or advice in this book.

Material in this book appeared previously in *Age Erasers for Men* (Rodale, 1994), *Age Erasers for Women* (Rodale, 1994), *The Doctors Book of Food Remedies* (Rodale, 1998), *The Doctors Book of Home Remedies for Preventing Disease* (Rodale, 1999), *The Doctors Book of Home Remedies for Seniors* (Rodale, 1999), *Growing Younger* (Rodale, 1999), *Healing with Vitamins* (Rodale, 1996), *Nature's Medicines* (Rodale, 1999), and *Seniors Guide to Pain-Free Living* (Rodale, 2000).

This edition published by Barnes & Noble, Inc., by arrangement with Rodale Inc.

Printed in the United States of America
Rodale Inc. makes every effort to use acid-free ∞, recycled paper ♻.

Cover Designer: Joanna Williams
Interior Designer: Christopher Rhoads

ISBN 0–7607–3371–6

2 4 6 8 10 9 7 5 3   paperback

CONTENTS

INTRODUCTION

You've probably heard the old saying that "Getting old is tough, but it sure beats the alternative." Well, that's true enough, but here's a corollary worth considering: Getting older doesn't have to be *that* tough, nor is it inevitable that you'll face a gradual physical and mental decline along the way.

There's no such thing as an "aging process." There aren't any rules that say you'll have trouble walking at this age or lose your memory skills at that age. Sure, we all know people who seem to begin a rapid slide downhill in their fifties, but if you think about it, you probably also know people in their seventies and eighties who have tremendous energy and enthusiasm—women and men who are in great shape, not just "for their age," but for any age.

Theories about aging are changing rapidly as scientists learn more about human potential. One thing already is quite clear from their studies: Aging is inevitable—there's no way to stop the clock—but a gradual decline in good health and good looks isn't. In fact, many of the problems we blame on aging really have nothing to do with aging. Memory problems, deep wrinkles, diminished strength and vitality, waning sexual desire. None of these is the natural side effect of reaching the age of 40, 50, 60, or 70 years old. Rather, they're often tied to things like poor diet, a lack of exercise, stress, bad reactions to medications, and too much exposure to the sun. You can control each of these things.

Yes, it's true; you can lead the pack, staying strong and active well past middle age. Or, you can fall into line with those who accept the notion that aging and decline are inseparable. But make no mistake, you have a choice: You can take an active role and hold on to your looks, your vitality, and your sexuality, or you can let a little bit of each slip away with each birthday.

The earlier you start wrestling with the hands of time, the better. The problems that lead to aging are cumulative, and the sooner you start correcting them, the more likely you'll be to control them in the long run.

But that doesn't mean you should give up if you're well into middle age and you've been lax about your health up to now. It's never too late to rev up your anti-aging forces. In fact, a study at Tufts University in Medford, Massachusetts, showed that people in their nineties were able to increase their leg strength by as much as 200 percent when they started lifting weights.

If they can do it, so can you.

Inside the pages of this book, you'll find the advice you need to redefine your personal agenda for the coming years and change your thinking about what it means to age in the new millennium. You'll discover all you need to know to combat the forces that can make you look and feel older than you are—not just facts but practical, simple steps you can take right now to start turning back the clock.

If you're ready to take an active role in your future health, read on. And if you need a quote to live by, forget that stuff about aging being tough. Here's a better thought from noted anthropologist Ashley Montague: "The goal of life is to die young—as late as possible."

Part 1
Aging and the Age Erasers

THE ONSLAUGHT OF FATHER TIME

Make the Years Treat You Right

Pepper Herman plays killer golf, drives a sports car, and zips back and forth between her home in Charlottesville, Virginia, and voice-over jobs for ad agencies in Wilmington, Delaware, and Philadelphia.

Her hair is long and dark. Her skin is smooth. People tell her that she looks a lot like Cher.

Oh, and one other thing: Pepper Herman is 60.

Back in her thirties and forties, Herman started to create the vibrant, energetic woman she is today. You can do that, too.

The Real Age Makers

Aging today is not like it was for our parents.

Lots of us had mothers and fathers who put on an extra 10 pounds at age 30. They got wrinkles at 35, dry skin at 40, joint stiffness at 45, high cholesterol at 50, heart disease at 55, memory loss at 57, and osteoporosis at 60.

We don't have to.

Why?

Because today we know that a low-fat diet prevents the weight gains and increases in cholesterol associated with aging.

We know that staying out of the sun and using sunscreen prevents the proliferation of wrinkles.

We know that alpha-hydroxy acids—acids found in fruit and milk—prevent baggy skin and the dry, patchy skin that comes with age spots.

We know that exercise—particularly water aerobics and swimming—delays the onset of arthritis.

We know that aerobic exercise, a low-fat diet, aspirin, and relaxation exercises prevent the progression that leads to clogged arteries and heart disease.

We know that working crossword puzzles and reading the op-ed section of a newspaper can counteract the memory loss that results from an aging brain.

And we know that weight-bearing exercise and getting enough calcium can prevent our bones from thinning, which leads to osteoporosis.

In other words, we know that although overweight, wrinkles, dry skin, arthritis, high cholesterol, heart disease, memory loss, osteoporosis, and a whole host of other things could rob us of our youth, the real age maker is not physical: It's the mindset that allows us to veg out in front of the television, eat high-fat foods, smoke, skip vegetables, bake in the sun, and forget to play and challenge ourselves.

Aging, for the most part, is what we do to ourselves.

The Biology of Aging

"The human body is designed to last 110 years," says Ben Douglas, Ph.D., professor of anatomy at the University of Mississippi Medical Center in Jackson and author of *AgeLess: Living Younger Longer.* "Just like other members of the animal kingdom, our bodies are designed to last roughly five times the age of when we reach our sexual maturity. And with proper care, we should."

So what is it about aging that stops us? Let's take a look at our bodies, keeping in mind that much of what we call aging can be overcome.

Skin. In your twenties, accumulated sun damage may cause skin across your forehead to wrinkle. In your thirties, it may wrinkle between your eyes. By age 40, crow's-feet appear and by age 50, wrinkles will have started at the corners of your mouth. Your skin will grow thinner, drier, and less elastic with time—mostly because of a dwindling supply of connective tissue and hormones that begins in the forties.

Cardiovascular system. After age 25, there's a small but steady decline in your cardiovascular system's ability to deliver oxygenated blood throughout your body during exercise. Typically, a person's aerobic capacity drops 5 to 10 percent a decade between the ages of 25 and 75, which, as a practical matter, means that you get winded easier as you get older. The heart itself shrinks and beats at a slower rate. Blood vessels narrow and become less flexible. Systolic blood pressure—the top number on a blood pressure reading—increases about 20 to 30 percent between the ages of 30 and 70.

Muscles. After the age of 45 or so, your muscles begin to shrink as fat deposits expand. Muscle strength declines approximately 30 percent between the twenties and seventies, while muscle mass declines up to 40 percent.

Bones. Minerals—particularly calcium—are constantly being added and withdrawn from your bones throughout life. Deposits exceed withdrawals until around age 35. After that, there's a steady decline in bone strength and density. This particularly is an issue for women. Partly because women's skeletons are smaller than men's to begin with, and partly because hormonal changes after menopause accelerate bone loss, women are more likely to develop osteoporosis. For women, the risk of hip fractures starts to increase in the forties, then doubles every 6 years thereafter. In fact, researchers estimate that a woman is likely to have lost 30 percent of her peak bone mass by the time she's 70—making her increasingly prone to breaks.

Joints. A little stiffness in the knees, hips, and neck begins somewhere in the forties. It gradually gets worse until your doctor diagnoses it as arthritis somewhere in your sixties. The disks between your vertebrae begin to degenerate and your spine stiffens somewhere in your seventies.

Metabolism. Starting around age 20, your body's engine starts to slow down. This means the number of calories your body needs gradually declines. By the time you're 70, you need 500 fewer calories a day.

Brain. We start life with a fixed number of neurons designed to provide a lifetime of service. Although we lose some nerve cells throughout life, in the absence of any disease, nerve cells function, repair, regenerate, and make new connections during our entire lives. So what causes senility? Most of what we think of as senile behavior in older folks is caused by disease—not the loss of neurons.

Immune system. After age 60, the gradual decline in the immune system makes us more vulnerable to infection. If there's a bug around, we're more likely to get it.

Cholesterol. The amount of cholesterol in our blood—which is generated by the liver from saturated fats and cholesterol in our diet—tends to increase with age. It generally reaches a peak between the ages of 60 and 70 for women, about a decade earlier for men.

Hair. After age 30, if you're a man who is susceptible to male pattern baldness, you will start to lose hair. By age 50, man or woman, you're likely to have some gray hair. If you're a woman, after menopause there's a chance that you will have increased facial hair.

Eyes. When you start holding the newspaper at arm's length somewhere in your early forties, the lens in your eye is losing its elasticity, making it less able to focus on close objects or shift from near to far. By age 65, you may begin to develop cataracts and by age 80, you may need three times as much light to see as clearly as you do now.

Ears. Your ability to hear begins to decline in your sixties if you're a woman. For men, the decline moves at a faster pace.

Nose. Your ability to smell declines gradually after age 45.

Mouth. Your ability to sense subtle distinctions between flavors is reduced as the number of tastebuds on your tongue declines.

The Age Erasers

Despite what you've just read, very little of what we call aging has to happen. Somewhere around age 40, for instance, Pepper Herman realized that if she wanted to maintain her youthful body and energetic personality into her

Why Men Die Younger

When it comes to longevity, women may be tougher than men from the moment of conception.

The reason remains a mystery, scientists say. But they note that although 170 male embryos develop for every 100 female embryos, only 106 boys are actually born for every 100 girls.

More baby boys also die during infancy and childhood, so that by the time reproductive hormones start to flow during adolescence, the ratio of boys to girls is roughly one to one.

After that, the guys seem intent on leaving the planet. They are twice as likely to die from an unintentional injury as women and nearly three times as likely to die from suicide or murder.

Part of the reason for the early demise of so many men is the social expectations that encourage men to perform hazardous jobs, experts say. That's why men are 29 times more likely than women to fall to their deaths from a ladder, 23 times more likely to get killed by machinery, or nearly 20 times more likely to be electrocuted.

Of course, as women gain more opportunities in the workplace, they'll probably also have an equal opportunity to be smashed, mangled, and zapped, so it's a good bet, experts say, that the discrepancies in death rates between men and women that are related to occupation will vanish.

sixties and seventies, she'd better develop a battle plan to fight off the encroachment of age.

Herman approached it in her usual way: She talked to her friends, visited doctors, and read everything she could get her hands on about maintaining a healthy body. Then she experimented to find what was right for her.

She started on an eating regimen that included beans, brown rice, broccoli, miso soup, and rice cakes along with tomatoes, green peppers, and chicken.

The diet was so successful that it made her look and feel about 10 years younger. "My cholesterol dropped from 300 to 167 and I lost weight," she admits. "But I didn't exercise, so my build still wasn't good."

Finally a friend dragged her to an aerobics class that was simultaneously trying to build "buns of steel," "super abs," and "power pecs." "It was awful," says Herman. "They all looked like movie stars, and I couldn't keep up. I could only do a quarter of what they did."

Exhausted, Herman decided that she might need exercise but not to that degree of intensity. "I found a local exercise class in which I felt more comfortable and went twice a week," she says. "I also started walking with my sister-in-law and playing golf."

"I started losing more weight, and toned and tightened myself up," she adds. "My body became better than it had been in my twenties and thirties."

Eventually, Herman says, she added a relaxation technique, popped some vitamins—especially vitamins C and E plus beta-carotene—chewed a calcium-enriched gum, earned her master's degree, hung out with creative people who stimulated her mind, got involved with political action groups, and seduced her husband on energizing trips to Santa Fe, Anguilla, Vermont, and anywhere else that took her fancy.

The result? The Pepper we have today: the prototype of an exciting, seemingly ageless woman—a woman who smashes every previous generation's concept of "old."

Not everyone can become such a dynamo, of course. But everyone can hold aging at bay by changing the way they think about getting old.

To stay young, says Mary M. Gergin, Ph.D., associate professor of psychology at Pennsylvania State University's Delaware County campus, "We need to liberate ourselves from outdated notions of aging. We need to be unafraid and daring and willing to take risks. And we need to be willing to break the mold of aging."

Once we do, says Dr. Gergin, we need to use the age-erasing secrets that most suit our own individual needs.

Which ones? We'll explore the answer to that question throughout this book, but here's a sample of strategies you might want to consider.

Get out and sweat. If there's anything close to a genuine youth drug, it's sweat. "There's nothing science can do for you that could be of more benefit than exercise," says William J. Evans, Ph.D., director of the nutrition, metabolism, and exercise program at the University of Arkansas for Medical Sciences in Little Rock.

A single classic experiment vividly illustrates his point. In the late 1960s, a Swedish physiologist named Bengt Saltin asked five young men, two of them athletes, to lie in bed for 3 weeks while he monitored their bodies' physiological responses to prolonged disuse.

The result? In the space of 21 days, doing nothing reduced the men's aerobic capacity so dramatically that Saltin concluded it was equivalent to almost 20 years of aging.

Fortunately, subsequent research found that exercise could not only reverse Saltin's results, it could actually reverse the results of age. In one study, for example, 11 healthy men and women from 62 to 68 years old were put on a moderately strenuous walking program for 6 months, and it boosted their aerobic capacity an average of 12 percent. When they continued the program for another 6 months, at double the intensity, their aerobic capacity climbed an additional 18 percent.

Many other physiological changes that were normally associated with aging can also be prevented or delayed with moderate exercise. What does "moderate" mean? About 20 minutes of aerobic activity, three times a week, should do the trick.

Researchers at Tufts University in Medford, Massachusetts, put a group of elderly volunteers on an 8-week strength training program and found that women as old as 96 were able to increase their muscle size and strength by more than 200 percent.

Other researchers have found that weight-bearing exercises such as walking, jogging, and dancing can keep bones strong and help prevent osteoporosis.

And still other researchers have found that exercise can prevent the age-related increases in weight, triglycerides, cholesterol, and diastolic blood pressure—the bottom number in a blood pressure reading.

In a study at the University of Pittsburgh School of Medicine, researchers recorded weight, triglycerides, cholesterol, and blood pressure for 500 women between the ages of 42 and 50 both at the beginning of the study and then again 3 years later. In the years between measurements, diastolic blood pressure, weight, triglycerides, and total cholesterol levels went up for everyone. But the women who exercised the most gained the least weight and had healthier blood cholesterol levels.

How much exercise is necessary to keep your body youthful into your sixties and seventies?

"For years, exercise zealots kept saying that you had to work out for 30 to 40 minutes, three times a week, in order to get any benefit," says Dr. Evans. "But there's now good evidence that fairly low-level activity is also beneficial."

Low level means taking the stairs when you could take the escalator, he adds. It means parking the car far from the entrances of malls, supermarkets, workplaces—in short, anywhere you go. It also means walking 10 minutes in the morning or at lunch and another 10 minutes around dinnertime or before bed.

"It all adds up," says Dr. Evans. And the bottom line is that it will erase many of the problems that make you old before your time.

Eat veggies for longevity. Florets of broccoli, a heap of steamed carrots, or a few ruffled leaves of kale may not seem important in the larger scheme of life. But these unassuming vegetables are actually "longevity foods"—clean-burning, high-octane fuels that can prevent many causes of premature aging.

Broccoli, brussels sprouts, carrots, and most leafy green vegetables are packed with beta-carotene, the vitamin A–producing substance that has been shown to block cancer and prevent heart attacks.

Kale and other green vegetables are loaded with calcium, the mineral your body needs most to maintain its youthful bone strength.

And all vegetables have almost no fat or cholesterol, which will help keep age-related weight gains, high blood pressure readings, and clogged arteries at bay.

Feast on fruit. Nutrients called antioxidants—vitamins C and E and beta-carotene—turn out to be key players in what could be described as an "anti-aging diet." Contained in fruits, nuts, and some vegetables, antioxidants are the body's defense against what scientists call free radicals—highly reactive molecules zinging around the body doing all sorts of cellular damage. They are implicated in the initiation of cancer, heart disease, and even aging itself—so much so that some scientists feel that the aging process is produced largely by a lifetime of tiny cellular nicks, dents, and bumps caused by free radicals as they oxidize various cells.

Antioxidants—as their name suggests—provide the body with a natural defense against these free radicals. That's why nutritionists frequently recommend that you eat foods that are rich in vitamins C and E and beta-carotene.

Sources of vitamin C include citrus fruits, red bell peppers, and cabbage. Other good sources are strawberries and tomatoes.

The best sources of beta-carotene are carrots, spinach, broccoli, and lettuce.

Vitamin E is found mostly in nut oils such as hazelnut, sunflower, and almond—all of which weigh in at more than 100 calories per tablespoon. You could eat the nuts themselves, of course, but you'd have to eat so many to get much vitamin E that you'd be munching all the time—not to mention getting all that fat, too. As a result, many people prefer to get their vitamin E from a supplement.

Commit yourself to life. "The scientific literature is absolutely unequivocal on one point," says Dr. Evans. "People who have meaningful lives and something that gives them a sense of purpose—a fulfilling career, involvement in community or church work—live longer and live healthier than those who don't."

Walk in the moonlight. You may call the effects of sun on your skin tanning, but dermatologists call it photoaging. This is because exposure to the ultraviolet rays in sunlight literally causes the wrinkles, speckles, uneven pigments, and age spots that we generally attribute to aging skin. With enough exposure, the skin thickens, sags, and develops a harsh, leathery texture. And the fairer your complexion, the more extensive the damage.

You'll also look older than you really are. Dermatologists studied 41 white women, ranging in age from 25 to 51, who'd lived in Tucson, Arizona, for at least a decade. Some were inveterate sun worshippers; others stayed pretty much indoors.

The women's faces were photographed, without makeup, in unflinching close-ups. Then the photos were shown to a panel of judges who were asked, "How old do these women look?"

For the women who were in their twenties and early thirties, there was no difference in perceived age between those who'd exposed themselves to a lifetime of tanning and those who'd shunned the sun. But among the older women (median age 47), the story wasn't so pretty. In fact, the women with sunbaked faces were perceived to be fully 5 years older than those who'd kept out of the sun.

What's more, since studies have shown that long-term sun exposure increases your risk of cataracts, too much sun can age your eyes as well.

This is why experts say you should stay out of the sun as much as possible and learn to love big shady hats. Wraparound sunglasses and a sunscreen with a sun protection factor, or SPF, of 15 will also help shield your eyes and skin from the sun.

Avoid smoke. Want to save money, look younger, and stay healthier? Then stay away from tobacco.

Smoking not only increases your risk of lung cancer, emphysema, and a host of other internal ailments, it produces "smoker's face." This includes wrinkles at the mouth, nose, and eyes that are exclusively from the facial contortions necessary to drag on a cigarette.

Work those neurons. The best way to keep your mind alert, your intellect sharp, and your memory keen is to keep your brain active. That's because brain cells have tiny branches that grow and spread when used—just like the roots of a plant when it's watered—or wither and die when not used.

Researchers have found that the brain cells of rats housed in an intellectually stimulating environment—meaning rat toys and other rats—are more densely packed with these brain cell branches than animals kept in toyless, joyless isolation.

The same may be true in humans. Studies indicate that when one or another area of the brain is used intensively, that area explodes with growth. The area of the brain devoted to understanding words, for example, is much larger in college grads than in high school grads. And the reason is probably because college students spend more time working with words.

In short, keeping your mind working—pursuing an advanced degree, reading on a wide variety of topics, learning a new language, or in any way providing the brain with mental stimulation—keeps your neural filaments jangling well into old age.

ANTI-AGING FOODS

Grazing in the Garden of Youth

Pablo Picasso once said, "It takes a long time to become young." He could easily have added, "And a lot of food."

Yes, food.

There's no longer the slightest doubt that eating the right foods is one of the keys, if not *the* key, to preventing heart disease, cancer, and other age-related diseases. But now there's scientific evidence that a healthy diet can actually delay—or in some cases, even reverse—the aging process itself. Pretty amazing, don't you think?

The right diet can encourage your body to produce "youth hormones" that control the ebb and flow of the body's anti-aging mechanisms, says Vincent C. Giampapa, M.D., president of the American Board of Anti-Aging Medicine and president of Longevity Institute International, a company based in Montclair, New Jersey, that provides personalized anti-aging programs through member physicians. The result is increased energy; stronger immunity; improvements in memory, vision, and hearing; more muscle; and denser bone.

Eating right can also help your cells repair and replace themselves more quickly, transport energy, and get rid of waste and toxins more efficiently. Just as important, diet can help protect your DNA, the genetic blueprint that tells your body's 50 to 60 trillion cells how to do their jobs.

Take a Bite Out of Aging

According to Dr. Giampapa, the goal of a "longevity diet" is to return your body to its youthful efficiency, which it can do in three ways.

Boost your youth hormones. The most important hormones for keeping you young are human growth hormone (hGH), which is released by the pituitary gland and converted in the liver to another anti-aging hormone called insulin growth factor (IGF-1), and dehydroepiandrosterone (DHEA), which is produced by the adrenal glands.

Starting in your twenties, your body slows down production of these hormones by about 10 percent every decade. By age 65, you are making only 15 to 20 percent of the hGH and 10 to 20 percent of the DHEA that you did when you were in your twenties.

With fewer youth hormones around, says Dr. Giampapa, chemical messages don't come and go as efficiently, which reduces the ability of your cells and organs to maintain and repair themselves. So you experience loss of muscle and bone density, lowered immunity, and more illnesses, including diabetes and cancer.

Situation hopeless? Not quite.

"Increasing the body's production of these hormones can slow the aging process significantly," says Dr. Giampapa. "And it can be done primarily through diet."

Stem free-radical damage. Your cells use oxygen to produce energy. In the process, they generate free radicals—unstable oxygen molecules that damage cells and DNA. Free radicals are also produced by pollution, by the pesticides in the food supply, and by a diet high in chemical additives, refined starches and sugars, artery-clogging saturated fat found in meat, whole-milk dairy products, tropical oils, and foods like cookies and crackers that contain hydrogenated or partially hydrogenated oils.

Your body is good at fending off free radicals when you're young. But as you grow older, you start to lose some of that fight as the damage caused by years of exposure starts to take its toll. You begin to need help from antioxidant nutrients such as vitamins C and E, the minerals zinc and selenium, and the plant chemicals (phytochemicals) in many fruits and vegetables, which join forces with our bodies' internal defense systems.

Replenish your "cellular soup." Each of your cells contains a substance called cytoplasm, which is made up of fluid, nutrients, and other materials that help make energy and fight free-radical damage, says Israel Kogan, M.D., director of the Anti-Aging Medical Center in Washington, D.C.

The typical American diet is loaded with chemical additives, pesticides and fertilizers, and other toxic substances, all of which encourage the formation of free radicals, says Dr. Kogan. When your diet is free of these toxins, you protect your cells from free-radical damage, give your cytoplasm the nutrients it needs, and help your cells to function at their peak.

A "clean" diet also helps return your body to the right level of acidity (pH), which is tremendously important in building up your cellular soup, says Dr. Giampapa. That's because your body makes hormones, repairs cells, and generally works most effectively at a neutral pH.

Check the Index

So how do you boost—or even hang on to—your youth hormones? One way is to skip the cherry-cheese Danish and enjoy the cherries straight. That's good advice for all the obvious reasons, but for a not-so-obvious one as well: Sugary pastries like that cherry-cheese Danish have what is known as a high glycemic index.

The glycemic index measures how quickly a food raises your blood sugar levels after you eat it and how quickly your levels return to normal.

Foods with a low glycemic index, like cherries, along with most fruits and vegetables and whole grains, encourage youthful levels of hGH and IGF-1, according to Dr. Giampapa.

They travel slowly through your digestive system, so sugar enters your bloodstream a little at a time, says Shari Lieberman, Ph.D., a nutrition scientist and exercise physiologist in New York City. This slow, steady rise in blood sugar promotes a stable release of insulin, the hormone that moves energy (glucose) from your blood to your cells.

When your insulin levels stay steady, your body produces less cortisol, often called the stress hormone, says Dr. Giampapa. That's good. Low cortisol levels encourage your body to produce DHEA as well as the hormones made from it.

By contrast, you digest high-glycemic foods, such as cornflakes, rice cakes, white potatoes, and white rice, more quickly. As a result, your blood sugar rises rapidly, triggering a flood of cortisol. High insulin and cortisol levels reduce your output of DHEA and the hormones made from it.

You can discourage these youth-stealing spikes in insulin and cortisol by eating mostly foods with a low to medium glycemic index, says Dr. Giampapa.

Aim Low

As you may have guessed by now, low-glycemic foods tend to be high in fiber and complex carbohydrates, while high-glycemic foods contain virtually none. Here's how to make your diet more "complex."

Eat heavyweight bread. Buy whole-grain bread that contains at least 3 grams of dietary fiber per slice, says Dr. Lieberman. It will have a much lower glycemic index than white bread or even low-calorie whole-wheat bread.

Rule of thumb: The heavier the loaf, the better. "The bread I eat? You can eat it or use it as a paperweight," says Dr. Lieberman. (While dense bread contains more calories, it also fills you up, leaving you more satisfied.)

Pass on the lightweight cereal. Puffed wheat, puffed rice, and cornflakes may be light on calories, but as low-fiber, high-glycemic foods, they send blood sugar through the roof, says Dr. Lieberman. Choose an unsweetened cereal that contains at least 3 grams of fiber per serving, such as Nabisco Shredded Wheat.

Pick beans. Dried beans score low on the glycemic index and are an excellent source of protein, says Dr. Lieberman. While virtually all dried beans are also a good source of fiber, black-eyed peas, chickpeas, kidney beans, lima beans, and black beans are fiber champs, containing 6 to 8 grams of fiber in a ½-cup serving.

Yam it up. Sweet potatoes have a lower glycemic index than white potatoes, so enjoy them often, says Dr. Lieberman. They're great mashed, for example. Or, for mouthwatering "fries," slice sweet potatoes into thin strips, coat them with a tablespoon of olive oil and a sprinkling of paprika, and bake them at 400°F for 40 minutes.

Make mixed-up meals. Consume high-glycemic foods, such as white rice, with a high-protein food, such as chicken. The mix of carbohydrates and protein will keep your blood sugar from rising too quickly, which will slow your body's release of insulin.

The Fat Factor

Is there anyone who doesn't slow down when she wheels her shopping cart past a display of sticky buns?

If you need a good reason to keep walking, here it is: Eating less pastry and other foods high in saturated fat can help you maintain or increase your levels of youth hormones, according to Dr. Giampapa.

On the other hand, a steady diet of saturated fat switches off production of hGH, IGF-1, and DHEA. "We don't know why saturated fat has this effect, but it does," says Dr. Kogan.

You can encourage your body's production of youth hormones by getting no more than 10 percent of your daily calories from saturated fat, says Dr. Giampapa. In other words, if you consume 1,800 calories a day, no more than 180 of them (about 16 to 20 grams) should come from saturated fat.

As you trim the saturated fats from your diet, replace them with foods high in monounsaturated fats, such as nuts, avocados, and canola, olive, and peanut oils, says Dr. Giampapa.

Monounsaturated fats tend to reduce harmful low-density lipoprotein (LDL) cholesterol and raise beneficial high-density lipoprotein (HDL) cholesterol. That's not only good for your heart, it's good for your youth hormone levels, too. The higher your HDL levels, the better equipped your body is to make DHEA, estrogen, and testosterone, says Dr. Giampapa. (That's because these particular hormones are actually made from cholesterol.)

Olive oil is perhaps the best-known monounsaturated fat. And it can do more than lower LDL cholesterol. It contains several compounds, such as polyphenols, that are powerful antioxidants. These substances keep the LDL cholesterol in your bloodstream from being damaged by free radicals, making it less likely to stick to artery walls.

The Zorba Diet

Fish, nuts, olive oil—Zorba the Greek would have no problem getting 30 percent of his daily calories from monounsaturated fats, as Dr. Giampapa suggests. The tips below can help you eat like Zorba.

Go a little nutty. The people in Mediterranean countries eat a lot of nuts, a primo source of monounsaturated fats. Follow their example and toss a small handful of raw almonds, walnuts, or sunflower or pumpkin seeds on salads, rice dishes, or veggies, suggests Dr. Lieberman. In a 10-year study of 86,016 women ages 34 to 59 conducted by researchers at the Harvard School of Public Health, women who ate 5 ounces of nuts a week were 35 percent less likely to have heart disease, most likely because of the nuts' beneficial effects on cholesterol.

Get hooked on fish. Eat fish such as salmon, tuna, cod, haddock, herring, perch, or snapper once or twice a week, suggests Dr. Lieberman. These fish, caught in the deepest and coldest waters of the North Atlantic, are rich in omega-3 fatty acids, substances that have been shown to raise HDL cholesterol. (Omega-3's also help make eicosanoids, hormonelike substances that encourage our bodies to make hGH, says Dr. Giampapa.)

Feast on a fatty fruit. Toss a few chunks of avocado into your salads or add a few slices to a sandwich in place of cheese. Avocados are rich in oleic acid, the same monounsaturated fat found in olive oil. Since avocados are high in calories and contain about 30 grams of fat apiece, enjoy them in moderation, says Dr. Lieberman.

Protect olive oil. Buy small bottles of olive oil with long, narrow necks. And after you use the oil, cap the bottle tightly and refrigerate it. "These steps limit the oil's exposure to oxygen, which will keep it from turning rancid and discourage the formation of free radicals," says Robert Goldman, D.O., Ph.D., cofounder of the American Academy of Anti-Aging Medicine, a Chicago-based society of physicians and scientists who believe aging is not inevitable, and coauthor of *Stopping the Clock*.

Refrigerated olive oil will solidify. When you're ready to use it, run the bottle under warm water for a few minutes, then pour off the reliquefied oil that forms at the top.

What about Meat?

Just like Mom always said, meat is an excellent source of protein. And what was good for you when you were growing up is still good for you now that you're growing older.

Your body uses the protein in meat and other high-protein foods to make amino acids. These substances help your body make its own proteins, which are used to regulate hormones, grow new tissue, and repair or replace worn-out tissue.

Unfortunately, meat tends to be high in saturated fat. So you may be wondering: If I cut back on meat, will I lose out on protein? No, says Dr. Giampapa. You can get the protein you need from food without consuming meat at all.

A wide array of plant foods, including beans and grains, are excellent sources of protein, says Dr. Lieberman. Some, such as soy and the grain quinoa (pronounced "KEEN-wah"), are considered "complete" proteins because they contain all of the nine essential amino acids people need to stay healthy. But your body will make its own complete proteins if you eat enough calories and a variety of plant foods, such as nuts and seeds, grains, and fruits and vegetables.

Get the Protein, Forgo the Fat

The bottom line? It's absolutely okay to eat meat as long as you don't eat Fred Flintstone-size portions every day and you get the majority of your protein from plant sources, says Dr. Lieberman. Here's how to get the protein you need without the saturated fat.

Toss back a soy cocktail. Soy foods such as soy milk and tofu are an excellent source of protein. But if you don't enjoy these foods, drink one of the delicious soy shakes available in health food stores, suggests Dr. Lieberman. "They're a great way to consume high-quality protein every day or a few times a week."

Before you select a soy shake, read its label, advises Gregory Burke, M.D., professor and interim chairperson in the department of public health sciences at Wake Forest University School of Medicine in Winston-Salem, North Carolina. While some brands are low in fat and contain natural sweeteners, others are loaded with sugar and fat.

Get keen on quinoa. The beadlike, ivory-colored seeds of this plant are usually eaten like rice. But you can also cook it in fruit juice and eat it for breakfast, use it as a substitute for rice in pudding, or make a cold salad of quinoa, beans, and chopped vegetables. Its soft texture and somewhat bland flavor make it easy to add to other foods, such as soups and pasta dishes. You'll find quinoa in health food stores.

Use the palm computer. To avoid eating too much meat at any one meal, use this simple guideline of Dr. Giampapa's: Don't eat more meat than you can fit in the palm of your hand. And aim to eat four handfuls of vegetables to every one handful of fish or lean meat.

Wok meat into your diet. Adding a small amount of steak or pork to a vegetable stir-fry lets you savor the flavor of meat for a fraction of its saturated fat and calories, says Dr. Lieberman.

The Toxic Avengers

Free radicals hit your body 10,000 times a day. Adding injury to injury, these little molecules actually burn holes through the membranes that surround cells, the better to penetrate and vanquish them.

Faced with this onslaught of malicious marauders, hell-bent on crippling your cells and mutating your cellular DNA, your body could use a little help. That's where antioxidants come in. These common vitamins such as C and E and minerals such as zinc and selenium neutralize free radicals.

So do phytochemicals, substances in common fruits, vegetables, and other plant foods. Phytochemicals also seem to fight a plethora of age-related diseases, from arthritis to cancer.

To give just a few examples, ellagic acid, a compound found in berries (with strawberries and blackberries containing the most), may help prevent cellular changes that can lead to cancer. Lutein, found in dark green vegetables like spinach and kale, has been found to cut the risk of macular degeneration nearly in half. Indole-3 carbinol, found in broccoli, cabbage, and other cruciferous vegetables, may help prevent breast and cervical cancer.

In short, every juicy berry, steamed broccoli floret, or spinach salad you consume helps sheath your body in nutritional armor to stem free-radical damage and help prevent age-related diseases.

Great Ways to Ambush Radicals

The way you choose, store, and cook antioxidant-rich fruits and vegetables can boost their protective effects. Here's how to get the most from their anti-aging powers.

Choose the antioxidant all-stars. Wondering which vegetables will give you the most antioxidant bang for your buck? Wonder no more. Researchers at the Jean Mayer USDA Human Nutrition Research Center on Aging at Tufts University in Boston analyzed 22 common vegetables, then calculated the ability of each to neutralize free radicals. The winners included kale, beets, red bell peppers, brussels sprouts, broccoli florets, potatoes, sweet potatoes, and corn.

Follow Popeye's lead. Consider eating more spinach and strawberries, too. Their high levels of antioxidants may prevent or even reverse the effects of free-radical damage to the brain, helping to keep it sharp as you age, according to another study conducted at the Jean Mayer USDA Human Nutrition Research Center on Aging at Tufts University.

Researchers fed 344 rats extracts of strawberry or spinach, vitamin E, or a control diet. After 8 months, they tested the test animals' long- and short-term memories. The rats that consumed the daily equivalent of a large spinach salad performed better when made to run a maze than those fed a normal diet, strawberry extract, or vitamin E. However, the spinach and strawberry extracts and the vitamin E diet all slowed signs of aging in the rats in other tests. The spinach extract, in particular, is speculated to have protected different types of nerve cells in various parts of the brain against the effects of aging.

Choose high-octane olive oil. Cold-pressed, extra-virgin olive oil contains more antioxidants and phytochemicals than yellow olive oil, says Dr. Lieberman. That's because it is extracted by literally crushing the olives, rather than by using heat and chemicals.

Don't be put off by this oil's greenish hue. "Yellow olive oil is yellow because it's been processed and heated, which removes all the good stuff," says Dr. Lieberman. While you'll pay more for extra-virgin oil, it's healthier (and, according to many folks, tastier) than less expensive varieties.

Seek the color purple. If you see broccoli that's so dark it's almost purple, put it in your shopping cart. That purply color means it's packing a motherlode of beta-carotene. If it's yellow, don't buy it—it's lost its vital nutrients.

Quick-cook veggies. Steam rather than boil your vegetables, advises Dr. Lieberman. "Steaming locks in their antioxidants and phytonutrients," she says. When you boil them, you leave their protective substances in the water.

Simplify salad prep. No time to peel, slice, and dice salad fixings? Do it once a week, suggests Dr. Giampapa. Every Sunday, prepare a huge bowl of dark green lettuce, along with carrots, peppers, and other fixings. Store them separately in airtight plastic bags or containers to limit their exposure to oxygen.

Is That a Toxin in My "Soup"?

As mentioned earlier, your cells are filled with a broth of nutrients and other substances called cytoplasm. It's where the action is—where cellular machinery makes energy, synthesizes proteins, and disarms free radicals.

It's hard for cells to get the fuel they need to perform these important jobs from the typical American diet, say anti-aging experts. Foods high in fat and sugar and processed foods containing additives and preservatives sic free radicals on your hapless body. These chemicals build up in your body, gradually weakening your cellular machinery.

What's more, sugary, fatty foods laced with preservatives and additives tend to turn to acid in your blood, upsetting your body's delicate pH balance, says Dr. Giampapa. A steady diet of them acidifies your cellular soup, causing cells and tissues to age before their time.

Just as cars run smoother and cleaner on high-octane fuel, people run best on foods that don't contain additives and preservatives, and that keep the body close to a neutral pH, says Dr. Giampapa. These foods are—you guessed it—fruits, vegetables, legumes, and whole grains.

Put Your Diet into Rehab

The cleaner and more natural your diet, the more nutrients your cells get—and the more efficiently they are likely to work, says Dr. Giampapa. The strategies below can help put your diet into detox.

Eat naked produce. Make an effort to buy organic fruits and vegetables whenever you can, says Dr. Goldman. It's easier to find organic produce than it used to be, he says. "Many supermarkets now carry organic fruits and vegetables alongside the commercially grown variety, and some food chains (such as Fresh Fields, Bread and Circus, and Whole Food Markets) carry only organic food." Make sure that you wash organic produce to remove as much bacteria and dirt as possible.

Buy boxed organics. If you can't find organic fruits and vegetables, consider buying other organic products, says Dr. Lieberman. "I buy organic cereal, organic milk, and organic juice and eggs," she says. "If you can get even 20 percent of your diet organic, that's 20 percent less of a toxic burden on your immune system."

Whip white-sugar cravings. When a craving for a slice of coffee ring or another sugary, fatty food strikes, eat a cold sweet potato, says Dr. Lieberman. "Its natural sweetness may be enough to satisfy your craving for white sugar." If this trick works for you, bake up a mess of them and have them on hand for those times when you get the "craves."

Soy: The Food for Future Youth

"Soy is a superfood," says Dr. Lieberman. "You might even call it a youth food because it has such potential to stave off age-related conditions from menopausal symptoms to osteoporosis to breast cancer."

Skeptical? Think about the robust health and super-longevity of people in Asian countries, where soy is a dietary staple. Compared to Americans, Asians who eat a traditional soy-rich diet have fewer heart attacks; are less likely to develop breast, colon, and prostate cancers; and suffer fewer hip fractures. Asian women going through menopause don't have as many hot flashes. And the Japanese, as a population, have the longest life expectancies in the world.

Adding soy to your diet is easy. The new generation of soy foods actually tastes good, with none of the beany flavor or unpleasant aftertaste that characterized soy products of the past. Your family will never suspect that you're serving them soy in those delicious new burgers, hot dogs, or sausage or that you're sneaking tofu or soy milk into their favorite dishes. And afterward, you'll feel great for having treated yourself—and your family—to a delectable serving of good health.

As mentioned earlier, soy is an excellent source of low-calorie, high-quality protein, as well as other nutrients that older bodies need, such as iron, calcium, and B vitamins like thiamin, riboflavin, and niacin.

But that's not all. Nestled in the heart of soybeans are substances called isoflavones, which are part of a group of plant substances known as phytochemicals. The isoflavones in soy, called phytoestrogens, may be the key to soy's disease-fighting powers, says Dr. Burke.

The average Asian consumes 50 milligrams of isoflavones a day—the amount in 2 to 3 ounces of soy, says Dr. Burke. Consuming these minuscule amounts may afford you the protection that many Asians enjoy from many of the illnesses of aging, including the ones below.

Cancer. In animal and test-tube studies, the phytoestrogen genistein slows the growth of cancer cells. How? Researchers don't know. But they do know that genistein and another phytoestrogen, daidzein, act as weaker versions of the estrogen that women produce naturally.

It is well known that estrogen can fuel so-called hormone-dependent cancers of the breast and uterus. Dr. Burke says it may be that soy phytoestrogens compete with natural estrogen for molecules on the surfaces of cells that recognize and bind to estrogen. If soy phytoestrogens fill these receptors, the more potent natural estrogen can't, thereby helping to prevent cancer.

High cholesterol. Soy may lower both "bad" LDL and total cholesterol levels without reducing "good" HDL cholesterol. In one large study conducted at the University of Kentucky in Lexington, the LDL cholesterol of people who consumed about 2 ounces of soy protein a day plunged 12.9 percent, and their total cholesterol dropped 9.3 percent. Their levels of "good" HDL cholesterol stayed steady.

No one knows exactly how soy might lower cholesterol. But one theory is that soy phytoestrogens help transport LDL cholesterol from the bloodstream to the liver, where it's broken down and excreted. Phytoestrogens may also keep LDL from turning rancid (a process known as oxidation), making it less likely to clog the walls of your arteries.

Osteoporosis. Soy phytoestrogens appear not only to repair bone but actually to build it. In one study, people who consumed 40 grams of soy protein (containing high concentrations of isoflavones) a day for 6 months significantly increased the thickness of the bone in their lower spines. And there's another reason to bone up on soy: Animal protein seems to speed up the body's excretion of calcium. Apparently, soy protein doesn't, says Dr. Burke.

Menopausal symptoms. Sometimes isoflavones block a woman's natural supply of estrogen, and sometimes they actually supplement it. This is a boon for women in menopause, when declining levels of estrogen and progesterone can trigger hot flashes and night sweats. In one study, women who consumed 60 grams of soy protein a day for 12 weeks cut their rate of hot flashes by nearly half.

By now, the soy revolution has probably reached your supermarket. With tofu in the produce section, soy milk in the dairy case, and soy-based frozen yogurts next to the Häagen-Dazs, it has never been easier to add soy to your diet. But if you haven't yet joined the revolution, read on to get acquainted with these commonly available soy foods.

Tofu. The mother of all soy foods comes in three varieties, one as versatile as the next. Firm tofu is solid, so it's often stir-fried, grilled, or added to soups and stews. Soft tofu, which has a creamy consistency, and silken tofu, which has a custardlike texture, can be mashed or pureed and added to blender drinks, dips, dressings, and puddings. Don't be put off by its taste. Standing alone, tofu is bland, but it takes on the flavors of other foods that it's mixed with.

Tempeh. Pronounced "TEM-pay," this traditional Indonesian food is made of cooked, fermented whole soybeans. The result is a chunky, tender cake with a smoky or nutty flavor. Tempeh is a tasty, low-fat alternative to meat—in fact, many people marinate it and grill it, just like a steak. Tempeh can also be added to soups, casseroles, or chili.

Soy milk. This creamy liquid comes from soybeans that are soaked, finely ground, and strained. It's a good source of protein and B vitamins, and many brands are fortified with calcium. Lots of folks pour it over their breakfast cereal or use it in cooking. And since soy milk comes in a variety of flavors, including vanilla and chocolate, some people drink it straight. Because it isn't dairy milk, look for "soy beverage" or "soy drink" on the labels when you are purchasing soy milk.

Many people have come to enjoy soy foods. Other people—well, it might take a little longer. If you fall into the latter category, take the stealth approach to soy, in which you sneak the stuff into already familiar dishes. These ideas will get you started.

Cook up some pudding. You could get 30 to 50 milligrams of isoflavones by consuming 1 cup of soy milk or ½ cup of tofu or tempeh. Or you could savor some creamy pudding. Pudding mixes are made to be blended with firm tofu. One brand, Mori-Nu, contains 30 milligrams of isoflavones per ½ cup. Or simply add 2 cups of soy milk to your favorite fat-free pudding mix.

Savor a smoothie. For another quick dessert, blend ½ cup silken tofu with ½ cup each fresh berries, nonfat yogurt, and skim milk. Add a dash of vanilla or honey if you like.

Dig into pizza. "Soy can transform pizza from everyone's favorite 'fun' food into serious nutrition," writes Patricia Greenberg in her book *The Whole Soy Cookbook*. Start with a homemade crust that contains soy flour, add tomato sauce and shredded soy mozzarella cheese, then top it with crumbled soy sausage or soy pepperoni. Delicious.

Kick back with a latte. Microwave 1 cup of vanilla soy milk for 60 seconds, then add 1 teaspoon of instant coffee. No need for sugar—vanilla soy milk is sweet. This elegant beverage packs 30 milligrams of isoflavones.

Go nuts. If you're hooked on roasted peanuts, try soy nuts. They are a concentrated source of isoflavones and a tasty, high-protein alternative to other roasted nuts, says Patricia Murphy, Ph.D., professor in the food science and human nutrition department at Iowa State University in Ames. "They taste somewhat like peanuts and make a great snack."

Slip soy into sweets. Bake with soy flour, suggests Dr. Murphy. Just ½ cup contains 30 to 50 milligrams of isoflavones. When baking quick breads and muffins, replace one-quarter to one-third of the total flour with soy flour. In yeast-raised recipes, use only 15 percent soy flour, or just a little more than ⅛ cup. (Soy flour is gluten-free, so expect yeast-raised breads to be denser in texture.)

You can find soy flour in natural food stores. Keep it in the fridge or freezer; soy flour goes bad more quickly than processed white flour.

Play hide-the-tofu. If you're exploring the countless delicious ways to prepare tofu, take a bow. But if you just want to hide the stuff, add cubed tofu to soups, stews, chili, and spaghetti sauce.

Take a powder. Add 2 to 3 tablespoons of powdered isolated soy protein (ISP) to milk, juice, or health shakes, suggests Dr. Burke. Available at health food stores, ISP is a simple way to get soy protein *and* isoflavones. Pass up ready-made soy shakes, however. "They tend to contain a lot of sugar and fat and may not be as healthy as you think," he says.

Get out the ketchup. Try the new breed of soy hot dogs, burgers, and sausage (as well as the many soy cheeses and yogurts), suggests Dr. Burke. While these products contain few or no isoflavones, they are still lower in total and saturated fat and cholesterol than their full-fat counterparts. "And that's still to your benefit," he says.

YOUR ANTI-AGING ARSENAL

It's More Than Just Food

When your parents were young, people who ate more vegetables than meat, exercised regularly, and took other anti-aging steps were considered, well, a bit strange. The all-American way to age was to accept that you would get sick—"old" people always did—and that a kindly, wise Marcus Welby–type would make all of your medical decisions for you.

Not anymore. This generation has a new focus: preventing age-related diseases before they strike.

The weapons? Food, as we've already mentioned, but there's a whole wealth of other age-erasing elements you can draw upon. Here are three of the best.

Aerobic Exercise

Aerobic exercise, the type that makes you breathe harder and gets your blood pumping faster, is "the best anti-aging medicine in the world," says Andrea Z. LaCroix, Ph.D., professor of epidemiology at Group Health Cooperative of Puget Sound in Seattle. Lifelong exercise may add as much as 7 years to our life spans. Studies suggest that regular exercise may boost our bodies' levels of antioxidants, preventing the free-radical damage that gums up our works.

When you walk briskly, swim, bike, hike, or do some other form of aerobic exercise, you produce some tremendous short- *and* long-term profits. Here are some of the immediate youth-enhancing benefits exercisers can cash in on.

Boosts metabolism. All that heart-pounding, lung-filling exercise burns a lot of calories and elevates your metabolism, says Miriam E. Nelson, Ph.D., director of the Center for Physical Fitness at Tufts University School of Nutrition Science and Policy in Boston and author of *Strong Women Stay Young*.

Without exercise, your metabolism begins to slow by 2 to 5 percent per decade after you hit your thirties.

Why is metabolism so important? Because it's what helps you control your weight. As it slows, so does your body's ability to use up the calories you eat before they're converted to fat, Dr. Nelson says. Exercise for at least 30 minutes every day, and you'll maintain or even *lose* weight by giving your metabolism a daily boost.

Boosts energy. Try this the next time you're falling asleep at your desk: Go take a brisk 10- to 15-minute walk. Chances are that you'll feel refreshed and energized when you return. "After it's over, you feel like your energy level is really surging," says John Duncan, Ph.D., an exercise physiologist at Texas Woman's University Center for Research on Women's Health in Denton. A number of things probably go on in your body to create that energy boost, he says. One is that your brain releases feel-good chemicals called endorphins—the same ones that, in excess, create the "runner's high" that marathoners often experience.

Reduces stress. Studies show that exercise is a great stress buster. And the best part is that you don't have to run a 4-minute mile to take that load off your shoulders. Researchers at the University of Georgia in Athens found that anxious college students cut their anxiety in half just by leisurely riding an exercise bike for 20 minutes.

Makes falling asleep E-Zzz. If you've been counting more sheep than a shepherd lately, you're not alone. Women age 40 and older are especially prone to insomnia as they begin to experience the hormonal changes that usher in menopause. Aerobic exercise can improve your sleep by reducing stress, tiring you out, and regulating your body temperature.

The best time to exercise for improved sleep is in the late afternoon, according to Peter Hauri, Ph.D., co-director of the Sleep Disorders Center at the Mayo Clinic in Rochester, Minnesota. The body goes through a cycle of rising and falling temperatures throughout the day. When your temperature is at its lowest point, it's easiest for you to fall asleep. Vigorous exercise in the afternoon can boost your body temperature for up to 5 hours, so your temperature will drop just in time for bed.

The worst time to work out is less than 1½ hours before you normally hit the sack, when your body temperature will still be elevated. But everyone is different, adds Dr. Nelson. As long as you cool down adequately before tucking yourself in and you don't have problems sleeping, exercising at night is fine.

Revs up your sex drive. If your libido is in low gear, exercise may give it a turbo-boost. Experts say that aerobic exercise can put the sizzle back in your sex life in a number of ways. First, it reduces stress.

When we're more relaxed, we're often more interested in having sex, says David Case, Ph.D., a research specialist in the department of psychology at the University of California, San Diego.

Exercise can also make you feel better about your body as you find yourself becoming more fit. The more attractive you feel, the friskier you usually are, he says. And finally, exercise has been found to boost the levels of the hormone responsible for sex drive in men, according to a study done by Dr. Case and colleagues at the University of California, San Diego. And that effect may be similar in women, Dr. Case says.

Eases menstrual cramps. When cramps hit, most women probably aren't in much of a mood for a jog. But women who exercise regularly experience fewer and less painful menstrual cramps. "We're not sure exactly how exercise helps, but it may be that fit women have tighter abdominal muscles, and that may be beneficial somehow," says Mary Lang Carney, M.D., medical director of the Center for Women's Health at St. Francis Hospital in Evanston, Illinois. Exercise also relaxes us and produces those "happy hormones" called endorphins, which may help relieve the discomfort as well.

Treats you to a natural facial. Exercise can give your face a rosy radiance. The glow probably occurs after exercise because of the extra blood your heart pumps throughout your body, explains Priscilla Clarkson, Ph.D., professor of exercise science and associate dean of the University of Massachusetts School of Public Health in Amherst. What's more, people who exercise regularly may feel better about themselves. And when you're happier, your face tends to exude that charisma, she says.

So it's clear. The immediate benefits of aerobic exercise are remarkable. But its long-term benefits are even more impressive.

Regular exercise increases your vitality, endurance, flexibility, and balance—all things that tend to decline as we age. Fit people not only live longer, they also function as well as unfit people 20 years their junior. But the most significant benefit of exercise is undoubtedly its role in disease prevention. "If you look at a list of all the health problems that occur as you age, exercise has been shown to reduce almost all of them," Dr. Clarkson says. "There's no pill, no medicine that can do that, but exercise can." Here are just some of the conditions exercise can counteract.

Heart disease. Regular aerobic exercise helps prevent heart disease by improving several risk factors: It lowers blood pressure and cholesterol, controls weight, reduces stress, and improves cardiovascular fitness, says Elizabeth Ross, M.D., a cardiologist at Washington Hospital Center in Washington, D.C. The link between exercise and heart health is so strong that even people who already have heart disease can lower their risk of having a heart attack by exercising.

Cancer. Exercisers have a lower risk of developing breast and colon cancer. An 11-year study of more than 1,800 women (average age 75) conducted by James R. Cerhan, M.D., Ph.D., and researchers at the Mayo Clinic in Rochester, Minnesota, found that those who walked, gardened, or did housework several times a week cut their breast cancer risk to half that of inactive women. Those who did more vigorous activity—such as swimming or running—at least once a week were 80 percent less likely to develop breast cancer. And when it comes to colon cancer, in 1996 the Surgeon General's report concluded that physical activity protects against it.

Diabetes. People who exercise regularly have a significantly lower risk of developing type 2 diabetes. A 6-year study of more than 8,600 subjects, conducted by researchers at the Cooper Institute for Aerobics Research in Dallas, found that those who were least fit had a four times greater risk of developing diabetes than those who were most fit.

Stroke. Regular exercise can cut your stroke risk in half, according to a recent study conducted by researchers at the Harvard School of Public Health. Swimming 5 hours a week, gardening 6 hours a week, or walking an hour a day for 5 days a week are all ways of dramatically reducing your chances of having a stroke.

Depression. Exercise can help relieve mild depression by raising levels of feel-good substances in the brain and by reducing stress, according to June Primm, Ph.D., a clinical psychologist and associate professor of pediatrics and psychology at the University of Miami School of Medicine. In fact, several studies have shown that aerobic exercise is just as effective as psychotherapy at treating mild depression.

Osteoporosis. Regular exercise can help prevent osteoporosis, the disease that causes bones to become so weak that they easily break. A study of nearly 240 post-menopausal women between the ages of 43 and 72 found that those who walked about a mile a day (7.5 miles a week) had denser bones than women who walked less than a mile a week.

Arthritis. At one time doctors told patients with arthritis *not* to exercise. But now we know that exercise—especially walking—can actually ease arthritis pain. A study at Wake Forest University in Winston-Salem, North Carolina, assigned elderly people with arthritis of the knee to do aerobic exercise, strength training, or no exercise. After a year, those who did best were in the aerobic exercise group. They reported less pain and disability than the nonexercise group and were able to walk, climb stairs, and get in and out of the car more easily.

Anti-Aging Supplements

Phosphatidylserine. It doesn't exactly spell P-R-O-M-I-S-I-N-G, does it?

It looks more like one of those unpronounceable ingredients listed on the label of a hair shampoo. But actually, it's brimming with promise. This natural supplement is on the cutting edge of anti-aging medicine. It has been shown to renew brain cells and sharpen mental performance.

Where can you find this exotic stuff? (It's pronounced "foss-fuh-TID-ill-SEER-een," by the way.)

It's sitting on a shelf at your local health food store or just a click away on the Internet, along with other exciting, cutting-edge anti-aging substances that you may not know much about yet. Among them are alpha-lipoic acid (ALA), coenzyme Q-10, and melatonin, to name just a few.

"I'm sure these supplements seem somewhat mysterious," says Ronald Klatz, M.D., D.O., author of *Brain Fitness* and president of the American Academy of Anti-Aging Medicine, a Chicago-based society of physicians and scientists who believe aging is not inevitable. "After all, we've known about the role of vitamin C in good health for the past 30 years, and vitamin E for longer than that. These are quite new."

What makes these substances so special?

For one thing, many of them are potent antioxidants, says Dr. Klatz. Only antioxidants can neutralize free radicals, the unstable oxygen molecules that punch holes in cell membranes, destroy vital enzymes, damage cellular DNA—and, ultimately, lead to the diseases of aging.

For another, their antioxidant power is, in some cases, many times more powerful than better-known antioxidants such as vitamins C and E. Some actually recycle vitamins C and E, giving them new life in the endless war against free radicals. Still others dissolve in both fat and water, enabling them to neutralize free radicals wherever they occur, from our watery blood to our fatty brains.

These new substances have the potential to extend life span and stave off age-related degenerative diseases, says Dr. Klatz. Future youth is out there!

Here's a primer on some supplements that have longevity experts and medical researchers buzzing.

Alpha-lipoic acid. An antioxidant made by the body, ALA also helps break down food into the energy needed by your cells. It helps the body recycle and renew vitamins C and E, making them serviceable again. And unlike many antioxidants, which dissolve only in fat or only in water, ALA fights free radicals in both the fatty and watery parts of cells, protecting both from free-radical damage. "Lipoic acid can zip in and out of any cell in the body, even those in the brain," says Lester Packer, Ph.D., professor of molecular and cell biology at the University of California, Berkeley.

Clinical studies suggest that ALA may help prevent the nerve damage, caused by free-radical attacks, that frequently accompanies diabetes. In one German study, intravenous ALA significantly reduced pain, tingling, and numbness in the feet of people with diabetes.

Note: If you have diabetes and are being treated for symptoms of nerve damage, Dr. Packer suggests that you talk to your doctor before taking ALA supplements.

Bioflavonoids. Bioflavonoids are a group of plant pigments that give fruits and flowers some of their color. Some bioflavonoids act as powerful antioxidants, "many of which are more potent than better-known antioxidants such as vitamins C and E," explains Shari Lieberman, Ph.D., a nutrition scientist and exercise physiologist in New York City.

Bioflavonoids may help lower the risk of heart disease. In 1996, a Finnish study found that women who ate the most flavonoids had a 46 percent lower risk for heart disease than those who ate the least.

Bioflavonoids keep the tiny disks in our blood (called platelets), which help blood clot, from clumping together and forming clots that can block the arteries. They also keep harmful low-density lipoprotein (LDL) cholesterol from oxidizing and sticking to artery walls.

Some bioflavonoids can stop cancer before it starts. To give just a few examples, quercetin, found in apples, yellow and red onions, and tea, has been shown in test-tube studies to discourage the growth of tumors and prevent malignant cells from spreading. And rutin, found in buckwheat, helps reduce cancer risk through its action as an antioxidant.

Coenzyme Q-10. An antioxidant made by your body, coenzyme Q-10 helps make ATP (adenosine triphosphate), the fuel that allows your cells to do their jobs. Every cell in your body contains this antioxidant, but it's most concentrated in heart-muscle cells, which require the most fuel. People have plenty of coenzyme Q-10 until they hit age 40. After that, levels take a nosedive.

Coenzyme Q-10 may help prevent or treat many common forms of heart disease, says Peter Langsjoen, M.D., a staff cardiologist at Mother Francis Hospital and the East Texas Medical Center in Tyler. "It provides such dramatic improvement; it's unthinkable for me to practice medicine without it."

Research shows that people with various types of heart disease are deficient in coenzyme Q-10, and that the more severe the heart disease, the lower these levels drop. This substance appears to improve the heart's ability to contract. And because it's a powerful antioxidant, coenzyme Q-10 also helps prevent "bad" LDL cholesterol from sticking to the walls of the arteries and clogging blood vessels.

Coenzyme Q-10 is used to treat a variety of heart conditions, from heart pain (angina) to cardiomyopathy (any noninflammatory disease of the heart muscles). Some studies suggest that this antioxidant helps treat angina by allowing heart muscle cells to use oxygen more efficiently. In a small study of 19 people with cardiomyopathy conducted by Dr. Langsjoen, those who took 100 milligrams of coenzyme Q-10 a day along with their conventional therapy did far better than those who got conventional therapy and a placebo.

Coenzyme Q-10 also helps treat congestive heart failure, which occurs when the heart is too weak to pump blood through the body. In a large study conducted by Dr. Langsjoen, 58 percent of people taking coenzyme Q-10 improved by one New York Heart Association classification (the standard doctors use to assess heart patients' conditions), 28 percent improved by two classes, and 43 percent stopped using one or more drugs.

Note: In rare occurrences, people who were taking the blood thinner warfarin (Coumadin) had a slight decrease in the effectiveness of the drug after they started taking coenzyme Q-10. Also, if you have heart disease, consult your doctor before taking coenzyme Q-10, says Dr. Langsjoen.

Flaxseed oil. This polyunsaturated vegetable oil is a rich source of omega-3 fatty acids. Studies have repeatedly suggested that omega-3's lower blood levels of cholesterol and triglycerides and reduce the stickiness of platelets, thus reducing the risk of heart attack or stroke. Other studies have found that omega-3's raise high-density lipoproteins (HDLs), the "good" cholesterol that helps whisk artery-clogging LDL out of the blood. While fish oils are the best-known sources of omega-3's, flaxseed oil contains twice the amount of omega-3's as fish oils do.

Researchers have conducted numerous studies on flaxseed to study its potential in preventing and treating cancer, particularly breast and colon cancer. In animal studies, flaxseed helps keep breast cancer from starting and slows the growth of breast tumors already in place.

Research suggests that the cancer-fighting substance in flaxseed is lignan precursors, compounds that the body converts into lignans. These are estrogenlike compounds that may prevent breast cancer by taking up estrogen receptors on breast cells, thereby blocking stronger, cancer-causing estrogen.

Lignans also act as antioxidants and contain other beneficial plant chemicals. An accumulating body of research suggests that they may help protect against age-related chronic conditions such as heart disease.

Note: Due to its high calorie content, you could gain weight if you don't figure flaxseed oil into your total calorie intake.

Ginkgo. This herb, which is extracted from the fan-shaped, leathery leaves of the ginkgo tree, helps the brain function more efficiently. Already used in Germany to treat dementia, ginkgo enhances blood circulation so more nutrients reach brain cells, enabling them to work more efficiently. In European studies, ginkgo has also been found to improve mental performance and short-term memory.

While there's no proof that taking ginkgo now will prevent Alzheimer's disease later, a growing body of research suggests that a concentrated extract of this herb improves the mental functioning of people who already have the disease.

In one of the biggest studies, researchers found that among people with Alzheimer-type dementia and those with dementia caused by blood-vessel disease of the brain, those taking ginkgo were better able to think and interact with others than were those taking a placebo.

Note: You should be cautious about using ginkgo if you are taking herbs that help prevent blood clotting such as garlic, ginger, and feverfew. Also, don't take it if you're currently using aspirin, warfarin (Coumadin), or an MAO inhibitor drug.

Melatonin. Melatonin is a hormone secreted by a pea-size gland, called the pineal gland. Melatonin is a powerful antioxidant, says Russel J. Reiter, Ph.D., a cellular biologist at the University of Texas Health Science Center at San Antonio, author of *Your Body's Natural Wonder Drug: Melatonin,* and editor of the *Journal of Pineal Research.*

As such, it protects against age-related diseases such as cardiovascular disease and cancer, which may be linked to free-radical damage.

But there's more. Unlike many other antioxidants, melatonin is able to cross what's called the blood-brain barrier, which means that it penetrates the brain more easily than some other antioxidants, says Dr. Reiter. So it's better able to fight the free-radical damage in the brain.

Other evidence suggests that melatonin may also slow the progression of Alzheimer's disease. "Much of the dementia associated with aging, including Alzheimer's disease, is due to loss of neurons as a result of free-radical damage," says Dr. Reiter. "While very high doses of vitamin E, a well-known antioxidant, given for long periods of time can slightly delay Alzheimer's, a study on a pair of identical twins found that as little as 6 milligrams of melatonin taken every day for 3 years substantially reduced the progression of Alzheimer's disease."

In some laboratory studies, melatonin has also been found to prevent the growth of cancer cells and to slow the growth of some tumors.

Note: Since melatonin makes you drowsy, don't drive or engage in any activity that requires you to be alert after taking it, says Dr. Reiter. Before you start using melatonin, talk with your doctor. Though rare, interactions with prescription medications can occur.

Pycnogenol. A trademarked supplement derived from the bark of the French maritime pine tree, pycnogenol (pronounced "pik-NA-je-nal") contains about 40 bioflavonoids with antioxidant powers. Its active ingredients—a class of flavonoids called proanthocyanidins, also found in grape seeds—make it a potent antioxidant. Pycnogenol also recycles vitamin C and, indirectly, vitamin E, making them effective again, says Dr. Packer.

Pycnogenol reduces the risk of heart disease by keeping platelets unstuck so that they can't adhere to artery walls and by keeping LDL cholesterol from oxidizing, says Dr. Packer.

Pycnogenol also strengthens the body's smallest blood vessels, called capillaries, and prevents free-radical damage to blood vessels. And pycnogenol suppresses the overproduction of nitric oxide (NO) by immune system cells, which has been linked to rheumatoid arthritis and Alzheimer's disease, says Dr. Packer.

Phosphatidylserine. This substance is a phospholipid, a kind of a fat concentrated in the nerve cells of the brain. Phosphatidylserine improves memory and age-related brain changes, says Timothy Smith, M.D., an expert in anti-aging medicine in Sebastopol, California, and author of *Renewal*. It also helps regenerate damaged nerve cells, so they can send and receive their "messages" more effectively.

Researchers at Stanford University and at Vanderbilt University in Nashville studied the effects of phosphatidylserine in 149 people between the ages of 50 and 75 with "normal" age-related memory loss. The most memory-impaired people reversed an estimated 12-year decline in memory. In other words, the average scores attained by 64-year-olds rose to match the average scores of 52-year-olds.

Vitamin C. An antioxidant nutrient, vitamin C is found in citrus fruits, strawberries, broccoli, kiwifruit, and other fruits and vegetables. Studies suggest that people who consume a high-C diet have lower rates of cancer, heart disease, and high blood pressure. There's also evidence that vitamin C supplements may help stave off cataracts and may help thicken bones during the early postmenopausal years and in women who never used estrogen-replacement therapy.

Note: Taking more than 1,000 milligrams of vitamin C a day can cause diarrhea in some people. If this happens to you, immediately stop taking vitamin C. If you want to take more than 1,000 milligrams, start with 250 milligrams and increase the dose every few days as your tolerance increases.

Vitamin E. An antioxidant nutrient, vitamin E is found in nuts, seeds, and vegetable oils. Research suggests that vitamin E's antioxidant power may help pre-

vent heart disease and cancer, boosts the immune system, and possibly helps nor-
malize blood sugar levels in people with diabetes.

Vitamin E also seems to slow the progression of Alzheimer's disease. Researchers at Columbia University and other centers gave 341 people with moderately severe Alzheimer's disease 2,000 international units (IU) of vitamin E a day
for 2 years. At the end of the study, researchers concluded that vitamin E had
slowed the mental deterioration of those people by about 25 percent, mainly in
their ability to perform everyday tasks such as dressing, using the toilet, and
eating.

Recent studies have found that our bodies absorb the natural form of vitamin
E (d-alpha tocopherol) more effectively than the synthetic kind (dl-alpha tocopherol). You'll pay more for the natural kind, however.

Note: If you are taking anticoagulant drugs, use vitamin E only with medical
supervision.

Water: The Fountain of Youth

The Spanish explorer Juan Ponce de León sailed halfway across the world
looking for the fountain of youth. He never found it. We, on the other hand, can
make it appear instantly by turning on the kitchen tap.

Sound like magic? Not really. Today we know something that Ponce de León
didn't: The power of that fountain lies in simple, fresh, clean water.

Your body needs water for all the basic processes of life, which include everything from transporting nutrients to regulating internal temperature. But drinking
plenty of water—at least eight 8-ounce glasses a day—can give you benefits above
and beyond the basics. It can also help you maintain healthy, younger-looking skin
and prevent certain diseases and conditions that can make you feel far older than
your years.

If you want to keep your skin smooth, supple, and radiant, water is one of the
secrets you're looking for. "Healthy skin is about 10 to 20 percent water," says
Diana Bihova, M.D., clinical assistant professor of dermatology at New York University Medical Center in New York City. If your skin loses more than half its
moisture, it becomes dry and flaky. Even fine lines become more pronounced.
Over time, dry skin can age more quickly.

One way to fight back is by using moisturizers. When you moisturize your
skin, it plumps up and looks smoother, and fine lines seem to disappear.

The problem is that time makes the going tougher. Our skin gets drier as we
get older. Around age 30, oil and sweat glands slow their production and skin is
less able to retain moisture, says Dr. Bihova. And as women get closer to menopause and estrogen levels drop, their skin may dry out even more.

That's where water comes in. Drinking plenty of water is important. Whether
you sip it or soak in it, water moisturizes your skin. But that's not all you need to
do. "Drinking an ocean of water is not, by itself, going to repair your dry skin,"

says Dr. Bihova. And simply slathering on lotion won't end your dry skin dilemma either. Here, Dr. Bihova shares some secrets to getting the most from moisture.

Keep your cool. Just as washing a sinkful of dishes in hot water leaves your hands dry and pruny by the last plate, bathing or showering in steamy-hot water may have you hankering for hand-and-body lotion hours later. That's because hot water can dry out your skin. To save face, try soaking or showering in lukewarm water instead of hot.

Switch your soap. Washing with harsh soaps can leave your skin feeling like sandpaper—so stick to gentle cleansers like Cetaphil. They cleanse your skin without irritation and leave behind a moisturizing film. Buy cleansers with ingredients such as water, glycerin, sodium lauryl sulfate, cetyl alcohol, and stearyl alcohol.

Time it right. The best time to moisturize is right after a shower or bath, when your skin is still wet and the moisture can be sealed in.

Water the air. Dry winter air wicks moisture away from your skin, leaving it dull and dry. But running a humidifier adds moisture to the air and prevents water loss through your pores.

Water not only lubricates your skin, it keeps everything inside your body flowing smoothly as well. "Most people are minimally dehydrated, and that can impact practically everything a person does," says Felicia Busch, R.D., a nutritionist in St. Paul, Minnesota, and a spokesperson for the American Dietetic Association. You can lose 1 to 2 percent of your body weight in water without ever feeling thirsty. And once you have lost that much water, your body can't function at its best. You start to feel tired, unfocused, weaker, and slower. You may even get a headache—all things that make you feel sluggish and older than you really are.

A well-watered body has what it needs to stay young and healthy. Here are some ways you can use water to help you feel your best.

Keep your colon healthy. Drinking the standard eight glasses a day may lower your risk for colon cancer. Researchers have found that women who drink more than five glasses of water a day have about half the risk of colon cancer as those who drink two or fewer glasses.

Stay regular. Older people are five times more likely to be constipated than younger folks. And chronic constipation can lead to uncomfortable and painful conditions like hemorrhoids or diverticulitis.

To keep your bottom end feeling as young as a baby's bum, drink up. Having enough water in your pipes can help prevent and relieve constipation, especially if you eat a high-fiber diet. That's because water softens your stools so that they can move more easily through your system.

Slim down. Drinking lots of water keeps you trim—first, by helping you burn fat more efficiently. And second, if you drink it right before meals, it fills you up, so you eat less.

Beat bladder infections. Almost half of the 16,000 women surveyed by *Prevention* magazine and the American Medical Women's Association a few years ago had experienced a bladder infection and had tried drinking plenty of water to treat it. Eight out of 10 said it worked for them. Doctors say that all those fluids may help by flushing infection-causing bacteria out of your system.

Stave off kidney stones. When you don't drink enough water, wastes that are normally dissolved and removed in your urine may become concentrated in crystals, which could lump together to form a kidney stone.

Prevent muscle soreness. When you're physically active—whether you're doing work around the house, gardening, or playing tennis—water can ward off the day-after aches that make you feel all washed up. If you're slightly dehydrated, your body taps the water that's stored in your muscles. That can decrease your strength and increase your risk of microscopic muscle damage, which shows up as soreness the next day, says Scott Hasson, Ed.D., chairperson of the department of physical therapy at the University of Connecticut in Storrs.

How much water do you need?

A good rule of thumb is to drink a glass of water before and after physical activity as well as a half-cup every 15 to 20 minutes during the activity, he says.

Staying hydrated is especially important for women because their bodies store less water than men's, says Busch. That's because women have less muscle, which holds a lot of water, and more fat, which doesn't. As a result, a woman's well runs dry more quickly than a man's, so you have to be more faithful about replenishing what you lose each day. Women who are pregnant or nursing need to drink even more water, Busch adds—at least 10 to 12 glasses a day.

Still others need extra water to keep their skin supple and their bodies working at their best. Here's how to know if you are getting your fill.

Check the conditions. You need to drink more than the average eight glasses a day if you're sick, if you live in a hot climate, if you spend a lot of time inside heated or air-conditioned buildings, if you do a lot of public speaking (like a teacher), or if you're larger than average, Busch says.

Drink before you're thirsty. You can't use thirst to determine when you need to fill up, because you can lose as much as 5 percent of your body's water supply before feeling thirsty, Busch says. To prevent this, try water breaks: when you first wake up, when you get to the office, at break times, before meals, and before bed. One glass of water at each of these times will keep you well-hydrated on regular days.

As you get older, your sensitivity to thirst decreases, so it becomes even more important to drink throughout the day, whether you're thirsty or not, adds Joanne Curran-Celentano, Ph.D., associate professor of nutritional sciences at the University of New Hampshire in Durham.

Clear things up. Check the color of your urine. "It should be almost clear, a pale yellow," says Lucia Kaiser, R.D., Ph.D., a nutrition specialist at the University of California, Davis. If it's not, you need to drink more fluids.

If downing 2 quarts of water a day sounds like more than you can stomach, don't dry-dock just yet. These tips from our experts will help you get a handle on staying hydrated.

Call in a substitute. All eight glasses don't have to be water. Other beverages like milk, juice, seltzer, and sparkling water can also count toward your daily intake. So can foods that contain lots of water such as soups and juicy fruits like watermelon, cantaloupe, grapes, and oranges. But don't count beverages that contain alcohol or caffeine; they actually cause you to lose more water than you take in.

Punch up the flavor. If water's too plain for you, try flavored water or squeeze in fresh fruits like lemon, lime, orange, or pineapple. Or toss frozen-juice ice cubes into your water—they add flavor as they melt. For soft-drink fans who miss the carbonation, try adding sparkling water to ¼ cup of juice.

Sip before you snack. People often think that they're hungry when they're actually thirsty. So have a drink first; it may take care of your hunger pangs.

Measure it out. Fill a 64-ounce pitcher and try to empty it by the end of the day.

Keep it close. Have a glass or bottle of water with you when you're at your desk, outdoors, in your car, or at the gym.

Take it slow. Sipping rather than gulping will prevent you from feeling bloated.

Make a pit stop. Every time you pass a water fountain, take a drink.

Part 2
Battling the Age Robbers

AGE SPOTS

What to Do
When the Damage Is Done

Ours is a culture with little appreciation for spots. None of us likes getting a spot on our record, on our reputation, or on our shirt. And we certainly don't like seeing spots when we're looking into a mirror!

But as we age, many of us do begin to see spots, especially on our hands and faces. And whether we call them liver spots, age spots, or sun spots, the reaction is likely the same: We want a spot remover.

The Sources of Your Spots

Technically known as lentigines, age spots are the result of excess pigment being deposited in the skin during years of exposure to ultraviolet rays. The exposure could have come from a tanning booth, a sunlamp, or years of going outdoors without sunscreen. In response, your skin has tried to protect itself by producing an overabundance of melanin—the pigmented cells in your skin—only it does so in uneven patches.

Certain substances may make you more susceptible to sun damage and related age spots, says Karen E. Burke, M.D., Ph.D., a dermatologic surgeon and dermatologist in private practice in New York City. These substances include:

- Chemicals called psoralens, which are present in foods such as parsley, limes, and parsnips. Psoralens can make your skin more sensitive to sunburn and lead to age spots.
- Drugs such as the antibiotic tetracycline (Achromycin), some diuretics (water pills), and antipsychotic medicines such as chlorpromazine (Thorazine).
- Fragrances and lotions that contain musk or bergamot oil. When applied to sun-exposed areas, these ingredients can make your skin more susceptible to sun damage, says Dr. Burke.

Is It Skin Cancer?

Age spots are harmless, and if you choose to ignore one, nothing will happen to you. Ignore a melanoma, however, and it can kill you.

Melanoma is a nasty form of cancer that appears as a discoloration on the skin. How can you tell a melanoma from an age spot?

Use this alphabetical checklist to help spot these potential killers, suggests Thomas Griffin, M.D., a dermatologist at Graduate Hospital of Philadelphia and clinical assistant professor of dermatology at the University of Pennsylvania School of Medicine in Philadelphia.

- *A* **is for asymmetry.** Be concerned if a brown spot or mole develops an irregular shape. Age spots are usually round.
- *B* **is for border.** Look for a jagged one; age spots are usually even.
- *C* **is for color changes.** It could mean trouble if a dark area arises within a mole or brown spot, or if an area within a mole or brown spot begins to lighten. Age spots are usually one color.
- *D* **is for diameter.** A brown spot that gets larger than a pencil eraser could be a melanoma.

If any of these characteristics are present, or if you're at all uncertain whether something is an age spot or a melanoma, get yourself to a doctor quickly, Dr. Griffin says. Though melanoma is dangerous, it's also curable if caught early.

An Ounce of Prevention

You can put the little spot factories in your skin out of business right now, doctors say, but it will take vigilance and preventive steps like these to keep them from gearing up again.

Keep yourself coated with sunscreen. Wearing sunscreen—all the time—is by far your best protection from age spots. "Start using an SPF 15 or higher sunscreen on a daily basis," says John E. Wolf, Jr., M.D., professor and chairman of the dermatology department at Baylor College of Medicine in Houston. What's SPF? It stands for sun protection factor. SPF 15, for example, means you can stay out in the sun 15 times longer before burning than you could without the sunscreen.

"Apply it to the backs of your hands and to your face first thing in the morning, before you put on any moisturizer or makeup," says Dr. Wolf. "When you wash your hands, don't forget to reapply your sunscreen. If you see the beginnings of age spots, switch to a higher SPF sunscreen than the one you are currently using."

And remember that if you're not prepared to use sunscreen every day, year-round, there's really no point in treating your age spots, says Nicholas Lowe, M.D., clinical professor of dermatology at the UCLA School of Medicine. Without daily sunscreen, "in a number of months your skin will be back in the same shape," he says.

Wash away sun-sensitive chemicals. Wash your hands thoroughly after handling foods that contain psoralens and reapply sunscreen before going outdoors again, says Dr. Burke.

Save your scents for the shadows. Apply your perfume or lotion to areas of your skin that will not be exposed to sun, Dr. Burke suggests.

Natural Spot Removers

Once spots have formed, there is an assortment of natural treatments you can try that may fade your age spots, if not remove them completely.

Wipe them away with Retin-A. Originally developed as an acne medication to unplug clogged pores, tretinoin (Retin-A) has found resounding success as an anti-aging ointment. Though not a fountain of youth, the vitamin A acid works to eliminate fine wrinkles, blemishes, and age spots by stimulating cell turnover in a metabolic process that still is not entirely understood, says Retin-A creator Albert Kligman, M.D., Ph.D., professor of dermatology at the University of Pennsylvania School of Medicine and an attending physician at the Hospital of the University of Pennsylvania, both in Philadelphia.

To remove an age spot, dermatologists often recommend applying the strongest dosage of Retin-A that you can tolerate directly on the spot. The area will proceed to peel, and after a few months, the spot should diminish and possibly even disappear.

In a 10-month study of 58 people with age spots, researchers at the University of Michigan Medical Center in Ann Arbor found that the majority of people treated with Retin-A had lighter age spots after 1 month. After 10 months, 83 percent of those treated with Retin-A had lighter age spots, and 32 percent had at least one spot disappear altogether.

Retin-A can be even more effective when used in combination with other treatments, says John F. Romano, M.D., clinical assistant professor of dermatology at New York Hospital-Cornell Medical Center and St. Vincent's Hospital, both in New York City.

"I often have people apply glycolic acid in the morning and Retin-A at night. Or I may combine it with a bleaching cream," says Dr. Romano.

Retin-A cream comes in a variety of concentrations, the weakest being 0.025 percent and the strongest being 0.1 percent. It's available only by prescription, so you'll need to work with your dermatologist to find the dosage that's right for you.

And because Retin-A continually sloughs off the outermost, dead layer of skin, it can not only eliminate existing spots but also nip new spots in the bud. The downside of this process is that an area of skin previously sheltered from evaporation and the elements is exposed. That's why a common side effect of Retin-A is dry, sun-sensitive skin that can be irritated and scaly. Though this effect typically diminishes with time, if you're using Retin-A, you'll likely need a moisturizer. Sunscreen is also a must once you start using Retin-A.

Protect your skin with vitamin C. If vitamin D is the sunshine vitamin, then vitamin C is the sunblock vitamin, say some researchers—many of whom also proclaim it the healthy skin vitamin.

"In general, vitamin C is important for keeping the skin younger looking," says Lorraine Meisner, Ph.D., professor of preventive medicine at the University of Wisconsin Medical School in Madison. She recommends a safe daily vitamin C intake of about 300 to 500 milligrams to maintain skin quality.

Medical researchers have also found vitamin C to be of some help when applied topically. It has been shown to significantly reduce the amount of so-called free radical damage that occurs from sun exposure. Free radicals are naturally occurring unstable molecules that steal electrons from your body's healthy molecules to balance themselves. Unchecked, they can cause significant tissue damage. Antioxidants such as vitamin C neutralize free radicals and protect the healthy molecules from harm.

"Since vitamin C prevents skin damage from sun exposure, it's reasonable to suspect that it can also prevent the consequences of that damage, including wrinkling and age spots," says Douglas Darr, Ph.D., director of technology development at the North Carolina Biotechnology Center in Research Triangle Park. Dr. Darr advocates using topical vitamin C in addition to sunscreen.

One such topical vitamin C product is Cellex-C, a 10-percent vitamin C lotion. It's available without a prescription from dermatologists, plastic surgeons, and licensed aestheticians (full-service beauty salon operators). For optimum sun protection, the lotion should be applied once a day, along with a sunscreen, according to Dr. Meisner, one of the developers of Cellex-C.

Control damage with vitamin E. Vitamin E, an antioxidant vitamin added to everything from nail polish remover to shampoo, is also helpful in preventing sun damage.

Researchers have shown that vitamin E oil can prevent inflammation and skin damage if applied within 8 hours of sun exposure. Because vitamin E itself produces free radicals when exposed to the sun's ultraviolet light, however, researchers recommend that you apply the oil following, not before, sun exposure.

You can buy vitamin E oil or vitamin E-fortified creams over the counter in drugstores. Research has shown that if the cream or oil contains at least 5 percent vitamin E, it can also be effective in reducing post-sun damage.

You can also reap some of vitamin E's sun-protective properties by taking supplements, adds Dr. Burke. "It's highly effective as an anti-inflammatory agent, and it reduces sun damage to the skin," she says. Dr. Burke recommends that people take 400 international units of vitamin E in the form of d-alpha-tocopherol daily.

Seek sun protection from selenium. You might want to boost your dietary intake of the antioxidant mineral selenium as well, says Dr. Burke.

"Selenium can prevent solar damage, pigmentation, and dark spots," says Dr. Burke. She recommends daily supplements of 50 to 200 micrograms of selenium in the form of l-selenomethionine. Note that selenium can be toxic in doses exceeding 100 micrograms, so if you'd like to try this therapy to protect your skin, you should discuss it with your doctor.

Answers in the Beauty Aisle

If your spots don't respond to natural removers, there are a few stronger options you can try.

Bleach them away. It takes time, but a hair bleaching product that's about 12 percent hydrogen peroxide may help fade smaller age spots. Dr. Burke suggests dabbing on the peroxide with a cotton swab. Test the peroxide on a very small age spot once every 3 days for a week, and then gradually adjust the frequency to accommodate your individual level of tolerance. Do not use peroxide on large areas of skin without seeing your doctor. If you develop a burn of any sort, see your doctor immediately.

Apply a fade cream. Another option is one of the fade creams available. You may remember hearing the ads for "Porcelana, the Fade Cream" when you were a kid. It's still around—and it just may work. Porcelana and other creams, including Esotérica and Palmer's Skin Success, contain hydroquinone, which interferes with your skin's production of melanin. Dr. Burke says these products work slowly, however. Prescription-strength hydroquinone preparations might work faster.

Peel or freeze them. A dermatologist can try trichloroacetic acid, which is often used for chemical peels and is quite effective on age spots. It would be a good choice for just a few spots that aren't too dark, says Dr. Wolf. Another alternative is freezing the spots with liquid nitrogen. With these treatments, which must be done in a doctor's office, there is some risk that the chemicals will do their job too well, leaving de-pigmented white spots where the age spots have been removed, he says.

Zap them with laser treatment. Wielded by a highly skilled physician, a laser is the high-tech solution to age spots, says Dr. Lowe. It's also the priciest. "The great thing about laser treatment for this problem is that in the hands of an expert, you don't run the risk of having white spots where the dark spots had been," he says. Ask your dermatologist whether laser treatment is available. Does it hurt? Only for an instant. And the pain is similar to a rubber band snapped against your skin, Dr. Lowe says.

AGING

Eating Back the Years

When Maud Ferris-Luse was born, Grover Cleveland was still president, the telephone was still a toy for the rich, and the major source of transportation had four legs. One hundred fifteen years later, Ferris-Luse was still around, having outlived all her contemporaries and establishing a record as the oldest person on Earth.

Most of us can expect to live about 75 years. While that's just a drop in the bucket for the likes of Ferris-Luse, it's still almost 20 years longer than the average life span just a few generations ago.

Every year, people are living just a little bit longer. This is partly because of our success in battling childhood diseases, like polio, as well as adult conditions, such as heart disease and diabetes. But it's also because scientists are unlocking the secrets of aging itself. We're finding out why our bodies break down and how to put the brakes on our own destruction. In the process, we're expanding not only our life spans but also what scientists call our health spans—the number of years that we can expect to live in robust good health.

"Once we can understand and manage the ways in which our bodies generate harmful molecules, which are major factors in biological aging, we will be able to reach out and grasp that 120-year life span," says William Regelson, M.D., professor of medicine at the Virginia Commonwealth University, Medical College of Virginia School of Medicine in Richmond.

The Power of Antioxidants

Researchers have identified one of the most important contributors to heart disease, wrinkles, cancer, arthritis, and many of the other problems of aging. "We rust," says Dr. Regelson.

Ironically, the same air that gives us life is what causes iron to rust, fruit to turn brown, and our bodies' cells to break down and age. Through a series of chemical changes, oxygen molecules in our bodies lose electrons, making them unstable. These unstable molecules are called free radicals.

In frantic attempts to stabilize themselves, free radicals pillage electrons from healthy cells throughout your body. Every time they steal an electron, two things happen: A healthy molecule is damaged, and more free radicals are created. Unless this process is stopped, an increasing number of cells are damaged every day, and our health pays the price.

To keep this destructive process under control, nature created an enormous arsenal of antioxidants, which are compounds that can stop free radicals from doing harm. Antioxidants come between free radicals and your body's healthy cells, offering up their own electrons and preventing yours from being pillaged.

Even though the body naturally produces antioxidants, studies clearly show that the antioxidants in foods and vitamins offer superior protection. Here are three of the strongest antioxidants.

Beta-carotene and C. More than 50 studies have demonstrated that high intake of foods rich in beta-carotene reduces the risk of cancer. More than 40 studies have indicated that vitamin C does the same. These two nutrients also have been shown to be very effective against heart disease.

The quickest way to get vitamin C naturally is to have a glass of grapefruit juice, an orange, or a half-cup of sweet red peppers, each of which provides more than 100 percent of the Daily Value (DV). For beta-carotene, deep green or bright orange fruits and vegetables are your best picks. One sweet potato or large carrot delivers between 12 and 15 milligrams, nearly double the basic amount experts recommend.

You also can boost your intake of these nutrients through supplements. "Nobody really knows what the optimum levels are," says Denham Harman, M.D., Ph.D., professor emeritus of medicine at the University of Nebraska College of Medicine in Omaha. "But I recommend daily doses of 1,500 to 2,000 milligrams of vitamin C, along with 25,000 international units (15 milligrams) of beta-carotene every other day." Note that some people may experience diarrhea from taking high does of vitamin C.

Vitamin E. Like vitamin C and beta-carotene, vitamin E has been shown to be very effective against age-related illnesses including cancer and heart disease. It's a bit trickier to get your daily intake of this essential nutrient from foods, though. Vitamin E is found mainly in high-fat foods, such as vegetable oils, that are best to avoid. You can get quite a bit of vitamin E in wheat germ, with ¼ cup providing 4 milligrams, 20 percent of the DV. Nuts and seeds are also good sources of vitamin E. You can supplement the amount of vitamin E in these foods by taking 200 to 400 international units in pill form.

Phytonutrients. Even though beta-carotene and vitamins C and E are essential antioxidants, they're not the only ones. Fruits and vegetables are loaded with plant compounds called phytonutrients, which also have powerful antioxidant abilities.

Eat Less, Live Longer

Even though we may need to eat more of certain foods in order to live longer, researchers are finding that the opposite can also be true: People who eat a little less sometimes live a little more.

Research has shown that laboratory animals on a restricted-calorie diet have lower blood pressure, higher levels of healthful high-density lipoprotein (HDL) cholesterol, and lower levels of potentially dangerous blood fats called triglycerides than their all-you-can-eat companions, says George Roth, Ph.D., a scientist at the Gerontology Research Center of the National Institute on Aging in Baltimore. In fact, the lean eaters outlive their gluttonous kin by about 30 percent.

"We believe that one of the ways in which calorie restriction works is by shifting animals' metabolisms to a survival mode so that they use the energy they take in most efficiently," says Dr. Roth. "Right now, we are testing calorie restriction on primates, which will give us a better indication of how well it will work in people." So far, all the signs, such as lower blood pressure and cholesterol levels, are indicating that it will be beneficial, he says.

The research is still preliminary, so it would be a mistake to start cutting calories if you're already at a healthy weight. But it does seem likely that cutting unnecessary calories from your diet will help stretch your life span a little further, says Dr. Roth.

In a study at the University of Michigan in Ann Arbor, researchers found that people who got the most glutathione, a phytonutrient found in avocados, grapefruit, winter squash, oranges, tomatoes, and potatoes, had lower blood pressure and cholesterol levels and maintained healthier weights than folks who got the least.

"Getting enough of all of these antioxidants won't guarantee that you'll live to be 150. But they will help you reach your maximum life span, and with some people only living to 60, adding another 15 years is quite nice," says Richard Cutler, Ph.D., former research chemist at the Gerontology Research Center of the National Institute on Aging in Baltimore and founder of Genox Corporation, which investigates strategies for stopping free radical damage.

How Eating Habits Affect Aging

While it's important to eat the right foods to prevent aging, you also need to adjust your eating *habits*. As the years pass, your nutritional needs can change dramatically.

"We produce less saliva as we age, so food isn't as easy to digest and swallow," says Susan A. Nitzke, R.D., Ph.D., associate professor in the nutritional sciences department at the University of Wisconsin in Madison. "We experience changes in taste and appetite, so we eat less. We also have less stomach acid, which means that we don't digest foods or absorb nutrients as well as we used to."

In a study of 205 older adults, many of whom had weakened immune systems, researchers in Newfoundland, Canada, found that almost a third of them were low in iron, zinc, folate, vitamin B_{12}, or protein—or a combination of these nutrients. But the problems were easily corrected. Once the folks began getting the necessary nutrients, they had significant jumps in levels of disease-fighting immune cells.

"I've seen people who thought they were having trouble with senility and who supposedly couldn't take care of themselves anymore. What they really had were nutritional deficiencies," Dr. Regelson says. Here's how to get more key nutrients in your diet.

Load up on zinc. Zinc is an essential mineral for maintaining a healthy immune system. It's also one of the nutrients that requires adequate amounts of stomach acid in order to be absorbed. When acid levels decline, getting enough zinc can be a problem, says Dr. Nitzke. This is especially true in people who are taking antacids, she adds.

The easiest way to get all the zinc your body needs is to have a plate of steamed oysters. Just six shelled morsels deliver 77 milligrams of zinc, 513 percent of the DV. Crab is also good, with 3 ounces providing 7 milligrams, 47 percent of the DV.

Battle aging with the Bs. Many older people have trouble getting enough B vitamins, which your nerves and brain need to stay healthy. "As we age, the lining of the stomach changes, making it harder to absorb these nutrients," says Dr. Regelson. "After age 55, it's particularly easy to be deficient in vitamin B_6."

Potatoes and bananas are your best sources of B_6. One potato provides 0.5 milligram, 25 percent of the DV, and a banana has 0.7 milligram, 35 percent of the DV. To get more folate (also a B vitamin), you need to eat greens and beans, particularly pinto and kidney beans. A half-cup of either of these beans provides over 100 milligrams of folate, more than 25 percent of the DV. Spinach is another good source of folate, with 1 cup containing as much as an equal amount of beans. Finally, you can get plenty of vitamin B_{12} in meats and other animal foods. Clams are a top performer: 20 small steamed clams provide an astonishing 89 micrograms of vitamin B_{12}, 1,483 percent of the DV.

Concentrate on calcium for strong bones. As bones get older, it's essential to get extra calcium to prevent them from becoming brittle, says Dr. Nitzke. This can be a problem for people who are lactose intolerant. But, Dr. Nitzke says, "most people can eat moderate amounts of dairy without trouble" even if they are sensitive to mild products.

Low-fat milk, skim-milk cheese, and yogurt are your best sources of this bone-building nutrient. One cup of fat-free yogurt contains 415 milligrams of calcium, 41 percent of the DV. Skim milk is also good, with one glass providing 302 milligrams, 30 percent of the DV.

Tap into the power of iron. Iron is a key ingredient in keeping your immune system functioning. A deficiency may lead to a host of conditions, from colds to fatigue to listlessness and restless leg syndrome. However, iron is another mineral that can be tough to get in the correct amounts. Some people don't get enough, while others get too much, says Dr. Nitzke. To be safe, she recommends having your doctor do a blood test for anemia. If it turns out that you do need more iron, you won't have any trouble getting it. Lean meat and seafood contain an abundance of iron, she says. Cream of Wheat and other fortified cereals are also good sources, with 5 milligrams of iron per serving, 29 percent of the DV.

ARTHRITIS

Slowing Joint Wear and Tear

An estimated 37 million Americans have arthritis, but often it's not whom you'd expect.

Sure, you might understand if it was one of your parents or grandparents. After all, about half the people over age 60 have some form of arthritis, making it the single most common chronic condition among older Americans.

But despite its reputation for being as much a part of growing old as gray hair, arthritis can strike younger people, too.

"Many people aren't surprised to hear that arthritis is the single leading cause of disability in people over age 45," says Paul Caldron, D.O., a clinical rheumatologist and researcher at the Arthritis Center in Phoenix. "But they are surprised to learn it's the single leading cause of disability among all ages."

A Burden to Body and Mind

At best, arthritis can slow down your movements and cause some pain; at worst, it can cause agony and even debilitate to the point where a person may need hospitalization or around-the-clock care, says Jeffrey R. Lisse, M.D., director of the division of rheumatology and associate professor of medicine at the University of Texas Medical Branch at Galveston. The pain of arthritis can also make you lose sleep and hamper your sex life. It can lead to weakness in the cardiovascular system, because people with arthritis often become sedentary when exercise is too painful. Also, it even can lead to depression, which Dr. Lisse says is "almost universal among arthritis patients."

Different Types, Same Symptoms

Most people know arthritis causes painful, stiff, and sometimes swollen joints. But the condition can also affect muscles and tendons, which may not swell but

47

still hurt. And while technically there are more than 100 different forms of arthritis, the two most common are osteoarthritis and rheumatoid arthritis.

Osteoarthritis, which affects about 16 million Americans, is the most widespread. It often is caused by a breakdown in the cartilage in joints because of joint stress, excessive weight, or injury, often sports-related. "That's not to say that if you play sports, you'll get arthritis. But those who have experienced repeated injury to a joint, no matter how minor, have an increased chance of getting osteoarthritis," says Dr. Caldron.

Osteoarthritis typically is localized to a certain area, such as the fingers, knees, feet, hips, or back. It usually strikes people in their forties and fifties.

The other major form of arthritis is rheumatoid arthritis. It usually strikes people in their twenties and thirties and is three times more likely to affect women than men.

"What's really sad is that many people have significant pain and loss of function, and there's nothing you can do to prevent it, since we don't know what causes it," says Arthur Grayzel, M.D., vice president of medical affairs for the Arthritis Foundation. Unlike osteoarthritis, rheumatoid arthritis occurs because of chronic inflammation in the joints. It is thought to be the result of an immunity disorder.

Reducing the Damage

You may not be able to prevent either type of arthritis, but you can lessen its aging effects on you by following these steps.

Get in shape. "Being overweight is a major risk factor, especially for arthritis of the knees and hips," says Dr. Grayzel. "Even when you're in your twenties and thirties, you should try to keep your weight close to the normal range for your height. If you're 20 percent overweight or more, you're a prime candidate for osteoarthritis."

Any weight loss helps, he says. "If you lose just 10 pounds and keep it off for 10 years, no matter your current weight, you can cut your risk of osteoarthritis in your knees by 50 percent."

Get physical. Regular exercise to build your muscles and flexibility can keep osteoarthritis at bay or lessen its effects. Exercise also is recommended for rheumatoid arthritis, although workouts should be under a doctor's supervision and emphasize range-of-motion exercises.

"Exercise improves strength and flexibility, so less stress is placed on the joints, and they can move easier and more efficiently," says John H. Klippel, M.D., clinical director of the National Institute of Arthritis and Musculoskeletal and Skin Diseases in Bethesda, Maryland. "Inactivity, on the other hand, actually encourages pain, stiffness, and other symptoms."

Weight lifting is particularly helpful because it builds muscle tone, which is especially important for arthritis sufferers. Building the abdominal muscles can reduce back pain and strengthening the thigh muscles helps with knee pain, advises Dr. Grayzel. Meanwhile, aerobic exercise such as running, bicycling, and swimming is also good for improving flexibility.

There's one important point to keep in mind, though: When a joint is swollen and inflamed, continuing to use it doesn't help. "Don't exercise through pain," says Dr. Grayzel. "You'll just hurt more." Instead, when your joints or muscles begin to hurt, skip a day or two of exercise.

Avoid nutritional triggers. Since there's some evidence that rheumatoid arthritis is triggered by a faulty immune system, and the immune system is affected by what you eat, it makes sense that a change in diet might make a difference in how you feel.

"Diet is critical in the treatment of this form of arthritis," says Joel Fuhrman, M.D., a specialist in nutritional medicine at the Amwell Health Center in Belle Mead, New Jersey. "In populations that consume natural diets of mostly unprocessed fruits, vegetables, and grains, autoimmune diseases are almost nonexistent. You don't see much crippling rheumatoid arthritis in rural China, for example, because the people there eat differently than we do."

More is involved than just getting more fruits, vegetables, and grains. Some people are sensitive to certain foods—like wheat, dairy foods, corn, citrus fruits, tomatoes, and eggs—that can switch on the body's inflammatory response.

Since there are so many things that can exacerbate the pain of rheumatoid arthritis, knowing which foods, if any, to avoid can be difficult, says David Pisetsky, M.D., Ph.D., co-director of the Duke University Arthritis Center in Durham, North Carolina, and medical adviser to the Arthritis Foundation. He recommends starting a food diary so that you can keep track of what you were eating around the time a flare-up occurred. If you discover a pattern—for example, you remember eating tomatoes shortly before an attack—you'll have an idea of what to avoid in the future. Once you've identified a possible culprit, stop eating that food (or foods) for at least 5 days, he says. Then try the food again and see if your symptoms return.

Try a vegetarian diet. The proteins found in meats may occasionally play a role in causing arthritis pain, so it makes sense that following a vegetarian diet would help relieve it. Research bears this out.

In a study at Norway's University of Oslo, 27 people with rheumatoid arthritis followed a vegetarian diet for 1 year. (After the first 3 to 5 months, they could eat dairy products if they wished.) They also avoided gluten (a protein found in wheat), refined sugar, salt, alcohol, and caffeine. After a month, their joints were less swollen and tender, and they had less morning stiffness and a stronger grip than people who followed their usual diets.

Say no to fat. These days it's difficult to think of any illness that isn't made worse by a diet high in saturated fats. Arthritis, it appears, is no exception.

In one study, 23 people with rheumatoid arthritis were put on a very low fat (10 percent of calories from fat) diet for 12 weeks. They also walked 30 minutes a day and followed a stress-reduction regimen. People in this group experienced a 20 to 40 percent reduction in joint tenderness and swelling; many of them were able to cut back on arthritis medications. People in a second group who didn't follow the diet showed no such improvement.

"We think that the diet caused most of the improvements in joint swelling and tenderness," says study leader Edwin H. Krick, M.D., associate professor of medicine at Loma Linda University in California.

A diet low in saturated fats reduces the body's production of prostaglandins, hormonelike substances that contribute to inflammation, says Dr. Krick. In addition, a low-fat diet may hinder communications sent by the immune system, thereby interrupting the body's inflammatory response. "Interrupting those chemicals can help the joints get better," he says. "One way to accomplish that is by consuming a low-fat or largely vegetarian diet."

Some doctors recommend limiting dietary fat to no more than 25 percent of total calories, with no more than 7 percent of these calories coming from saturated fats.

Fish for relief. Even though it's generally a good idea to cut back on fats, there is one type of fat that you may want to include in an anti-arthritis diet. The omega-3 fatty acids, found primarily in cold-water fish such as mackerel, trout, and salmon, reduce the body's production of prostaglandins and leukotrienes, both substances that contribute to inflammation.

In one study, researchers at Albany Medical College in New York had 37 people with arthritis consume high doses of fish oil. After 6 months, these people reported having fewer tender joints, less morning stiffness, and better grip strength than those who consumed less or no fish oil.

To get the healing benefits from fish, you need to take an omega-3 fatty acid supplement, or eat fish two or three times a week, says Joanne Curran-Celentano, R.D., Ph.D., associate professor of nutritional sciences at the University of New Hampshire in Durham. Fish rich in omega-3's include salmon, bluefin tuna, rainbow trout, halibut, and pollack. Canned fish such as mackerel, herring, sardines, and tuna are also high in omega-3's.

Vitamin Cures

Along with a change in diet, increasing your intake of vitamins may help alleviate the symptoms of arthritis. Here are two vitamins that seem to play important roles.

Use E to ease painful joints. Joints damaged by osteoarthritis don't get as hot and swollen as joints hit with rheumatoid arthritis, but they are somewhat inflamed. That's one reason doctors sometimes recommend vitamin E for osteoarthritis. Vitamin E fights inflammation by neutralizing the biochemicals that are produced during inflammation.

In a study by Israeli researchers, people with osteoarthritis who took 600 international units of vitamin E every day for 10 days had significant reductions in pain compared with when they were not taking vitamin E. "Vitamin E also apparently stimulates the body's deposit of cartilage-building proteins called proteoglycans," says Joseph E. Pizzorno, Jr., N.D., a naturopathic physician and president of Bastyr University in Bothell, Washington.

Doctors recommend 400 to 600 international units of vitamin E, amounts that are considered safe, says Jonathan Wright, M.D., a doctor in Kent, Washington, who specializes in nutritional therapy and is the author of *Dr. Wright's Guide to Healing with Nutrition*. These large amounts are available only by supplementation.

Selenium, a mineral that increases the effectiveness of vitamin E, is often added to the osteoarthritis formula in amounts of about 200 micrograms a day. "That amount is considered safe, but you won't want to take much more than that without medical supervision," says Dr. Wright.

Harness the power of C. Researchers at Boston University School of Medicine studied the eating habits of people with osteoarthritis of the knee. They found that the condition was three times less likely to increase in severity among people who got more than 200 milligrams of vitamin C a day.

The researchers aren't sure why vitamin C seemed to make such a difference, says study leader Timothy McAlindon, M.D., assistant professor of medicine at the medical school. Since vitamin C is an antioxidant, it may protect the joints from the damaging effects of free radicals, unstable molecules that can cause joint inflammation. "Vitamin C may also help generate collagen, which enhances the body's ability to repair damage to the cartilage," he says.

Dr. McAlindon recommends that people get at least 120 milligrams of vitamin C a day in their diets, twice the Daily Value. "That's the amount in a couple of oranges," he says. Other fruits and vegetables rich in vitamin C include cantaloupe, broccoli, strawberries, peppers, and cranberry juice.

BACK PAIN

Coping with a Common Ache

No matter whether it occurs after a lifetime of pushing, pulling, and prodding, or simply comes as a bolt out of the blue—golf legend Lee Trevino developed an excruciating case of it after he was struck by lightning during a tournament—back pain is one of life's most common and debilitating afflictions.

"Other than the common cold, back pain is the most frequent reason people go to see a physician or miss work," says Stephen Hochschuler, M.D., cofounder of the Texas Back Institute in Plano and author of *Treat Your Back without Surgery.* "It can strike very suddenly. One thing is certain: It's not a very pleasant experience."

In fact, at least 70 percent of Americans will suffer from back pain at some point in their lives. Of those, 14 percent will have severe pain that lasts at least 2 weeks, and up to 7 percent will suffer chronic pain that can last for more than 6 months, according to Gunnar B. J. Andersson, M.D., Ph.D., professor and associate chairman of the department of orthopedic surgery at Rush-Presbyterian-St. Luke's Medical Center in Chicago.

The Age of Opportunity

Most people experience their first bouts of back pain between the ages of 30 and 45, says Dan Futch, D.C., chief of the chiropractic staff at Group Health Cooperative HMO in Madison, Wisconsin.

"Those ages are the window of opportunity for back pain," he says. "About the same time you start getting gray hairs, you'll probably start noticing twinges of pain in your back."

The thirties and forties are the years when arthritis and other types of natural degeneration in the small joints of the back begin to catch up with us, agrees Robert Waldrip, M.D., an orthopedic spine surgeon in private practice in Phoenix. Spinal stenosis, for example, a narrowing of the canal in the vertebrae that surround the spinal cord, puts pressure on nerves in the low back and causes pain. In other cases, the problem is a herniated disk. Disks are small pads made of a tough, elastic outer covering (called the annulus) and a soft center. The disks act like shock absorbers between the vertebrae. Over time, a disk can herniate, meaning that the annulus has torn and the soft center has extended out to press against a nerve root, causing horrible pain. Poor posture also increases strain on the back and can aggravate arthritis and lead to disk problems.

But by far, the most common cause of back pain is muscle strain. As we get older, many of us exercise less. As a result, the muscles in the abdomen and back that support the spine weaken and get out of shape, says Alan Bensman, M.D., a physiatrist at Rehabilitative Health Services in Minneapolis. So things that you used to do with ease, such as hauling a bag of groceries out of your car, lifting a baby out of a crib, or raking the leaves, suddenly make you feel like you have a dozen knives sticking in your back.

Keeping Your Spine Sublime

If you have back pain so intense that you can't move, see your doctor. Also, seek medical care if the pain spreads to your legs or buttocks, if your legs or feet feel numb or tingly, if you lose control of your bladder or bowel movements, or if you also have a fever or abdominal pain. If you're pain is less intense, there are many simple steps you can take to reduce the pain or prevent it altogether.

Do an early morning stretch. "I tell my patients to always start off their days by stretching while they're still in bed," Dr. Bensman says. "Remember that you've been lying prone for 8 hours, and if you jump right up, you may be looking at a sore back." So before you get up, slowly stretch your arms over your head, then gently pull your knees up to your chest one at a time. When you're ready to sit up, roll to the side of the bed and use your arm to help prop yourself up. Put your hands on your buttocks and slowly lean back to extend your spine.

Keep in shape. Walking and other aerobic exercises such as swimming, biking, and running keep your back healthy by conditioning your whole body. They strengthen the postural muscles of the buttocks, legs, back, and abdomen. Aerobic exercise also may help your body release endorphins, hormones that subdue pain. Try doing an aerobic workout for 20 minutes a day, three times a week, says Dr. Futch.

Lose weight. For every 10 pounds you drop, you eliminate 200 pounds of stress on your spine and other joints.

Take a break. Sitting puts more strain on your back than standing. If you must sit at your desk for an extended time or you're traveling by plane, train, or car, change position often and give your back a break by standing up and walking around every hour or so, says Augustus A. White III, M.D., professor of orthopedic surgery at Harvard Medical School in Boston and author of *Your Aching Back*.

Let your luggage lie. At the end of a trip, instead of leaping out of the car or airplane and grabbing your bags, take a couple of minutes to stretch, Dr. Bensman suggests. Slowly bring your knees toward your chest and gently swing your arms around to loosen up stiff muscles. Avoid lifting with overstretched arms and try to keep the bags close to your body. Consider getting a collapsible luggage carrier with wheels.

Kneel, don't bend. Avoid bending over at the waist to pick up something. That creates tension in the back and increases your risk of injury, Dr. Futch says. Instead, use long-handled tools and kneel on a cushion or knee pad to garden, vacuum, or do other "low-level" activities.

Let your legs do the work. If you're lifting something—no matter if it weighs 5 pounds or 50—bend your knees, keep your back straight, and lift with your legs. "The legs are much stronger than the back and can lift a lot more weight without strain," Dr. Futch says.

Test the load first. "How many of us have strained back muscles when we tried to pick up boxes that we thought were empty but were actually filled with encyclopedias?" asks Joseph Sasso, D.C., president of the Federation of Straight Chiropractors and Organizations. Always nudge a box with your foot or cautiously lift it an inch or so before really trying to heft it. If it's too heavy for you, ask for help.

Turn your back on heavy lifting. If you can't find someone to help you move a heavy object, try this maneuver as a last resort: If the object is sitting at table height, turn your back to it to drag or lift it. You can also use this technique for raising windows. This position reduces the pressure that would be exerted on your spine by forcing you to use your legs for leverage.

Straighten up. Maintaining good posture is one of the best ways to prevent back pain, Dr. Futch says. To improve your posture, try this: Stand against a wall, making sure that your shoulders and buttocks touch the wall. Slip your arm into the space between your lower back and the wall. If there is a point where your hand isn't touching both your back and the wall, tilt your hips so that the extra space is eliminated. Hold that position for a count of 20 while looking in a mirror to see what your posture looks like. Try to sense what it feels like, so you can maintain that posture for the rest of the day. Do that exercise once a day for 3 weeks to ensure that good posture will become a habit.

Wear the right shoes. Worn-out shoes are terrible shock absorbers that allow the force of every step to rattle your legs, jostle your knees, and aggravate your back, says Daniel Handel, M.D., president and medical director of the Forest Park Institute Center for Pain Management in Fort Worth, Texas. If your shoes are worn, get a new pair or at least replace the insoles. Also, avoid wearing shoes with heels that are more than 1 inch high, Dr. Handel warns. High heels are the worst shoes for your back because they exaggerate the natural curve in your lower spine and can trigger back pain.

Check your mattress. Your mattress should provide proper support, be level, and not sag. If you feel like you're sleeping in the middle of a pita bread, it's probably time to get a new mattress, Dr. Sasso says.

Brace your lower back. A lumbar roll, a round foam-rubber pad that can be purchased at most medical supply stores, can help you maintain the natural curve

Four Steps to Quick Relief

Aside from drugs, immediate relief from back pain boils down to four fundamental steps, says Stephen Hochschuler, M.D., cofounder of the Texas Back Institute in Plano and author of *Treat Your Back without Surgery.*

1. Stop what you are doing. "It's hard to believe, but some golfers will hurt their backs on the second hole, yet continue to play to the last green. "That's simply not smart," he says. If you think you've hurt your back, stop immediately, no matter what you're doing.

2. Lie down in a comfortable position. Often, lying on your back with pillows under your knees or lying on your side with pillows between your legs will help ease the pain during the first 12 to 24 hours, he says.

3. Get up and go. Even though rest is important, too much of it—even during the first 24 hours—can weaken back muscles and worsen your pain. So at least once an hour while you're awake, get up and do something physical. Even a mild stretch will help.

If your pain worsens while you are stretching, stop. But try again an hour or two later. The more you stretch, the better your back will feel, Dr. Hochschuler says.

4. Ice, then heat. Ice is a good treatment for the first 48 hours after back pain sets in because it helps numb the area and prevent swelling, Dr. Hochschuler says. You can simply wrap a bag of frozen vegetables in a towel and place it over the sore spot. Ice can be used once an hour, but don't apply it for more than 15 minutes at a time—excessive cold can injure your skin.

After 48 hours, you can place a warm, well-wrung towel on your sore back for 10 to 15 minutes, two or three times a day. Once the pain subsides, try to do a few stretches to keep your back limber after you remove the heat.

in the small of your spine and prevent lower back pain, says Hamilton Hall, M.D., director of the Canadian Back Institute in Toronto. Whenever you sit, stick the roll between your lower back and the chair.

Forgo tobacco. Smoking decreases blood flow to the back and can weaken disks, Dr. Bensman says. If you smoke, quit.

Putting Your Pain to Rest

So now you know how to head off back pain before it starts. But what do you do when you're in the midst of one of those razor-sharp twinges? For immediate relief, Dr. Hochschuler recommends the steps in "Four Steps to Quick Relief" on page 55. After that, here's what the experts recommend.

Take an over-the-counter medicine. Taking one or two aspirin or ibuprofen tablets every 4 to 6 hours can relieve pain and reduce swelling, Dr. Bensman says. Be sure you don't exceed the manufacturer's recommended dosage.

Try arnica for ache relief. Arnica is a good homeopathic remedy found in most health food stores and even some drugstores for acute back spasms, bruises, and other trauma, says Andrew T. Weil, M.D. director of the program in integrative medicine at the University of Arizona College of Medicine in Tucson and author of *8 Weeks to Optimum Healing*. Take four 30X tablets as soon as possible after the injury, and repeat every hour until bedtime. The next day, cut down your doses to four tablets every 2 hours. In the days that follow, take four tablets just four times a day. You may continue this treatment for 4 to 5 days.

Get manipulated. An analysis of 25 studies of spinal manipulation—the heart and soul of chiropractic treatment—found that manipulation does provide at least some short-term relief for uncomplicated, acute back pain. In a typical case, a chiropractor may do a series of thrusts with the heels of his hands along the troubled area of your spine to realign the vertebrae. Ask your doctor for a referral to a chiropractor in your area.

Eat your fill of pineapple. Pineapple is a good source of bromelain and papain, two enzymes that help flush toxins out of your body and relieve painful back inflammation, says David Molony, O.M.D., a doctor of oriental medicine in Catasauqua, Pennsylvania, and executive director of the American Association of Oriental Medicine. He recommends eating half a pineapple daily until your back pain subsides. Be sure to eat close to the core, because it is a rich source of bromelain.

BLADDER CONTROL

Taming a Nasty Nuisance

Your bladder, once as dependable as the Hoover Dam, has lost its reliability and now you're never sure when the floodgates will open and embarrass you beyond belief.

"The psychological impact of a bladder problem is tremendous. If someone between the ages of 30 and 50 begins to urinate more frequently, wets herself, or has other bladder problems that she associates with aging, I'm sure that she might think, 'This never used to happen to me. My god, I must be getting older. This is the first thing that happened to Aunt Millie when she started her downward slide,'" says Alan J. Wein, M.D., chairman of the division of urology at the University of Pennsylvania School of Medicine in Philadelphia.

But in reality, most bladder difficulties are not an inevitable sign of aging. In fact, urinary tract infections and incontinence, the two most common causes of bladder problems, can affect people at any age and can usually be treated effectively or cured, Dr. Wein says.

Here's a closer look at the causes of and remedies for these two nuisances.

When Bacteria Invade

It may begin with a severe pain every time you urinate. Soon you feel the unmistakable urge to go again, even if you went just a few minutes ago. And when you do go, a surprisingly small amount of urine trickles out. Sometimes your urine has a strong odor and you pass blood. In severe cases, you might also develop back pain, chills, fever, nausea, and vomiting.

More than likely, you have a urinary tract infection (UTI), a bladder problem that is most common among women, Dr. Wein says. At least 25 to 35 percent of women between the ages of 20 and 40 have had at least one UTI. Of those, nearly 20 percent will have at least one recurrence, says Penny Wise Budoff, M.D., clinical associate professor of family medicine at the State University of New York at

Stony Brook Health Sciences Center School of Medicine. Overall, women are up to 50 times more likely than men to develop UTIs.

That's because a woman's urethra, the tube that carries urine out of the bladder, is less than 2 inches long. Since it is so short, the urethra is vulnerable to invasion by bacteria that naturally live in the vagina and rectum. Sexual intercourse can drive bacteria up into the urinary tract, where these microorganisms can cause inflammation of the urethra, bladder, or kidneys.

Waiting too long to urinate is another common cause of UTIs. If you go for hours without urinating, you can stretch the bladder muscle and weaken it to the point that it can't expel all the urine. This residue of urine increases your risk of infection.

Once an infection strikes, your doctor will prescribe antibiotics, says Jonathan Vapnek, M.D., assistant professor of urology at Mount Sinai School of Medicine in New York City.

While your family physician can treat a UTI, you should see a urologist or gynecologist if you have blood in your urine, recurrent UTIs, or a history of kidney infections or stones, Dr. Vapnek says.

In some cases, women with UTIs may develop interstitial cystitis, a chronic disease that causes inflammation of the bladder. Women who have it often feel the urge to void up to 60 times a day. It has no known cause or cure, but its symptoms are often relieved by drugs such as steroids and antihistamines.

Although bladder infections should be brought to your doctor's attention, there are plenty of ways to prevent them in the first place. Here's how.

Drink plenty of water. Drinking at least eight 8-ounce glasses of water and other noncaffeinated beverages every day dilutes urine in the bladder, which makes it more difficult for bacteria to thrive, Dr. Budoff says.

Urinate often. Try to empty your bladder at least four to six times a day, Dr. Budoff says. That will help keep your bladder clear of bacteria. Going to the bathroom that often shouldn't be a problem if you drink plenty of fluids.

Try the cranberry juice cure. This age-old remedy got a shot of scientific validation from researchers at Harvard Medical School, who divided 153 women into cranberry juice drinkers and non-cranberry juice drinkers. Those who drank about 10 ounces a day of the tangy beverage experienced bladder infections only 42 percent as often as those who did not. The researchers speculate that cranberry juice may inhibit bacteria's ability to latch on to the bladder wall.

Consider your birth control method. Researchers at the University of Washington found a connection between recurrent UTIs and women who use diaphragms in conjunction with spermicide. Women who used this contraceptive method had much greater risk of having *Escherichia coli* bacteria, the most likely culprit to cause UTIs, in their urine. If you use a diaphragm with spermicide and suffer frequent UTIs, consider switching to another form of birth control, says Seth Lerner, M.D., assistant professor of urology at the Baylor College of Medicine in Houston. Consult with your doctor.

Battle bacteria with goldenseal. Goldenseal's anti-microbial and immune-stimulating properties help it fight the *E. coli* bacteria and make it a popular choice for treating infection in general, says naturopathic doctor Tori Hudson, N.D., professor at the National College of Naturopathic Medicine in Portland, Oregon. Take 500 to 1,000 milligrams of goldenseal root extract daily, but don't take it for more than 1 week. And do not take this herb at all if you are pregnant.

Practice good hygiene. Washing your hands before and after urinating may reduce your chances of a UTI, Dr. Budoff says. When wiping your bottom, do it from front to back. That will keep potentially harmful bacteria away from your urethra. For extra cleanliness, Dr. Budoff suggests using a large, moistened cotton ball to wipe from front to back.

Shower, don't bathe. Soaking in a tub filled with soapy water or bubble bath can irritate the lining of the urinary tract, particularly if you have a history of recurrent bladder infections, says David Rivas, M.D., a urologist at Thomas Jefferson University Hospital in Philadelphia.

Stick with cotton. Snug nylon panties can restrict airflow, trap moisture, and promote bacterial growth around the urethra, Dr. Rivas says. Instead, wear loose-fitting cotton undergarments that permit better air circulation. If you wear panty hose, be sure that they have a cotton crotch.

The Horror of Losing Control

A picture that slips off the wall and breaks. A knife that slips and cuts your finger while you're making dinner. These are accidents you can shrug off as a part of everyday life. But when you have trouble getting to the bathroom in time or experience an embarrassing leak when you cough, sneeze, or even lift weights at the gym—well, that's the type of accident that can make you feel old in a hurry.

"Some people think incontinence is a sure sign that they're becoming decrepit. It signifies a lack of control and suggests that other valued qualities of life, such as exercising, traveling, and even living independently, are at stake," says Katherine Jeter, Ed.D., executive director of Help for Incontinent People in Union, South Carolina.

But incontinence isn't necessarily a sign of aging, Dr. Lerner says. In fact, studies indicate that about one in four people between the ages of 30 and 59 has had at least one instance of incontinence. That's about the same rate as for people over 60.

"Incontinence isn't like gray hair. It's not inevitable," Dr. Lerner says. "It usually has an underlying physiological cause that may be treatable."

Older people tend to have incontinence for different reasons than younger ones, says Tamara Bavendam, M.D., assistant professor of urology and director of the Female Urology Clinic at the University of Washington Medical Center in Seattle. Arthritis, for instance, can make it more difficult for an older person to walk to a bathroom quickly. Older people are also more likely to take medications, and some drugs—such as those used to treat heart disease—can cause excessive urine production that overwhelms the bladder's capacity.

Of the major types of bladder leakage, stress incontinence and urge incontinence are the most common among people in their thirties and forties, Dr. Lerner
says. Stress incontinence in women may result when pelvic floor muscles are
weakened or damaged. This can occur because of pregnancy and childbirth, excessive weight, or decreased hormonal production. The bladder and urethra sag,
and the sphincter muscle can't completely close. So any abdominal pressure, such
as a laugh or sneeze or lifting a heavy object, triggers a leak.

Urge incontinence, which can be caused by UTIs or inflammation of the
bladder, occurs when irritated or overactive bladder muscles contract uncontrol-
lably. As a result, a person can feel a compelling need to urinate. If she hesitates,
she may lose urine before she gets to a bathroom, Dr. Bavendam says.

In another type of incontinence called overflow incontinence, a person feels
no urge to void, so the bladder fills to the brim and causes so much pressure that
the excess urine spills out. Diabetes is one of the primary causes of this type of
bladder leakage.

It's important to remember that incontinence is not a disease but a symptom
of an underlying ailment, says Deborah Erickson, M.D., a urologist and assistant
professor of surgery at the Pennsylvania State University College of Medicine in
Hershey. So if you have a leaky bladder, don't assume that you'll need to wear
adult diapers the rest of your life. More than likely, your doctor can help you.
Sometimes that may mean taking drugs that will tighten the sphincter muscle or
relax the bladder muscle to stop inappropriate bladder contractions. As a last resort, surgery can restore a sagging bladder to its natural position or make the urethra tight. But in most cases, simple remedies such as doing pelvic muscle
exercises or making changes in diet or bathroom habits relieve the problem. Here
are some ways to keep yourself dry.

Keep track. Keep a urinary log for a week or two before you see a doctor, Dr.
Vapnek suggests. Note what you eat and drink, when you go to the bathroom, and
when and where you leak. Were you coughing, or did you feel an urge and not
make it to the bathroom on time? The diary will help you and your physician track
down the problem.

Know your drugs. Some medications, including diuretics, antihistamines,
sedatives, and anticholinergics such as motion sickness drugs and over-the-counter
cold remedies, can weaken bladder control, Dr. Wein says. If you're taking any
drug, ask your doctor or pharmacist if it could be contributing to your problem.

Target your diet. Some people report that consuming coffee, tea, carbonated
soft drinks, artificial sweeteners, chocolate, tomatoes, hot spices, and other foods
and beverages makes their incontinence worse, Dr. Bavendam says. If you suspect a food may be contributing to your problem, try eliminating it from your diet
for a week and see what happens. If your symptoms improve, continue to avoid
that food, since it may have been irritating your bladder.

Stop smoking. People who smoke are 2½ times more likely to develop incontinence than those who don't, says Richard Bump, M.D., associate professor
and chief of the division of gynecologic specialties at Duke University Medical

Center in Durham, North Carolina, who studied incontinence among 606 smoking and nonsmoking women. He suspects that excessive coughing, which is common among smokers, weakens pelvic floor muscles and causes stress incontinence. Smoking may also irritate bladder muscles, so they contract more often and cause leaks. So if you smoke, quit.

Drink up. "A lot of people will cut back on their fluids in the hope that less in equals less out," Dr. Jeter says. But doing that may make you more, not less, likely to have problems, because highly concentrated urine irritates the bladder and causes it to contract to rid itself of that urine as soon as it can. Restricting fluids can also lead to dehydration, constipation, UTIs, and kidney stones. Drink at least six to eight glasses of water, juices, or other nonalcoholic, decaffeinated fluids a day, Dr. Erickson says.

Try it twice. If you feel like your bladder isn't draining completely, try double voiding. To do this, remain on the toilet until your bladder feels empty. Then stand up for 10 to 20 seconds, sit down, lean slightly forward over your knees, relax, and wait until your bladder empties completely, Dr. Jeter says.

Shed a few pounds. Excess weight strains the pelvic floor muscles and increases the risk of incontinence, Dr. Vapnek says. "People who are moderately overweight tell us that the loss of just 5 to 7 pounds means the difference between being wet and staying dry," Dr. Jeter says.

Exercise your muscles. Kegel exercises can strengthen the pelvic floor muscles and reduce your chances of a leak, Dr. Erickson says. To do Kegels, squeeze the muscles in your rectum as if you were trying to prevent passing gas. This should also tense the pelvic floor muscles. Feel the sensation of the muscles pulling upward. That's the sensation you want to achieve when doing these exercises. Squeeze the muscles, hold for a slow count of four, then relax for another count of four. Try to do 10 sets of Kegels each day. As these muscles become stronger, gradually increase the time you squeeze until you can hold the position for 25 to 30 sets of 10 seconds each. Your bladder control should improve within 3 to 4 weeks.

BODY IMAGE

Looking for, and Liking, the Real You

You look in the mirror at a trim forty-ish figure, but that's not what you see. You focus on all the "flaws" of aging. The chest *you* think is starting to look saggy. The hips *you* think are getting too big. The gray hair and wrinkles that *you* think make you look old.

The truth? It may be your mind that's betraying you, not your body.

"Body image has a total impact on how we feel about aging," says Mary Huntington Lehner, clinical director of the Rocky Mountain Treatment Center in Great Falls, Montana. "There's a direct connection between your self-esteem and your body image. The better your self-esteem, the better you'll feel about what is happening to your body as you journey through life."

Distorted Beliefs

Physical changes are natural as we grow older, but it can be tough to accept this fact in a society that worships youth and thinness. "In the eyes of society, when you're 20, you're hot; when you're 40, you're not; and when you're 60, you're shot," says Stanley Teitelbaum, Ph.D., a clinical psychologist in private practice in New York City.

This not-so-subtle vision is reflected in the ages and sizes of advertising models. Models have steadily become younger, thinner, and taller in the past 50 years. A generation ago, a model weighed only 8 percent less than the average person. Today, a model weighs 23 percent less. For perspective, consider that only 5 percent of women can achieve the same weight and proportions of today's models without dieting.

Even the clothing-store mannequins project an unreal image: The average American woman would have to lose 30 percent of her body weight to have similar proportions, says Debbie Then, Ph.D., a social psychologist in Stanford, California, who studies the effects of media on body image and conducts seminars on the topic.

The desire to meet the model's ideal is so intense that nearly half of all average-weight women actually consider themselves overweight, according to surveys conducted by Thomas Cash, Ph.D., professor of psychology at Old Dominion University in Norfolk, Virginia. Little wonder, then, that on any given day, 25 percent of all women are on diets, and up to one in seven women has an eating disorder.

These pressures to look thin, youthful, and sexy are clearly having an effect.

What Magazines Are Really Telling Us

Women's magazines love perfection. They tell us we can have perfect hair, perfect lips, perfect legs, perfect sex. They show us perfect models wearing perfect clothing and perfect makeup.

So how does all this perfection make us feel? Perfectly rotten, says Debbie Then, Ph.D., a social psychologist in Stanford, California, who studies the effects of media on body image and conducts seminars on the topic.

"Most women who look at those magazines know that they don't look like the models and never will," Dr. Then says. "Yet if you're constantly bombarded with those images, you might begin to consider yourself unattractive when in fact you're actually very good-looking."

In a small study, Dr. Then asked 75 women how they felt after reading their favorite women's magazines. Some said they were motivated to improve their appearances, but nearly 70 percent said the images in the magazines lowered their self-esteem and made them feel worse about their looks.

"I feel like every woman is at least 20 pounds lighter and 4 inches taller than I am," one woman wrote. "It really depresses me."

"It is impossible to look like the models unless I have a $5 million wardrobe, a personal airbrusher, a makeup artist, and I go on [a liquid diet] for 10 years," said another.

What to do? Well, a few women found what they considered the perfect solution: They stopped reading the magazines.

By most measures, a growing number of people believe looking young and attractive is important, but at the same time, more and more are displeased with their appearance.

Ann Kearney-Cooke, Ph.D., a Cincinnati psychologist in private practice who specializes in body image problems and eating disorders, and Ruth Striegel-Moore, Ph.D., associate professor of psychology at Wesleyan University in Middletown, Connecticut, conducted an attitude survey of 1,000 women. The doctors found that 68 percent of the women believed that being attractive is very important. In addition, 91 percent said they wanted to change their bodies.

What exactly do most women dislike about their bodies? Twenty percent are dissatisfied with their faces, 45 percent dislike their muscle tone, 32 percent would like to change their breast or chest sizes, and about 40 percent are dissatisfied with their overall appearance, according to Judith Rodin, Ph.D., author of *Bodytraps* and professor of psychiatry and medicine at Yale University School of Medicine in New Haven, Connecticut.

But the thing most women would change is their weight, because they believe men are attracted to thinner women. In a study of women who were asked to rate their body shapes against the body shape they believed was most attractive to men, women consistently rated themselves as far plumper than a man's ideal. However, their body shapes were actually closer to what men said they found attractive.

Although most people feel compelled to do something to maintain their looks, women in their thirties and forties may have the most difficulty doing it, says Susan Olson, Ph.D., director of psychological services at the Southwest Bariatric Nutrition Center in Tempe, Arizona.

"Women are in the middle of careers, raising children, and possibly caring for their aging parents. So it's hard to find time to focus on themselves," Dr. Olson says. "When they do, they all of a sudden realize they're getting older, and that's scary."

Feeling Better about Your Body

While body image can be a problem throughout the lives of many women— Dr. Kearney-Cooke has patients who at age 62 obsess about their appearance— worries about it usually level off for most women as they near their fifties.

"As women get older, they're more concerned about having healthy bodies than looking good," Dr. Kearney-Cooke says. "Instead of worrying if they can still fit into a size eight dress, they're more concerned that their backs will hurt tomorrow if they play golf today."

The ultimate reward for improving your body image at any age is that you'll feel more comfortable with yourself, and as a result, more people will want to be around you. "A good body image can definitely make you feel younger," Dr. Then says. "The more positive you are, the more outgoing you'll be. And that's important, because it's been shown that people who have more friends and acquaintances are healthier."

Here are some tips to help you develop a stronger self-image.

Take a look inside. "You aren't your body. You just happen to be in your body," Dr. Olson says. "Try not to look at yourself as just a physical being, because that's going to pass." Find other reasons for liking yourself, such as a solid career or a good sense of humor.

Find a role model. "I used to browse through magazines looking for pictures of women who had features similar to mine," Dr. Olson says. "They weren't perfect, but here they were in these magazines, and that made me feel better about myself." Find a picture of a woman you admire, cut it out, and put it on your mirror for inspiration.

Give yourself a hug. Dr. Olson suggests that each time you look in a mirror, say to yourself "I love you. I think you're absolutely beautiful." "That affirmation may seem ridiculous, but it's important, because you're not going to believe those words coming from anyone else until you believe them from yourself," she says.

Look back. Find a favorite picture of yourself from each decade of your life. "Looking at those pictures will help you realize that you were a better-looking person than you may have thought you were at the time," says Ann Meissner, Ph.D., a psychologist in private practice in St. Paul, Minnesota. "It will also make you think twice about how accurate your judgments are about yourself now."

Look ahead. Conjure up an image of yourself 5, 10, or 20 years from now. How do you look? How does it feel? Keep doing it until you find an image of yourself that feels comfortable, says Rita Freedman, Ph.D., author of *Bodylove*. "Look for role models whom you admire and think are attractive even though they are older and grayer. Put pictures of those people on your refrigerator, and use those images as something to look forward to and grow into."

Compare yourself to other real people. "When you go to a shopping mall or beach, specifically watch the people there. Chances are most of them aren't going to look like fashion models, and you'll end up feeling better about yourself," Dr. Then says.

Please yourself first. If you do decide to make changes in your body, do it for yourself; you'll enjoy it more. "As we get older, we cling to this idea that our physiques have to look like they did when we were 22. In fact, your friends and family probably don't care if you have the body of a 22-year-old. They just want you to have a decent 40-year-old body," says Mark Leary, Ph.D., professor of psychology at Wake Forest University in Winston-Salem, North Carolina.

Exercise the outer you. Regular exercise such as walking, bicycling, swimming, or weight training can help you stay fit—and improve your body image—when you do it for at least 20 minutes a day, three times a week, says Dr. Leary

Exercise the inner you. If you're working on changing your appearance, commit yourself to two other goals that aren't related to your body, Dr. Kearney-

Cooke says. For example, take a class or start keeping a journal to enhance your self-image. "It helps you see yourself as a whole person," she says.

Dress for success. "Appearance does count at any age, but you don't have to obsess about it. Just make the most of what you do have," Dr. Then says. "For health reasons, exercise, eat a balanced diet, maintain a weight that is right for your proportions, and practice good grooming. Wear clothes, makeup, and accessories that complement your figure, but realize that you don't have to look like a cover girl to have a happy, successful life. Try to be the best possible version of yourself."

BREAST SAG

Keeping Your Breasts Firm and Healthy

Turn to the right and look at your breasts sideways in the mirror. Now turn back to the front, lift your arms over your head and check again. Then turn to the left and check one more time.

Do you see sags and stretch marks that suggest you're beginning to age? Such signs are not uncommon in women in their late forties, doctors say. Yet while breast sag is most likely to occur after age 45, there is much you can do to prevent it with good breast care in the decades before. The first step: Understanding what causes your breasts to sag.

Gravity, Aging, and Hormones

There are two ways breasts may sag, doctors say: When large breasts sag, the nipples do a swan dive and head toward your waist; when small breasts sag, the nipples gracefully sink back toward your chest.

One way you look like a cow that needs milking. The other way you look like a boy. It may not be what God, nature, and Victoria's Secret intended, but sag can be the reality of the post-30 breast.

"Somewhere between the ages of 30 and 40, the elastic tissue in the breast begins to degenerate," explains Albert M. Kligman, M.D., Ph.D, professor of dermatology at the University of Pennsylvania School of Medicine and an attending physician at the Hospital of the University of Pennsylvania, both in Philadelphia. The breast fibers, which act like rubber bands and provide that resilient bounce as you walk, will still stretch. But they don't snap back quite as well. The result is saggy breasts with a few stretch marks thrown in for good measure.

Adding to the problem, hormonal changes—both during pregnancy and as you reach menopause—make breasts sag more.

During pregnancy, the hormones estrogen and progesterone, which are se-

Getting a Lift

When natural remedies fail, some women turn to a more radical cure to firm up their breasts: surgery.

Whether you're a good candidate for a breast lift is something you'll have to answer based on discussions with your doctor. But here is some information on your options.

"There are basically two kinds of lifting procedures we do in this country," says Robert L. Cucin, M.D., clinical instructor of plastic surgery at Cornell University Medical College in New York City.

"For smaller degrees of sagging, we can do what's called a doughnut mastopexy. You take some skin out from around the nipple's areola, then tuck the skin underneath where it gives you a modest degree of lift and tightening."

When sagging is more severe, American surgeons tend to use the inverted T, or anchor, mastopexy, says Dr. Cucin. The surgeon cuts around the nipple, straight down from the nipple to the bra line, then along the bra line in both directions for several inches. Excess skin and fat are removed, the nipple is repositioned and the remaining skin is drawn tight to support the breast. Scars will be about 9 inches long, and the amount of sensation left in your nipple depends on how much it's moved during the procedure.

creted by the ovary and the placenta, stimulate development of the 15 to 20 lobes of milk-secreting glands embedded in the breast's fatty tissue. These changes are permanent. And although the glands may be empty after they're no longer needed to produce milk, they will still add bulk and firmness to the breast.

Once menopause arrives, however, the drop in estrogen and progesterone signal the breasts that its milk ducts and lobes can retire. As a result, the breast shrinks, adds fat, and begins to droop.

Beating Breast Sag

Fortunately there are several ways to prevent, and sometimes reverse, the effects of aging on your breasts. Here are six steps that doctors recommend.

Build your pecs. "There's no way I know of to build up the breast's fatty tissue," says Sondra Lynne Carter, M.D., a gynecologist in private practice in New York City who treats patients with breast problems. "But you can build up the pectoralis muscles underlying the fatty tissues so that you get the same effect."

To prevent or reduce sag, get a couple of 2-pound weights—no heavier—and work those muscles five times a week, says Dr. Carter.

With a weight in each hand, extend your arms sideways, and do 15 small, backward circles about a foot in diameter. Widen the circles slightly and do another 15; widen them again and repeat. Slowly work your way up to 50 circles for each repetition.

Roll your shoulders. Put your weights aside and with your arms hanging at your sides, roll your shoulders backward, down and forward in a circular motion 15 to 20 times, says Dr. Carter. Do it 5 days a week. This strengthens the shoulders and upper chest and helps improve your posture.

Perform pushups. "Start off trying to do 10 pushups and work your way up to 20," says Dr. Carter. It may take up to 6 months, she adds. But you're more likely to do them regularly if you add one pushup at a time. Just get on your hands and knees, raise your feet 6 inches off the floor, and lower your upper body down to within an inch of the floor. Do these 5 days a week as well.

Get some support. Wearing a bra is a good way to prevent sagging, says Dr. Kligman. In fact, he suggests that any female over the age of 15 do so.

Get a style that has great support and allows minimal bounce, says Dr. Kligman. And wear it all day, not just when you work out.

Shrink the stretch marks. If you've just had a baby and the stretch marks on the top and sides of your breasts are red and inflamed, you can treat them with daily applications of tretinoin (Retin-A), says Dr. Kligman. Talk to your doctor about getting a prescription for the drug. Not only does Retin-A tighten the stretched skin, but there's some evidence that it also builds a new superstructure under the skin to help firm it.

Talk to your doctor about HRT. Hormone replacement therapy, or HRT, can halt breast sagging that occurs after menopause by helping to keep breast fibers from further degenerating, doctors say. It won't turn back the clock to your twenties, but it will keep your breasts from sagging more.

BURNOUT

Take Your Brain off Roast

Are you feeling as cranky and as easily irritated as an arthritic lap dog? Do you feel like you've lost your youthful resilience and you're fighting a losing battle with fatigue? Has your body become a playground for all manner of backache, chest pain, and headache?

Then you could be a victim of burnout.

While burnout can strike at any age, it is more common as you grow older, says C. David Jenkins, Ph.D., professor of preventive medicine and community health at the University of Texas Medical Branch at Galveston. "Burnout tends to drain people of the physiological and mental reserves that are, in youth, typically there to keep them going. It certainly can make you feel old before your time. Luckily, burnout does not necessarily age people or take years off their lives in a permanent fashion. It can be reversed."

But if you want to stop feeling decades beyond your biological age, you first need to know what's happened to you and why.

No Variety, No Relief

Many people assume that burnout is just a matter of doing too many things. Yet actually, it is not the number of activities in your life but rather a lack of variety among activities that causes burnout, says Faye Crosby, Ph.D., professor of psychology at Smith College in Northampton, Massachusetts, and author of *Juggling*. "Burnout does not occur by having too many pots boiling on your stove. Many times it occurs because you have only one pot boiling constantly and can never take it over to the sink to fill it up. Eventually, all the water boils away."

Variety is a basic human need, says Dr. Crosby, and it's a good way to vaccinate yourself against burnout. But you don't achieve variety merely by doing different activities. The activities have to answer different needs. "At work, our activities tend to be very agenda-oriented," Dr. Crosby says. "At home, our activities are much more socioemotional. They please us, they make us feel good, they answer emotional needs without having specific agendas."

Or at least they should. The problem starts when there's too much agenda and not enough emotional outlet. If home life is just another job—filled with routines like cleaning the house, handling paperwork, chauffeuring kids—you never have time to rejuvenate. To avoid burnout, you need to find time for hobbies, for cuddling with the family in front of the fireplace, for taking that relaxing walk.

Perfectionism Hurts

Another burnout-inducing extreme is the concept of all-around perfectionism. You know the type: the man who sets impossible goals and refuses to delegate any tasks. The woman who must be the perfect wife, mother, and professional.

"To be a perfectionist is to make unrealistic demands on yourself. You might be able to do it for a while, but in the long run, burnout is almost a certainty," says Herbert J. Freudenberger, Ph.D., author of *Women's Burnout* and *Burnout: The High Cost of High Achievement* and originator of the term *burnout*.

It's no coincidence then that one of the highest burnout ratios is found among air traffic controllers, a profession in which anything short of constant perfection could amount to a loss of life. So great is the pressure that by the time they reach their mid-forties, many controllers leave their jobs, says Dr. Jenkins, who participated in a definitive study of air traffic controllers and burnout. "And in fact, it seems that the professions most prone to burnout are the ones where constant vigilance is demanded and where the cost of mistakes is horrendous. Nurses who work in the intensive care wards of hospitals also come to mind," he says.

But not everyone who suffers from burnout is operating in an environment that demands such perfection. Some people do it to themselves simply by setting unreasonably high goals and viewing all harmless mistakes as catastrophes.

A Thirst for Recognition

Burnout can also occur when there is a lack of positive reinforcement and social support. If you never hear words of praise and rarely receive financial rewards at work, it can drain you. Likewise, if you feel your family takes you for granted at home.

The presence of positive feedback can make all the difference between emotional well-being and burnout. "Some years ago, Massachusetts General Hospital was experiencing a burnout problem among its nurses that manifested itself in a high job turnover rate," recalls Dr. Jenkins. "So they called in some of their psychiatrists and started a support therapy group, which met once or twice a week."

Within this group, people shared experiences with their peers, got a lot of gripes off their chests, and received praise and understanding from the psychiatrists. "In terms of employee turnover and increased satisfaction, the results were quite good," says Dr. Jenkins. "And all that was really applied was a little feedback and support."

Signs of Trouble

How do you know if you have burnout? One way to tell is to listen to your body. "One of the first signs we noticed in the air traffic controllers who were burning out was a sense of fatigue," says Dr. Jenkins. "And I'm talking about a pervasive mental and physical fatigue that a good night's sleep will not get rid of."

Chest pain, gastrointestinal problems, sleep disturbances, headache, back pain, and a higher incidence of minor illnesses such as colds are some of the body's other responses to burnout. So are skin disorders, adds Dr. Freudenberger. "I see a lot of burnout-induced acne and eczema."

On the mental front, a lack of resilience, characterized by a feeling of being whipped, can be a harbinger of burnout. "Our air traffic controllers called it bounce-back," says Dr. Jenkins. "They couldn't bounce back from a taxing period of heavy controlling and face the next period of activity with any sense of ease, comfort, and casualness. They were drained."

Irritability and depression are also possibilities for those who are burning out. "But more interesting is the development of a superperson personality," notes Dr. Freudenberger. "The person feels that he or she can handle everything, needs no help, and may actually become arrogant about it."

Rekindle Your Flame

Whether burnout has made you move, think, and feel like a cranky Methuselah on a bad day, or you just want to make sure that you never end up aging 30 years in as many weeks, the following tips will help you revitalize your life.

Listen to others. "The first step to curing burnout is to admit the problem exists," says Dr. Freudenberger. "But that's harder than it sounds, because of the denial mechanism people often use to cope with burnout. So listen to your friends and family members. Pay attention when they say you've changed. You may not notice it yourself, but burnout can be very apparent to those close to you as well as to co-workers who can see the transformation."

Diversify. "Just as a bank must diversify its holdings so that it doesn't have to depend on one source for its profits, people have to diversify their emotional portfolios," says Dr. Crosby. "This means looking at your activities and making sure that you participate in some that are goal-oriented and some where the aim is to feel good and have fun. I actually encourage people to list them in two columns. If you have two items in one column and 40 in the other, things are out of whack, and you need to do some account balancing."

Stop being perfect. The trick is to give yourself a little leeway when you can. "Take stock of your situation and see what mistakes you can and can't make," says Dr. Crosby. "Not every miscalculation you make is going to plummet the world into Armageddon. In other words, don't sweat the small stuff." And that goes for all activities, work-related and otherwise.

Know your needs. "If you know that you need positive feedback to replenish yourself, then don't just ignore that fact," counsels Dr. Freudenberger. "Actively solicit feedback from family and friends and in the workplace." Tell them that you would occasionally like to hear "Good job!" when you've done something well. Or find a support group that you can share your feelings, achievements, and gripes with. It doesn't have to be anything formal. A few people going through the same things as you will do just fine.

A corollary to this rule is: Ask for help. "Especially around the holidays," adds Dr. Freudenberger. "You're busy, things are hectic, and the last thing you need to be doing is scrambling around at all hours doing prep work by yourself." Enlist family members to help clean. When you invite people over, have them bring a salad or side dish.

Volunteer. "Volunteering is a very important anti-burnout device," says Dr. Crosby. "Whether you're at work or at home, worrying over a set of marketing reports, or putting up aluminum siding, you have to drop what you're doing, mentally change gears, and go interact with a whole new set of people in a whole new environment."

"It doesn't matter if you work in a soup kitchen twice a week, collect clothes, or deliver meals. You receive gratification that you are doing something for someone else," adds Dr. Freudenberger. "You may also receive some very important perspective on your life by seeing those less fortunate than you."

Take five. Dr. Crosby prescribes a 5-day vacation alone at least once a year. "It's especially important for women not only to get away from the office but also to get away from home," she says. That means leaving the spouse, the kids, the dog, the goldfish—everything—behind. They'll get on just fine without you for 5 days. "As a matter of fact," adds Dr. Crosby, "if you feel that the world will fall apart if you leave for 5 days, you have a good indicator that you are taking things far too seriously and are probably heading for burnout."

Take 15. "You also have to set aside some relaxation time during the course of the day," says Dr. Freudenberger. "And I mean every day, both at work and at home. When people tell me they can't do that, I make them actually take apart their days piece by piece, and they suddenly find all sorts of little opportunities for 15-minute breaks. And that's all it really takes."

Remove the red cape. Stop trying to be a superperson. "The trick is to allow yourself the occasional mistake—to recognize pressure release points where mistakes will not mean the end of the world," says Dr. Crosby. In other words, mismatched silver at the dinner party you're throwing isn't going to signal the end of civilization. And handing in that report a day late probably won't push the company into bankruptcy.

Bursitis
and Tendinitis

Easing Those
Overworked Joints

$\mathbf{Y}$ou're on the stairclimber for an hour. You shovel snow all afternoon. You wallpaper the kitchen over the weekend.

What do these things have in common? They're all terrific ways to get a raging case of bursitis or tendinitis. These painful conditions overlap so often that doctors frequently diagnose them as bursitis/tendinitis, because it can be hard to tell where one leaves off and the other begins.

And they happen most often to people in their forties, particularly those who haven't worked to maintain their flexibility. Without regular stretching, muscles and tendons get tighter and rub together more, increasing the risk of inflammation.

Once bursitis and tendinitis strike, they can make any movement painful—a sudden motion can feel as though you've just been jabbed with a red-hot poker. Here's why it hurts.

The No-Use Syndrome

To protect your body from damage, nature equipped it with bursae—tiny fluid-filled sacs that cushion the spaces where muscle passes over bone and where two muscles rub together. In your kneecaps and elbows, the bursae form cushions between skin and bone. But they can get inflamed—causing bursitis—when you injure or overuse a joint or when you accelerate your workout beyond what you're used to, says Pekka Mooar, M.D., director of the Delaware Valley Sports Medicine Center in Philadelphia.

When tendinitis strikes, it is not really your tendon but a ring of tissue around

74

the tendon where it attaches to a bone or muscle that hurts. The pain is caused by overuse of the tendon, which produces inflammation.

"We all get more aches and pains with age; there's no controversy about that," says Phillip E. Higgs, M.D., a reconstructive surgeon at Washington University School of Medicine in St. Louis. But if you stay limber over the years, a burst of effort is much less likely to bring on bursitis and tendinitis, he says.

In fact, it is too little exercise, not aging itself, that increases your risk of these painful ailments. That's what Dr. Higgs and his colleagues concluded after counting cases of bursitis and tendinitis in a study of 157 poultry workers and 118 data processors. Although the workers ranged in age from 20 to 71, the younger workers who got little exercise had nearly the same number of inflammations as older workers who didn't exercise much.

Bursitis and tendinitis vary a great deal from person to person, Dr. Higgs says. For example, 1 day of all-out sports may cause symptoms in one person, while another may not have trouble until after many years of work on an assembly line.

Where It Hurts Most

Shoulders, elbows, hips, knees, and ankles are especially vulnerable to bursitis and tendinitis. Women tend to get inflammation in the hips more than men do because their hips are set at a wider angle from the pelvis, putting greater stress on the hip joints. For men, shoulders are the usual problem area, because they tend to do more throwing or to have jobs that require a lot of overhead lifting.

Any activity that requires repetitive motion or pressure, from working on an assembly line to sewing, increases the risk.

Bursitis and tendinitis are also caused by overdoing a favorite sport. Tennis can do in elbows and wrists; swimming can irritate the shoulder bursae; running can aggravate ankles and Achilles tendons, particularly if you run on hard surfaces in the wrong shoes. And aerobics, particularly step aerobics, can cause hips and knees to flare up.

Bursitis is often missed as a cause of lower back pain, experts say. And it often accompanies the disorder called fibromyalgia, which causes muscle pain and stiffness throughout the body.

Fortunately, bursitis and tendinitis are very treatable. And you can do a lot to prevent them.

Safeguarding Your Joints

The most important way to protect yourself from bursitis and tendinitis is to get into condition gradually and to ease into vigorous exercise gently, says Stephen Campbell, M.D., a rheumatologist at Oregon Health Sciences University in Portland. Here are some suggestions.

Stretch before exercise. "In preparation for vigorous activity, you need to do more stretches of the muscles you'll be using," says Dr. Mooar. "Hold a slow, sustained stretch for 10 seconds, and don't bounce. Repeat the stretch three to five times before exercising." And don't do high-speed stretches, or you risk tearing muscle fibers or ligaments, he says. If you're unsure which stretching exercise is best for you, check with a trainer.

Start new activities slowly. If you take up a new sport, work at gradually increasing the strength and flexibility of the muscles you'll be using, says Dr. Mooar.

Pain-Free Workouts

There's no need to let bursitis or tendinitis spoil participation in your favorite sport. Just get into condition gradually—or if bursitis or tendinitis has already hit, stage a comeback carefully. Here's some advice for various activities.

Aerobics. Learn the routines at your own pace; don't push yourself. Always warm up and stretch before you exercise and cool down after, says Robert L. Swezey, M.D., medical director of the Arthritis and Back Pain Center in Santa Monica, California.

Tennis. To avoid wrist pain or tennis elbow, choose a large-handled racquet, decrease the string tension, and wear an elastic band around your forearm to support the muscles, says Stephen Campbell, M.D., a rheumatologist at Oregon Health Sciences University in Portland. If your shoulder is the problem, modify your serve to avoid vigorously swinging your arm over your head.

Running. Condition yourself very gradually before running longer distances, says Dr. Campbell. Don't run too vigorously if you're just starting, avoid hard surfaces, and wear shoes with soft soles and high-quality insoles and arch supports.

Swimming. Although swimming is very gentle on most joints, the shoulder can get too much of a workout, Dr. Campbell says. To prevent or heal shoulder bursitis or tendinitis, avoid the freestyle, or crawl, and butterfly strokes, he says. Use the breaststroke or sidestroke or a kickboard instead.

For any activity, after a bout of bursitis or tendinitis, it's crucial to wait until all the pain has gone before restarting vigorous workouts, says Dr. Campbell. When you have your doctor's okay to start again, exercise at a lower frequency and intensity and recondition your injured joint over weeks or months, he says.

If you choose tennis, for example, take it one set at a time at first. "Don't pick up a racquet and play lots of sets at once, because your shoulder is going to feel like it's falling off," he says.

Precondition your joints. If your job or hobby calls for repetitive motion, ask a trainer to recommend strengthening and endurance exercises targeted for that motion, Dr. Mooar says. "If you do this," he says, "you can stop bursitis and tendinitis from happening over and over." Many people develop chronic inflammation from reinjuring their joints, he says.

Support your body. Typing and filing can trigger problems in your wrists and back. Use a keyboard wrist rest for typing, says Dr. Campbell. And check that your chair is well-adjusted so that your back is supported and your arms and wrists are level with each other.

Take a break. "Incorporate rest into your work and training program," suggests John P. DiFiori, M.D., a sports medicine specialist in the department of family medicine at the University of California, Los Angeles, and a team physician in the department of collegiate athletics. How often? Try a 5-minute break every hour. And stretch during your breaks.

Go easy on your knees. There is little but a tiny bursa between your kneecap and the skin over it, says Dr. Mooar. So if you're doing housework or gardening on your knees, kneel on a piece of foam rubber or wear knee pads to cushion them. Many garden centers, sporting goods stores, and hardware stores carry foam rubber or knee pads.

Pay attention to pain. If you begin to feel even some slight tenderness or soreness in a shoulder, elbow, or knee (the three most common sites for bursitis and tendinitis), don't ignore it, says Dr. DiFiori. People who try to work through the pain often end up with chronic problems. Instead, reduce your activity and apply ice to the area three or four times a day, for 20 minutes each time.

Tips for a Quick Recovery

If you already have bursitis or tendinitis, the first question to ask yourself is, what have you done differently? "You're overdoing whatever it is," says Dr. Campbell. "First, stop doing it." Then:

Give yourself an ice massage. "Apply a paper cup full of ice to the painful area," says Robert L. Swezey, M.D., medical director of the Arthritis and Back Pain Center in Santa Monica, California. Rub the icy bottom of the cup into the sore spot for 2 to 5 minutes, three or four times a day, to control the inflammation, he says.

Alternate it with heat. After the ice, apply a microwavable heat pack or electric heating pad to soothe the pain, says Dr. Campbell. The microwavable packs are available at most pharmacies, he says.

Bundle up for bed. Wear a flannel shirt or a wool sweater at night to keep a painful shoulder extra warm. If you sleep sleeveless in a cool room, your morning stiffness and soreness will be greater.

Use the right pain reliever. Choose an aspirin or ibuprofen pain reliever for the pain, says Dr. Campbell. Aspirin and ibuprofen block the production of chemicals called prostaglandins, which contribute to swelling and pain in inflamed tissue. Acetaminophen won't control inflammation because it does not block prostaglandins.

Another option: Ginger. It's well known for its anti-inflammatory properties, says Jacob Schor, N.D., a naturopathic doctor in Denver and president of the Colorado Association of Naturopathic Doctors. "It's kind of a homestyle ibuprofen."

As a supplement, you can take ginger in tincture or capsule form. If you're in acute pain, take six 500-milligram capsules of the concentrated extract per day, says Dr. Schor.

Swing your shoulder. Sometimes bursitis in the shoulder progresses to a painful condition called adhesive capsulitis, or frozen shoulder. When this happens, the shoulder's range of motion is almost completely restricted, and the joint is nearly immobile. To avoid frozen shoulder, you need to start moving your shoulder as soon as the acute pain has passed, says Dr. Campbell. Lie facedown on a cushioned surface such as a bed and hang the affected arm over the side. Gently swing your arm like a pendulum, gradually increasing the range until you can swing it in a full circle. Do this for 15 to 30 minutes, three to five times a week, to restore your range of motion, he says.

Consider chiropractic care. If your pain won't quit, a technique called friction massage may clear up the problem, says Warren Hammer, D.C., a chiropractor in private practice in Norwalk, Connecticut. When inflammation is chronic, fibrous adhesions don't allow the bursae to glide smoothly. Friction massage can break down those adhesions, says Dr. Hammer, relieving the cause of bursitis pain. "Also, an inflamed tendon becomes thicker and shorter, which creates further inflammation in the bursa it's rubbing over," Dr. Hammer says. "The deep pressure of massage across the bursa and tendon can lengthen the tendon fibers again." Use ice to calm the inflammation before chiropractic treatment, he says.

CELLULITE

It's Fat—And Nothing Else

Ah, summer. Time to trade in baggy pants and bulky sweaters for leg-baring shorts and scarcely there swimsuits. Time to expose parts of your body that haven't seen daylight for 3 months or more. Time to show the world square inches of skin that have been under wraps all winter.

Or maybe not—if you feel self-conscious about signs of cellulite on your thighs, hips, or backside.

Cellulite usually appears around your 30th birthday. Besides making you look as though you have cottage cheese burbling under your skin, it can make you feel old—especially if you're standing next to a 19-year-old in a string bikini at the beach.

But relax. You're not alone.

"Ninety-nine percent of women develop at least some dimply fat after age 30," explains Donald Robertson, M.D., medical director of the Bariatric Nutrition Center in Scottsdale, Arizona.

Part of the problem is genetics. But much of it is simply because of aging. Sometime in a woman's thirties, a natural drop in estrogen levels, along with sun damage accumulated over the years, causes the skin to lose its elasticity, says Ted Lockwood, M.D., assistant clinical professor of plastic surgery at the University of Missouri-Kansas City School of Medicine. The skin sags a little here, bags a little there, and generally doesn't have the firm resiliency of youth.

At the same time, the supporting network of fibers that anchors the skin to underlying muscles is also starting to stretch. That, combined with the extra pounds most of us put on as we approach midlife, leads to cellulite, a fancy word for what is really just dimply fat and skin that has lost its elasticity.

Cellulite is mostly a problem for women. One reason men aren't affected is because they tend to gain weight around their midriffs rather than in their hips, thighs, and butt, where cellulite is most likely to show. Another is that men's skin is thicker and more elastic, so it holds the fat beneath it more firmly than women's does. And still another reason is that the fibers that anchor skin to muscle are structured differently in men than in women: While the fibers that support women's skin run in only one direction, men have tight, crisscrossed fibers that form a net to keep their fat firmly in place.

Life is not always fair.

What to Do about It

While you may not be able to avoid getting cellulite, you don't have to keep it. Cellulite is fat. And like other forms of fat, you can dump it. Here's how.

Burn it off. The best way to reduce cellulite—as with fat anywhere else on your body—is with aerobic activity that burns calories throughout the entire body. Pick an activity that gets your heart rate up and keeps it there for 20 continuous minutes, then do it at least three times a week.

Running, walking, bicycling, skating, dancing, and swimming—all of which stoke up the metabolism for efficient fat burning—are perfect.

What about those claims that you can get rid of cellulite by doing exercises that concentrate on specific parts of the body like the thighs and buttocks? Forget them. "Spot reducing doesn't work," says Susan Olson, Ph.D., director of psychological services at the Southwest Bariatric Nutrition Center in Tempe, Arizona.

Pump some weights. A good aerobic workout will help tone muscles. But building them up through weight training may also help hide dimpled skin. "Bulking your muscles can make a slight improvement," says Dr. Lockwood. "Just don't expect miracles." Check with a trainer at your gym for a program that will help you.

Reduce the fat in your diet. Besides exercise, eating a low-fat diet is the best way to keep so-called cellulite to a minimum. "A lot of cellulite comes from eating high-fat foods," says Maria Simonson, Sc.D., Ph.D., professor emeritus and director of the Health, Weight and Stress Clinic at Johns Hopkins Medical Institutions in Baltimore. "So the less fat you have in your diet, the less problem you'll have."

Try limiting your total fat intake to around 25 percent of the daily calories you consume, adds Dr. Simonson. You can track fat intake by reading product labels and staying away from high-fat fare such as cakes, cheeses, fried foods, and processed luncheon meats.

Massage it away. "A deep massage using the knuckles may help break up the dimples," says Dr. Robertson. When combined with weight loss and smart eating, a twice-weekly massage helps whittle down the most resistant fat pockets.

Cover it with cream. Rubbing any skin cream that contains alpha-hydroxy acids—essentially, acids made from fruits or milk—into your skin will give your body a smoother look. But remember: No cream or lotion will get rid of cellulite.

Camouflage it. Use a tanning cream to camouflage cellulite. The darker color will even out your skin tone and make the shadows cast by the lumps of fat beneath the skin less apparent.

Always wear sunscreen. You can't undo the years of sun exposure that paved the way for cellulite by zapping your skin's elasticity. "But by limiting your

Cellulite Products: A Big Fat Lie

Each year, Americans spend more than $20 million trying to get rid of cellulite with gels, creams, electrical currents, and other too-good-to-be-true products. Unfortunately, the only thinning these products do is to your wallet.

The Food and Drug Administration is now monitoring claims made by the manufacturers of these products, many of which are imported from France, where consumer protection is more lax. But those hawking cellulite products have long been able to promise too much, since *cellulite* is a marketing term—not a medical diagnosis.

A research team from the Health, Weight and Stress Clinic at Johns Hopkins Medical Institutions in Baltimore tested 32 cellulite removal products, says Maria Simonson, Sc.D., Ph.D., professor emeritus and director of the clinic.

Not a single one worked.

sun exposure or using a good sunscreen when you're outdoors, you can keep your skin from degenerating further," says Dr. Lockwood. The sun's skin-damaging rays are most harmful between 10:00 A.M. and 2:00 P.M., so it's essential to keep thighs and other vulnerable areas covered during those hours. And whenever you're in the sun, use a sunscreen with a sun protection factor (SPF) of at least 15.

CHOLESTEROL

The Less, the Better

When you consider that haggis, a favorite food in Scotland, is made of the innards of various animals mixed with animal fat, and that many of the people there never eat vegetables, it's easy to understand why the Scots have one of the highest mortality rates from cardiovascular disease in the world. Of course, Americans are more likely to eat hamburgers than haggis, but when it comes to cardiovascular health, we're only a few chest-clutching steps behind the Scots.

The reason, to a large extent, is high cholesterol. Having high cholesterol is one of the primary risk factors for heart attack, stroke, and other vascular diseases. Over half of American adults have cholesterol levels over 200, which is considered borderline high. Twenty percent of us have levels of 240—the standard for high cholesterol—or above.

If there's good news in these statistics, it's this: While elevated cholesterol puts you at higher risk of heart disease, it's a risk that you can control. By eating a low-fat, low-cholesterol diet, you can efficiently reduce the amount of cholesterol in your blood. Moreover, making even small reductions in cholesterol can add up to big health benefits. For each 1 percent that you lower your total cholesterol, you lower your risk of having a heart attack by 2 percent.

The Nature of the Beast

By itself, cholesterol isn't the toxic sludge you may think it is. Indeed, your body uses the cholesterol that you produce in your liver to make cell membranes, sex hormones, bile acids, and vitamin D. You couldn't live without it.

But it is easy to end up with too much cholesterol, since it also is found in animal foods, including meats, milk, eggs, and butter. When present in large amounts, this essential substance quickly becomes dangerous. This is particularly true of a form of cholesterol called low-density lipoprotein (LDL), the "bad" cholesterol.

As LDL cholesterol circulates in the bloodstream, it undergoes a process called oxidation. Essentially, this means that it spoils and turns rancid. Your immune system quickly spots the decaying LDL and reacts as it would to any invader. Immune cells gobble up the cholesterol molecules. Once engorged, the cells stick to the walls of the arteries, hardening into a dense, fatty layer called plaque. When enough plaque accumulates, there's less room for blood to flow. Eventually, blood flow may slow or even stop. When this occurs, it can lead to agonizing angina (chest pain), heart attacks, and strokes.

Your body has a mechanism for dealing with this threat. A second form of cholesterol, called high-density lipoprotein (HDL), transports the dangerous cholesterol out of the blood and to the liver for disposal. Normally, it does a good job. But when cholesterol levels get too high, the HDL can't keep up, and the LDL gradually rises to dangerous levels.

Ideally, you want to have high levels of HDL and low levels of the dangerous LDL. The national Cholesterol Education Program recommends keeping total cholesterol below 200 milligrams per deciliter of blood. More specifically, LDL should be below 130, and HDL should be above 65.

Turning the Tide

Experts say that you can dramatically lower your cholesterol by making some moderate lifestyle adjustments. With dietary changes alone, you can whittle away an average of 10 percent of your cholesterol reading—and perhaps even more. Margo Denke, M.D., assistant professor of medicine at the University of Texas Southwestern Medical Center at Dallas's Center for Human Nutrition and a member of the nutrition committee of the American Heart Association, says that the higher your cholesterol count, the greater impact a heart-healthy diet can have. For example, a person with a cholesterol reading of 280 may be able to steamroll 25 percent off the top by eating right. If longevity and anti-aging are your goals, that's a bottom line you can't afford to ignore.

To outmaneuver high cholesterol and the havoc it can wreak, give these cholesterol busters a try.

Switch fats. "Decreasing saturated fat is the most effective anti-cholesterol strategy you can use," says Karen Miller-Kovach, R.D., chief nutritionist at Weight Watchers International in Jericho, New York. That means eating less red meat, butter, cheese, whole milk, and ice cream, all which raise LDL and total cholesterol levels. On the other hand, consuming more monounsaturated fat, known as the good fat, can actually help decrease cholesterol.

"When you switch from a diet high in saturated fat to one high in monounsaturated fat and your weight stays about the same, your LDL cholesterol will fall while the HDL cholesterol remains stable," says Robert Rosenson, M.D., director of the Preventive Cardiology Center at Rush-Presbyterian-St. Luke's Medical Center in Chicago. "That's why olive oil is so popular, since it's high in monounsaturates." Other good monounsaturates include fatty fish, such as salmon and tuna.

Eat less cholesterol. Limiting the amount of dietary cholesterol you get from foods is the second most important step in lowering your risks. To cut back on cholesterol, try to eliminate organ meats (such as liver) from your diet. Limit the amount of lean meat and poultry to 3 ounces a day. And when it comes to eggs, limit your consumption of yolks to no more than two a week. Make your own cookies, cakes, and pies, and use egg whites and egg substitute when you bake or cook.

Finally, when you're going through the buffet line, reach with gusto for vegetables, fruits, and grains, which contain absolutely no dietary cholesterol. (Just steer clear of high-fat salad dressings, sauces, and butter.)

Fill up on fiber. Eating foods high in soluble fiber, including dried beans, lentils, citrus fruits, peas, and apples, can help lower your blood cholesterol by 5 to 10 percent. Plus, if you're eating more high-fiber fruits and vegetables, you'll probably eat a little less meat, reducing the amount of dietary cholesterol you consume.

Feel your oats. Oat bran has been on a roll as a cholesterol cure for years. But how much is hype and how much holds water? Researchers at the University of Minnesota in Minneapolis reviewed all the studies examining the power of oats and reached an artery-cleansing conclusion: Adding 1⅓ cups of oat bran cereal (or three packets of instant oatmeal) to your daily diet, will drop your cholesterol level by 2 to 3 percent. If your cholesterol level is already high, you'll reap even more benefits, with oat bran skimming 6 to 7 percent off the top.

Toast to moderation. A drink or two of any alcoholic beverage each day can raise the HDL component of your cholesterol. Even so, approach this cholesterol-fighting strategy cautiously. Alcoholic drinks are brimming with calories, so they can defeat your efforts at losing weight. And even moderate drinking may also increase a woman's chances of developing breast cancer.

Another option? Drink grape juice—the purple kind. Grape skin contains a cholesterol-lowering ingredient, according to Leroy Creasy, Ph.D., professor of pomology at Cornell University College of Agriculture and Life Sciences in Ithaca, New York.

Feast on garlic. Garlic contains a compound called allicin that changes the way the body uses cholesterol, says Stephen Warshafsky, M.D., assistant professor of medicine at New York Medical College in Valhalla. When Dr. Warshafsky analyzed data from five of the most reliable scientific studies of garlic and cholesterol, he found that eating one-half to one clove of garlic a day lowered cholesterol an average of 9 percent.

Try tofu. Soybeans and soy foods such as tofu contain compounds called phytoestrogens that researchers believe help transport LDL cholesterol to the liver, where it can be broken down and excreted. Phytoestrogens also may prevent LDL from oxidizing, making it less likely to clog coronary arteries. In fact, studies have shown that replacing protein from animal sources with about 1½ ounces of

Playing the Cholesterol Numbers Game

Once you've reached the ripe old age of 20, experts say that you're due for your first cholesterol test. After that, you should have one at least every 5 years.

One of the readings that this test will produce is your total blood cholesterol level. Here's a look at what that number means (all numbers refer to milligrams per deciliter of blood).

- Less than 200—desirable
- 200–239—borderline high
- 240 and above—high

Even if you are settled comfortably in the "desirable" range, you still need to have your cholesterol measured regularly, along with a check of your HDL (high-density lipoprotein) cholesterol, the good kind. Sometimes a high HDL level will help compensate for a total cholesterol number in the "borderline high" range (although you're still well advised to get your total cholesterol as low as possible). However, if your HDL reading is less than 35, it falls into the "low" category, and you need to work at raising it. Your best options are losing weight, exercising more, quitting smoking, and cutting back on how much sugar you eat.

And what about LDL (low-density lipoprotein) cholesterol, the bad kind? If your other tests reveal potential trouble, you should have your LDL level tested, too. Below 130 is generally considered desirable.

Finally, to help interpret what all these numbers mean, your doctor may determine your cholesterol ratio, which is the ratio between your total cholesterol and your HDL number. If this ratio is 3.5 to 1 or lower, you are doing just fine.

soy protein can lower total cholesterol by 9 percent. It lowers dangerous LDL cholesterol even more, by 13 percent.

Stock up on fish. Salmon, tuna, and other fish contain omega-3 fatty acids, which studies have shown may raise your beneficial HDL cholesterol. In addition, omega-3 fatty acids lower your triglycerides—blood fats that increase your risk of heart disease.

Get fit. This one won't surprise you: Exercise does a body good. And don't worry about having to go to extremes. "We've learned that even moderate aerobic exercise (brisk walking, jogging, swimming) raises HDL levels, although this often takes 6 months to a year to occur," says Dr. Rosenson.

Trim your waist. There are more than cosmetic reasons to chip away at unattractive fat around your middle. Dr. Denke has found that excess body weight can boost total and LDL cholesterol levels, while suppressing HDL levels. Losing weight produces the reverse effect.

Stop smoking. Smoking can lower your HDL reading, something that no health-conscious person can afford to do. But even if you're a chain-smoker, there's some encouraging news—if you're willing to toss out your cigarettes for good. If you stop smoking, says Dr. Rosenson, you can reverse the decline in your HDL level in about 60 days.

Boost your vitamin C. Research shows that increasing your intake of vitamin C may enhance your HDL cholesterol. In one study of 316 women and 511 men between the ages of 19 and 95, researchers for the National Institute on Aging in Bethesda, Maryland, found that the more vitamin C people got, the higher their HDL levels—but only up to a point. The study indicated that women who took 215 milligrams a day and men who took 346 milligrams a day increased their bodies' HDL to maximum levels. Doctors who recommend vitamin C for high cholesterol suggest taking 250 milligrams a day.

Neutralize with vitamin E. Vitamin E can help prevent LDL cholesterol from oxidizing and thus clogging your arteries. When your body has an adequate supply of E, the LDL particles harmlessly pass into the artery wall instead of forming plaque. Doctors who recommend vitamin E to prevent heart disease generally call for at least 100 international units a day. Up to 600 international units daily is safe, although people taking anticoagulants should not take vitamin E supplements.

DENTAL PROBLEMS

Teeth Can Last Forever

When you were young, a little dental neglect might have led to an occasional filling. But as you get older, ignoring your teeth can set you up for more serious problems, such as periodontal disease. If not arrested promptly, long-term neglect can eventually cause you to lose teeth entirely.

And when you get down to it, few things can age a person's appearance more quickly than bad or missing teeth.

As you grow older, damage to your teeth can take many forms.

• The teeth may start to show the telltale signs of years of indulgences. Coffee, red wine, tobacco, and food dyes can work their way deep into microscopic cracks in the tooth enamel, resulting in brown or yellowish stains.
• Years of chewing wears down tooth surfaces and actually shortens your teeth.
• Overaggressive brushing can wear down the transluscent enamel coating of your teeth so that the yellowish material underneath, called dentin, begins to show through.
• Gums recede with age and wear.
• As the gums recede with age, the root (which has no protective enamel) is exposed to decay.
• Gum disease may strike. This is a far greater concern for adults than even cavities. Bacteria can enter the tiny crevice between the gum and your teeth and linger, causing inflammation. As the inflammation simmers, bones, gums, and connective tissue may get eaten away, leaving you with less foundation to hold your teeth in place. All that simmering can also cause soreness and bleeding as well as bad breath.

A Daily Plan for a Perfect Mouth

If you want to keep a dazzling, healthy smile as you get older, it will take a new commitment to daily preventive care. That may mean spending more time brushing and flossing than you used to—and being more aware of the foods you eat. The first step is to catch up with the latest cleaning methods and keep an educated eye on what goes in your mouth.

Brush often, brush right. Brushing is your number-one defense against dental problems as you get older. "At a very minimum, be sure to brush after breakfast and before you go to bed at night," says Hazel Harper, D.D.S., associate professor of community dentistry at Howard University in Washington, D.C., and vice president of the National Dental Association. Of course, it's best to brush after every meal—with the right technique.

Done correctly, brushing removes the bacteria and plaque responsible for so many dental woes. Correct brushing, says Dr. Harper, means holding the brush with the handle in your palm and your thumb extended to act as a brace. This palm-thumb grasp tilts the brush at an angle, so bristles reach the gums and just underneath the gums as well as the tooth surfaces. Gently vibrate the brush in a small back-and-forth motion, covering only three teeth at a time. Then with a flick of the wrist, roll the brush against the sides of your teeth to sweep debris and bacteria away from the gum line. Finish up by brushing your tongue—your best antidote to bad breath, Dr. Harper says.

Use the right brush. Banish that hard-tufted, frayed thing from your toothbrush holder, says Dr. Harper. You need to use a soft-bristle toothbrush, and you should replace it every 3 months—sooner if the bristles start to fray, she says.

Pick a proper paste. Any toothpaste with the American Dental Association's seal of approval will do the job with a minimal amount of abrasion. If you tend to build up tartar, or hardened plaque, try a tartar-control toothpaste. Tartar feels like a rough coating on your teeth, says Richard Price, D.D.S., clinical instructor of dentistry at Boston University's Henry Goldman School of Dentistry. "These pastes reduce the amount of tartar you get, and the tartar that does build up will be softened and easier to remove," he says.

Remember to floss. Floss daily to ensure complete cleaning and healthy gums, says Dr. Price. Toothbrush bristles simply can't get into the crannies around teeth. It doesn't matter what type of floss you use—waxed, unwaxed, or flavored; just pick one that feels most comfortable.

Limit sweets. Sugary foods encourage large amounts of bacteria to flourish in your mouth. Over time, the bacteria and the acids they produce act almost like little dental drills, wearing away the surface of the teeth and allowing cavities to form. Even fruit juices, which many people drink as a healthful alternative to sodas, can be a problem. "Juice is a very concentrated source of sugar," says William Kuttler, D.D.S., a dentist in private practice in Dubuque, Iowa. In fact, researchers in Switzerland found that grapefruit and apple juices did slightly more damage to teeth than colas did. So try to limit your sweets, or brush as soon as possible after eating them.

Watch out for sticky surprises. While sweet foods can be a problem, sticky foods are even worse. They adhere to your teeth for long periods of time, making it easy for bacteria to remain in your mouth. But it's not always the foods you'd suspect that are the biggest danger. In the following pairs, which would you think are the stickiest: caramels or crackers? Hot-fudge sundaes or bread? Dried figs or puffed-oat cereal? Believe it or not, crackers, bread, and cereal are the most likely to cling for long periods. Your best defense is to brush after every single snack. But if you can't get to a toothbrush soon, it's best to avoid the stickier foods.

Eat tooth-boosting foods. Calcium-rich foods, such as low-fat milk and yo-gurt, fortify the bone that supports the teeth so they don't loosen over time. A glass of milk or a serving of yogurt each contains 300 milligrams of calcium, about 30 percent of the Daily Value. You can get smaller amounts of calcium from low-fat cheeses, turnip greens, bok choy, and curly endive. Foods that are rich in vita-mins A and C are also good for your teeth. Vitamin A is used to form dentin, a layer of bonelike material just beneath the surface of the teeth. Vitamin C helps your body produce collagen, a tough protein fiber that keeps gums strong. Car-rots, sweet potatoes, kale, and yellow squashes supply vitamin A, while broccoli, cantaloupe, and oranges are good sources of vitamin C.

Say cheese for dessert. It's an old custom in some cultures to serve cheese for dessert, and it might help cut cavities when you can't brush your teeth right after a meal. A few studies indicate that certain cheeses, particularly hard, aged ones such as cheddar and Monterey Jack, may reduce cavity-causing bacteria. Just a small slice will do the job—and not add much fat or cholesterol to your diet.

Rinse your mouth. Regardless of what you've just eaten, if you can't brush right away, the next best thing is to find a sink and swish a mouthful of water around your teeth, says Andrew M. Lewis, D.D.S., a dentist in private practice in Beverly Hills. Swishing will remove most debris and also dilute the acids formed by food particles.

Heavy-Duty Home Care

If your dentist has noticed new cavities or early signs of gum disease, don't give up on your teeth—take charge. There's a lot you can do to turn the tide at any age. Try these home treatments, with your dentist's guidance.

Use a fluoride rinse. "If you're prone to cavities, use an over-the-counter fluoride rinse every night," says Dr. Lewis. "You want to rinse and spit it out so that it's the last thing in your mouth just before you go to sleep." Fluoride actu-ally remineralizes teeth, making them stronger and less prone to cavities and root sensitivity.

Try an electric toothbrush. If you have trouble brushing thoroughly by hand or you have gum problems, an electric brush may help, says Dr. Harper. The gentle vibration of the brush head massages gums as it cleans the teeth, she says. And research at the University of Alabama School of Dentistry in Birmingham has proven that electric toothbrushes can significantly reduce gingivitis, an infection that can damage your gums, and if not stopped, your teeth.

Go with an irrigator. An oral irrigator, such as the Water Pik, can help clean debris from between teeth and under gums, but use it cautiously, Dr. Harper says.

Facts about Fillings

Your dentist tells you that you have a few cavities. "Whoaaaa," you say. "Have you inhaled too much of that laughing gas? I'm too old for cavities."

Sorry, but you're never too old for cavities.

Lots of people get them well into their later years, says Richard Price, D.D.S., clinical instructor of dentistry at Boston University's Henry Goldman School of Dentistry. One reason is that old fillings wear out. Although some may last decades, the average life span of silver fillings is about 9 years. Beyond that, they tend to chip, crack, and wear out.

"They're just replacement parts," says Dr. Price. "Any time you get a tooth drilled and filled, it will need to be drilled and filled for the rest of your life. It's like your warranty wearing out."

If you do need a filling—either a replacement or a new one—get ready to choose from a number of alternative materials.

Silver is by far the most common of the lot, because it's durable and affordable. Gold, though pricey, is super strong and especially good for jumbo cavities. Fillings made from porcelain, quartz, or acrylic, though not as durable as the metals, may be preferable for more visible fillings. They can be colored to match your own teeth.

"Sometimes irrigators aren't adjusted right, and the flow of water is strong enough to damage gum tissue," she says. Slow the flow if your gums feel sore or irritated after using your irrigator.

Get a regular checkup. No amount of zeal at the bathroom sink can substitute for regular dental checkups, Dr. Harper says. To keep your teeth looking younger, see a dental hygienist twice a year for cleaning and your dentist at least once a year for an exam.

DEPRESSION

The Sneaky Stealer of Youth

All of us get the blues at one time or another. They could be triggered by anything from the death of a family pet, to weight gain, to a losing streak by your favorite sports team. These gloomy feelings usually fade within short order, and you bounce back to your cheerful self. No problem.

But if you're in a funk day after day—particularly if you can't put a handle on why—that's a big deal. Depression can sap your energy, crumple your posture, add wrinkles to your face, and do a lot of other things that we associate with aging.

"Unquestionably, depression can make you look and feel older," says Harry Prosen, M.D., chairman of the department of psychiatry and mental health sciences at the Medical College of Wisconsin in Milwaukee. "Some people who are chronically depressed can look very old and have stooped shoulders, furrowed lines around the eyes, and all the other things that make a person look aged. I've seen some depressed people who look like they're in their sixties when they're actually 35 or 40."

Yet relieving the strain of depression may be all you need to make yourself look years younger. "It's amazing how quickly the signs of aging can lift once the depression lifts," Dr. Prosen says.

What's Getting Us Down

During our lifetimes, Americans have a 1 in 10 chance of suffering from a major depression, meaning having five or more known symptoms of depression for at least 2 weeks, including feelings of worthlessness or thoughts of death and suicide.

Women are twice as likely as men to be diagnosed as having major depression. That difference mystifies researchers, says Dan Blazer, M.D., Ph.D., professor of psychiatry at Duke University Medical Center in Durham, North Carolina. But heredity, biological differences, and a disparity in our society's expectations of how men and women should behave may contribute to the gap.

Are You Really Depressed?

Here's a list of symptoms, according to the American Psychiatric Association, that may help you determine the severity of a depression. If you have five or more of these symptoms in a 2-week span, or if you have felt depressed for more than 2 weeks, you should seek the help of your doctor or a qualified therapist.

• You feel sad most of the day and have lost interest in pleasurable activities, including sex.
• You feel tired or lack energy to do day-to-day chores.
• You feel restless and can't sit still.
• You either have insomnia or sleep more than usual.
• You have difficulty concentrating or making decisions.
• You have fluctuations in your appetite or weight.
• You feel hopeless, worthless, and guilty.
• You think about death and suicide.

"There's a theory of depression that revolves around anger," says Kimberly Yonkers, M.D., assistant professor of psychiatry and gynecology at the University of Texas Southwestern Medical Center at Dallas. "According to this theory, women tend to repress their anger, turn it inward, and, as a result, get depressed. Men, on the other hand, outwardly express their anger and rage by getting aggressive." However, it could also be that women are just more likely than men to talk about their emotions and seek treatment for depression, Dr. Yonkers says.

The Physical Price

Even mild sadness that lasts only 1 or 2 days can make you more susceptible to many of the illnesses and changes in appearance that are considered a part of aging. "Certainly, depression takes its toll on people physically. We don't know all the mechanisms that are involved, but we do know that the general well-being of the body is thrown out of whack when a person is depressed," Dr. Blazer says.

Decreased muscle tone is one of the most immediate physical changes that occurs when you begin to get depressed. "That causes muscles to sag and contributes to the sad facial expressions and poor posture that you see in depressed people," says Elmer Gardner, M.D., a psychiatrist in private practice in Washington, D.C.

But the changes caused by depression can be more than skin deep. Researchers believe depression can weaken the immune system, accelerate hardening of the arteries, and trigger some forms of arthritis.

If you're depressed, your immune cell activity can drop to the levels of a person who is 25 to 30 years older, says Michael Irwin, M.D., associate professor of psychiatry at the University of California, San Diego, School of Medicine. "Depression triggers a lowered immune response, but we still don't know to what extent that leads to sickness," Dr. Irwin says. "We do know, however, that the viruses that our natural killer cells help protect us against are more common in people who are depressed."

Depression can also stimulate atherosclerosis, a buildup of fatty deposits on artery walls that contributes to coronary heart disease, says George Kaplan, Ph.D., an epidemiologist and chief of the Human Population Laboratory of the California Department of Health Services in Berkeley.

Rheumatoid arthritis is yet another disease that can be aggravated or even triggered by depression, says Sanford Roth, M.D., a rheumatologist and medical director of the Arthritis Center in Phoenix. "It's not unusual for a person who suffers a devastating loss of a parent or spouse to develop a disease like rheumatoid arthritis," Dr. Roth says. "Because rheumatoid arthritis may be associated with a genetic root, these people probably had the potential to develop the disease all along. It just took a depressive episode to open it up."

Climbing into the Light

So now that you know depression can have a serious impact on how you age, what can you do to prevent or treat it? Plenty, doctors say.

Keep in mind that severe depression—one that persists for more than 2 weeks—may require a doctor's care and treatment with antidepressant drugs. But if your depression lasts a few days and doesn't appear to be interfering with your activities, here are a few suggestions that may perk you up.

Keep a goal in sight. "People who have dreams and visions of accomplishment are less likely to be depressed than those who don't have short- and long-term goals," says Dennis Gersten, M.D., a psychiatrist in private practice in San Diego. Write down a list of goals. Divide the list into sections that include things you want to do this week, this month, within a year, and within 5 years. Put the list in a prominent place, such as on your refrigerator, and check off the goals as you achieve them. Try to update your list at least once a month.

Stay busy. "If you can keep yourself busy, it will help, because staying active can prevent you from dwelling on whatever is making you feel unhappy," says Linda George, Ph.D., professor of medical sociology at Duke University Medical Center in Durham, North Carolina.

Laugh. Humor is your best ally against depression, Dr. Prosen says. Clip cartoons and funny articles out of newspapers and magazines and put them in a file you can flip through when you feel low.

Lean on family and friends. They've helped you survive bad relationships and other disasters; now they can help you through this bleak time. "That doesn't mean you're asking them to solve your problems for you," Dr. George says. "It just means you're asking them to listen, let you get things off your chest, and be supportive."

Put your negative thoughts on paper. Writing down your feelings when you're depressed can help you recognize faulty thought patterns and help you find ways to replace those thoughts with more uplifting ones, says Janice Peterson, M.D., a clinical psychiatrist at the University of Colorado Health Sciences Center in Denver. For every negative thought you write down, such as "I'm the worst person in the world," also write down a positive one, such as "I have imperfections, but I also have a lot going for me." After a while, the positive thoughts may replace the negative ones.

Stay away from alcohol. Although it may be tempting to drown your sorrows in a few glasses of wine, don't do it, Dr. Yonkers warns. Alcohol is a depressant that can drag you further into the dumps. "Excessive drinking will also disrupt your sleep and may drive your friends and family away from you just when you need their support the most," she says.

Sweat it out. "Exercise is a fabulous way to relieve depression," Dr. Gersten says. "Aerobic exercise such as walking, running, swimming, or bicycling cranks

Is It All in the Family?

You're not the only one who gets depressed. Grandma, Mom, Dad, and your brother all regularly tumble into a funk that they can't seem to shake. Coincidence, or is there something going on here?

"It's clear that people with family histories of depression are much more likely to suffer from depression than people who don't have family histories of depression," says Alan Mellow, M.D., Ph.D., assistant professor of psychiatry at the University of Michigan Medical School in Ann Arbor. "There is well-documented evidence that like cancer, diabetes, and high blood pressure, major depression has a genetic component."

Okay, so you can't choose your parents. But knowing that your family has a history of depression should help you understand why you may feel particularly on the downside more often than other people, Dr. Mellow says. If you are feeling unusually blue, especially if you have a family history of major depression, you should consider seeking counseling and asking about antidepressant drug therapy.

up your brain activity and can reverse the effects of even a major depression." He suggests exercising at least 20 minutes at a time, three times a week.

Keep the credit cards in your wallet. "Some people who get depressed try to break out of it with the credit card prescription," Dr. Yonkers says. "They think that if they go shopping and buy something, it's going to pick them up. But often they end up feeling guilty because they make major purchases they can't afford and that depresses them even more." If you are depressed and do go shopping, set a spending limit before you go, and pay in cash.

Be a good actor. A great way to fend off depression is to act happy for an hour, Dr. Yonkers says. Then try it for another hour and so on. By the end of the day, you might be surprised to find you're not faking it anymore.

Food and Mood

Researchers have been studying the link between food and mood for decades, but the connection is still uncertain. Studies have shown that for some individuals, poor diet can cause depression, according to Larry Christensen, Ph.D., chairman of the department of psychology at the University of South Alabama in Mobile and an expert on the effects of sugar and caffeine on mood. What you eat can lift your mood or, if you make the wrong choices, sink it. Moreover, what you don't eat can have as great an impact as what you do.

Cut back on sugar. While a sweet treat may temporarily boost your mood, the lift doesn't last. Some people notice a rebound effect and feel a little tired an hour or so after eating something sweet. This slump is especially pronounced in people who are depressed, Dr. Christensen says. To find out if sugar is contributing to your depression, cut out sweets and added sugar for a few weeks. If your mood improves, gradually reintroduce sweets to see how much you can tolerate.

Avoid the caffeine crash. Studies show that depressed people who depend on caffeine to get them through the day may be setting themselves up for a fall. Dr. Christensen advises his patients to eliminate coffee, tea, cola, chocolate, and pain relievers containing caffeine. "Depressed people who are sensitive to caffeine generally notice improvements after 4 days without caffeine," he says. Again, if you see improvement after abstaining, experiment to find your safe caffeine limit.

Go low-fat. Some research suggests that a low-fat diet may help stabilize your mood. In a 5-year study at the State University of New York at Stony Brook, 305 men and women followed a diet with only 20 to 30 percent fat. The people showed less depression and hostility after adopting the leaner diet—and lowered their cholesterol levels, too.

Boost your Bs. A healthy intake of the B-complex vitamins is important for anyone who wants to keep depression at bay, says Harold Bloomfield, M.D., a psychiatrist in Del Mar, California, and coauthor of *How to Deal with Depression*. "There's been a lot of evidence that if you're deficient in thiamin or riboflavin, over time it's going to lead to a depression of the whole functioning of the body, both physically and emotionally," says Dr. Bloomfield.

Another B vitamin that has been linked to depression is folate. Studies show that people who are clinically depressed often have low levels of folate in their bloodstreams.

The most convenient way to get all your Bs is to invest in a B-complex supplement, says Dr. Bloomfield. Look for a supplement that contains at least 10 milligrams each of thiamin, riboflavin, and B_6, and 100 micrograms of folic acid, he suggests, and take it twice a day.

Eat carbohydrates for a natural calm. For some people, comfort foods like pasta, potatoes, and bread can help ease feelings of depression, anxiety, and fatigue. These carbohydrate-rich foods have been shown to increase brain concentrations of the amino acid tryptophan, which the body converts to mood-boosting serotonin. "Women, particularly, may crave carbohydrates for their antidepressant effect," says Melvyn Werbach, M.D., assistant clinical professor of psychiatry at the University of California, Los Angeles, and author of *Healing through Nutrition* and *Nutritional Influences on Illness*. "This phenomenon does seem to exist, although not necessarily for everybody."

You can get an adequate amount of carbohydrates by eating a small portion of a carbohydrate-rich food such as a cup of low-fat yogurt, a baked potato, or a half-cup of raisins.

DIABETES

Disarming a Potential Killer

Sugar and spice are fine for nursery rhymes. But when the sugar is in your blood and the amount is too high, you probably have diabetes, a disease that afflicts nearly 15 million Americans.

Diabetes is the nation's fourth leading cause of death, claiming about 160,000 people each year. Over time, unmanaged diabetes can cause stroke, heart attack, blindness, and kidney failure even in young people, who normally don't face these problems.

It also causes nerve damage that could result in a loss of sensation in the legs and feet, making people with diabetes more susceptible to dangerous foot injuries. According to the American Diabetes Association, more than 54,000 diabetes sufferers lose their feet or legs to amputation each year because of the disease.

"Any time you change the chemistry of the blood, you're going to change virtually every system affected by the blood," says Steve Manley, Ph.D., a psychologist in private practice in Denton, Texas. "And that would be all of them."

Including your sexual organs. Since diabetes can debilitate both the neurological system and the vascular system, and you need good nerves and blood flow to function sexually, men may become impotent and women may lose the pleasure they once found in sex.

The Brain Drain

For many people, the aging effects of diabetes don't stop with the body. "When your blood sugar is out of control, it has an effect on your cognitive function," says Patricia Stenger, R.N., a diabetes counselor and senior vice president for the American Diabetes Association. "You may have slower response time, and you feel sluggish and fatigued."

Adds Dr. Manley, "In effect, diabetes kicks you into a grief reaction, because you have lost something. Some people feel helpless and hopeless that their bodies

97

somehow revolted against them. Some feel that they are no longer in control of their own destinies. They may lose belief, at least temporarily, that they are going to be okay at some point in the future. The disease begins to interact with their basic personalities."

Subtle Trouble

There are two types of diabetes. With type 1 (or juvenile) diabetes, which accounts for only 10 percent of cases, the body completely fails to produce insulin, a hormone secreted in the pancreas that's needed to convert food into energy. People with type 1 diabetes need daily injections of this hormone to keep their bodies functioning properly. Type 1 is often diagnosed during puberty, and the symptoms, which can mimic the flu, are sudden and very noticeable: extreme hunger and thirst, sudden weight loss, and extreme fatigue and irritability.

In the more common type 2 (formerly called adult-onset) diabetes, the pancreas produces insulin, but not enough. There may be some symptoms—slow-healing cuts or bruises, recurring skin, gum, or bladder infections, or slight tingling or numbness in the hands or feet. But many people don't notice these subtle changes or simply shrug them off. And that's exactly why over half of Americans with diabetes are unaware of their condition.

"Diabetes is a subtle disease that just creeps up on people—and with devastating results," says Xavier Pi-Sunyer, M.D., professor of medicine at Columbia University in New York City and past president of the American Diabetes Association. Therefore, it's important for you to get a blood screening for elevated glucose levels, especially if you have a family history of the disease, are overweight, are over age 40, or had a baby with a birth weight of over 9 pounds.

Beating the Odds

Although some people with type 2 diabetes require oral drugs or injections to stabilize their blood sugar levels, most can control the disease simply by adopting healthier lifestyles. Lifestyle change number 1: Control your weight.

"The best way to avoid diabetes is to watch your weight," says Audrey Lally, R.D., a certified diabetes educator and nutrition specialist at the Mayo Clinic in Scottsdale, Arizona. "That means eating a healthy diet that focuses on fruits and vegetables. Being overweight is the major risk factor for adult-onset diabetes. This is important for everyone but is essential if you have a family history of diabetes or you are a woman who had diabetes during pregnancy."

By committing yourself to lifestyle changes like this, you may be able to reduce your need for medication—and possibly get off and stay off diabetes drugs for the rest of your life, says James Barnard, Ph.D., professor of physiological science at the University of California, Los Angeles. Here are some suggestions that can help you avoid or control diabetes.

Eat right. For most people that means low fat and high fiber, with at least five servings of fruits and vegetables a day, says Lally. For each extra 40 grams of fat eaten per day—the amount found in one fast-food burger and a large order of fries—your risk of developing diabetes rises threefold, and if you already have diabetes, you face a greater chance of complications, finds a study in the *American Journal of Epidemiology.* The problem: Dietary fat readily converts to body fat, and body fat induces cells to resist insulin, says Frank Q. Nuttall, M.D., Ph.D., chief of the Endocrine, Metabolic and Nutrition Section of the Minneapolis Veterans Administration Medical Center.

Meanwhile, try to consume at least 25 grams of fiber daily from complex-carbohydrate foods. This will help slow glucose, a sugar your body produces, from entering your bloodstream. Fiber also keeps cholesterol low—important for people with diabetes, who face a higher risk of heart disease. The best sources of complex carbohydrates are potatoes, whole-grain breads, rice, pasta, legumes, oats, and barley.

Time it right. "If you have diabetes, you need to eat every 4 or 5 hours," says Lally. Grazing is best, since large meals make it tougher for your body to meet the increased demand for insulin. The key is to evenly distribute your food throughout the day, so no single meal overwhelms the pancreas.

Limit sugar and salt. Sugar is no longer forbidden for most people with diabetes. Still, you should eat sugary foods in moderation, because like all carbohydrates, sugar will raise your blood sugar level. If you really want to snack on ice cream, go ahead. But make up for it by cutting back on bread, pasta, or other carbohydrates at your next meal. Also try to limit your intake of salty foods. They can raise blood pressure, a danger for people with diabetes.

Neutralize stress. Studies by researchers at Duke University in Durham, North Carolina, show that when you're under stress, your body activates certain hormones that pump stored glucose into your bloodstream, raising your blood sugar level. Conversely, stress management and taking time to relax improve glucose control, a significant factor for those with diabetes. While joining a therapy group is one way to relax, others include meditation and yoga.

Get your heart pumping. In a Harvard University study, researchers found that exercise is an excellent way to help prevent type 2 diabetes. Those who exercised at least five times a week lowered their risk of developing diabetes by more than 40 percent. Regular aerobic exercise also can help if you already have diabetes. It not only helps control your weight but also makes cells more receptive to insulin. "You need to get your heart going and keep it going for at least 20 minutes," says Stenger. "You don't need to do anything fancy: A brisk walk is fine."

Keep in mind that people with diabetes need to exercise with care, says Greg Dwyer, Ph.D., professor of physical education at Ball State University in Muncie, Indiana. "The main concern for exercise and diabetes is the risk of hypoglycemia, or low blood sugar," he says. To avoid this, Dr. Dwyer suggests sticking to a routine that requires the same amount of exercise at the same time daily.

Pump some iron, too. Weight lifting also plays a role in improving glucose tolerance, the body's ability to metabolize sugar properly, according to a study by researchers at the University of Maryland College Park and Johns Hopkins University in Baltimore. Check with your doctor before starting a weight-lifting program. Resistance training may cause surges in blood pressure.

Take vitamins E and C. These two antioxidants tend to be in short supply among people with diabetes. Italian researchers have found that vitamin E helps improve the action of insulin. Good food sources include wheat germ, corn oil, and nuts, but you should take a supplement containing 400 international units each day.

Meanwhile, because those with diabetes are prone to vascular disease, they may need to increase their intakes of vitamin C, suggests Ishwarial Jialal, M.D., assistant professor of internal medicine and clinical nutrition at the University of Texas Southwestern Medical Center at Dallas. The Recommended Dietary Allowance is 60 milligrams a day, but Dr. Jialal suggests a minimum of 120 milligrams of vitamin C daily, the amount you'd find in a guava or a glass of orange juice.

Increase your chromium. The trace mineral chromium has been shown to improve your body's ability to regulate blood sugar. You can get more chromium in your diet by taking a supplement or eating foods such as broccoli, turkey ham, grapefruit, and fortified breakfast cereals.

Get a boost from magnesium. People with diabetes, especially those taking insulin or whose blood sugar is not well controlled, tend to come up short on magnesium, studies show. And magnesium offers a long list of potential benefits for people with diabetes. Low levels of magnesium have been linked to degeneration of the eye's retina, high blood sugar, high blood pressure, and clotting problems that can lead to heart disease. To get your Daily Value of magnesium, take a supplement, or eat foods such as baked halibut, oysters, and long-grained rice.

Pretend you have a headache. Aspirin can reduce the risk of heart attack and stroke among diabetes sufferers by as much as 20 percent, according to research conducted by the National Institutes of Health on 3,711 people with both types of the disease. "People with diabetes are much more likely to have cardiovascular disease, so the aspirin recommendation is even more relevant for them," says Frederick Ferris, M.D., chief of the Clinical Trials Branch at the National Institutes of Health in Bethesda, Maryland.

Most researchers recommend a daily dosage of one-half of an adult aspirin or one children's aspirin, but check with your doctor first. Aspirin therapy isn't suggested for people taking blood thinners or suffering from ulcers.

DIGESTIVE PROBLEMS

Calming the Pain and Rumble

As a kid, you could eat chocolate bars and cheese curls all night long. When you were single, nights out with friends meant spicy buffalo wings and jalapeño poppers—and never a hint of heartburn.

But these days your once cast-iron stomach is showing some signs of rust. Gas, bloating, cramps, diarrhea, constipation, and, yes, heartburn seem to have found a direct line to your door. What gives?

Apparently, your digestive tract. Like the rest of your body, it's starting to age.

"Just as it takes longer to recover from a cold or an injury as you grow older, the same happens to your digestive system. Things just kind of slow down, and the repair mechanisms aren't quite the same as they used to be," says William B. Ruderman, M.D., chairman of the department of gastroenterology at the Cleveland Clinic Florida in Fort Lauderdale. "You can't tolerate certain foods or the effects of alcohol as well as you used to. It certainly makes you feel your own mortality."

All those belches, rumbles, and other internal actions wear on more than just your digestive tract. "You may be hesitant to take a bus or go outdoors in case you have to go to the bathroom. You may not go to certain restaurants because you can't eat certain foods," says Devendra Mehta, M.D., a gastroenterologist and assistant professor of pediatrics at Hahnemann University Hospital in Philadelphia. "This can be very distressing at any age. But when you are young and have these problems, it disrupts your life."

Just because your innards may be out of kilter, however, it doesn't mean they have to stay that way. Whatever the problem, there is a fix.

Constipation: Get Yourself Moving

If you haven't been bothered by constipation, give yourself a few years. "Constipation gets a lot more common as you age," says Jorge Herrera, M.D., associate professor of medicine at the University of South Alabama College of Medicine in Mobile. "For one thing, as they get older, most people tend to eat less and be-

101

come less active." And many medicines that people tend to take as they age for conditions such as heart disease and diabetes also cause constipation, says Dr. Herrera.

Most people over age 30 can expect at least an occasional bout with constipation—and more as they get older. But here's how to keep problems to a minimum, no matter your age.

Eat in bulk. "If you're eating the typical Western diet with a lot of processed foods, that will lead to constipation," says Dr. Mehta. "But a diet with lots of roughage and fiber that centers on plenty of fresh fruits and vegetables is the most important thing you can do to treat or avoid constipation, especially as you get older."

Experts say you need at least five servings a day in order to get the recommended minimum of 25 grams of fiber—about twice what's actually consumed by the typical American. Besides fresh fruits and vegetables, good sources of dietary fiber include whole-grain breads and cereals, pastas, brown rice, beans, and bran.

Work out. Any type of exercise speeds up gastrointestinal transit time, the length of time it takes food to get from your mouth through the stomach and intestines. But researchers at the University of Maryland College Park found that people who undergo strength-training programs can improve their bowel transit times by about 56 percent compared with their pre-pumping days. It seems that the contractions of abdominal muscles done in weight lifting help "squeeze" the waste through the intestines more quickly. Researchers also believe that any type of exercise has an effect on motilin, a gastrointestinal hormone that's related to faster transit time. Exercise also improves blood flow to the intestines, which improves bowel movements.

Drink water. "One reason why constipation is more common as you age is that generally, the older people get, the less they drink," says Dr. Mehta. "And the less you drink, the harder and less frequent stools become." Even if you don't have a problem with constipation, you'll help keep yourself regular by drinking at least eight glasses of water or other nonalcoholic beverages each day.

Say good morning, joe. "A cup or two of coffee in the morning can help you stay regular," says Pat Harper, R.D., a nutrition consultant in the Pittsburgh area. The caffeine in the coffee stimulates the large intestine, causing it to contract, she says.

In fact, some doctors recommend that people who are constipated try drinking a cup of coffee rather than taking an over-the-counter laxative.

Keep in mind, though, that coffee (like tea and alcohol) is a diuretic, which removes the fluids from your body that you need to aid bowel movements. So if you try the coffee cure, limit yourself to a few cups a day.

Heartburn: Douse the Fire

Heartburn occurs when stomach acids, in a process called reflux, splash up into the esophagus, says Sheila Rodriguez, Ph.D., gastrointestinal laboratory director for the Oklahoma Foundation for Digestive Research in Oklahoma City. Eating too fast or too much is one common cause, but pigging out isn't the only reason for this all-too-common after-dinner ailment. Heartburn can also be the primary symptom of other conditions, such as gastritis, an inflammation in the lining of the stomach.

"It's not that the natural aging process contributes to heartburn per se, but the condition does seem to be more of a problem as you get older," says Dr. Mehta. One reason is that there's a clear association between heartburn and being over-weight—and most of us have gained a few pounds over the last few years.

But another, less obvious reason is bacteria. The same bacteria—*Helicobacter pylori*—that cause ulcers have been linked to heartburn symptoms in many people, says Dr. Mehta. Also, after age 40, our esophageal muscles start to weaken, which can contribute to reflux. No matter the reason, here's how to take the fire out of heartburn.

Eat smaller. Many people with heartburn problems find that grazing helps extinguish that internal blaze. When you eat four or five smaller meals instead of three massive squares a day, your stomach churns out less acid, says Frank Hamilton, M.D., director of the Gastrointestinal Diseases Program at the National Institutes of Health in Bethesda, Maryland.

Down it with water. Drinking lots of water—especially with meals—helps wash stomach acids from the surface of the esophagus back into your stomach, says Ronald L. Hoffman, M.D., a physician in New York City and author of *Seven Weeks to a Settled Stomach.*

Know the offenders. Certain foods are more likely than others to bring on the symptoms of heartburn. According to Dr. Rodriguez, onions, chocolate, and mints relax the lower esophageal sphincter, which allows stomach acids to wash up. Citrus fruits such as oranges and grapefruit, as well as tomato products, coffee, and fried or fatty foods, can also cause trouble because they can irritate the esophageal lining, adds Dr. Hamilton.

Sleep on a slope. If heartburn troubles you often, place wooden or concrete blocks under the headboard of your bed so that you sleep on an incline, advises William Lipshultz, M.D., chief of gastroenterology at Pennsylvania Hospital in Philadelphia. By raising the head of your bed 6 inches higher, it's harder for stomach acid to flow. That's because it would have to go uphill.

If you must lie flat, lying on your left side might produce less heartburn, says Leo Katz, M.D., a gastroenterologist at Jefferson Medical College of Thomas Jefferson University in Philadelphia. In tests, he found that people who ate the same heartburn-producing meal usually got more heartburn when they lay on their right sides compared with their left sides. "We think it has something to do with the anatomy of the stomach and gravity," he says.

Savor some seaweed. This unusual food can help form gels that bind up stomach acid, says Arthur Jacknowitz, Pharm.D., chairman of the clinical pharmacy department at West Virginia University School of Pharmacy in Morgantown. You can find seaweed in health food stores and Asian markets in the form of kelp, wakame, nori, and other varieties. Simply cut it into strips and add to soups, salads, or stews.

Note: If you are sensitive to sodium or have high blood pressure, rinse or soak sea vegetables to reduce the salt content before eating.

Lactose Intolerance: Drink Up—Safely

Dare to eat dairy? Perhaps not. As much as 70 percent of the world's population has some symptoms of lactose intolerance, meaning these people experience ill effects from milk, ice cream, and other dairy products. Symptoms include bloating, gas, stomach cramping, and diarrhea, which can curtail your activities and hamper your lifestyle. Besides making you feel older, the symptoms often get worse as you grow older.

By about age 8, many of us start losing an enzyme called lactase, which helps us digest lactose, the sugar that makes milk taste sweet. Without the lactase, much of the lactose passes along your digestive system undigested, possibly sending your colon into spasms and churning up gas. "By age 20, lactose-intolerant people pretty much lose the ability to digest milk," says Dr. Herrera. To avoid trouble, follow these tips.

Limit your exposure Many supermarkets sell reduced-lactose milk and reduced-lactose cheeses that can provide the bone-building benefits of the calcium in regular dairy products with much less of the lactose—70 percent less in some cases.

Take a supplement. A lactase supplement replaces the enzyme your body is missing, making it easier for you to digest dairy products. The supplements are available in many drugstores and supermarkets and can be stirred into milk or taken as a pill or caplet along with dairy foods.

Be a cocoa nut. Research suggests that cocoa slows stomach emptying, which reduces the rate at which lactose reaches the colon, says Dennis A. Savaiano, Ph.D., professor of food science/nutrition and associate dean at the University of Minnesota College of Human Ecology in St. Paul. So by drinking chocolate milk or having chocolate ice cream, you may avoid, if not lessen, symptoms.

Combine dining with dairy. Some people find they can go symptom-free if they have their dairy products with meals. That's because having food in your stomach slows the release of lactose into your intestines, says Douglas B. McGill, M.D., professor of medicine at Mayo Medical School/Mayo Clinic in Rochester, Minnesota. Still, it's not advisable to load up on several dairy products at one meal.

Choose the right yogurt. Yogurt may be one milk product you can eat without worry. But don't assume that all yogurt products are the same. "Some commercial brands add milk products, which can cause you problems," warns Dr. Mehta. So study the label before buying. Also, make sure you choose a brand whose label says it contains live active cultures. "As soon as the yogurt cultures pass into the intestine, they become active and start to break down the lactose," says Dr. McGill. Sorry, but frozen yogurt won't help, since there are too few bacteria to be helpful.

Irritable Bowel: Take Control

Here's a disease that some experts say might be as widespread as the common cold—and that causes even more misery. Doctors aren't sure what specifically causes irritable bowel syndrome (IBS) or even how to treat it. But IBS—sometimes called a spastic colon—is the diagnosis for people who are regularly annoyed with constipation, diarrhea, bloating, nausea, or abdominal cramps, either singly or in some combination and usually with abdominal pain.

The good news (if there is any) is that you will probably outgrow your problem. "IBS is more of a problem in those in their twenties to fifties," says Dr. Mehta. "But at any age, it has some significant aging effects." Many patients find themselves planning their lives around these symptoms, he says. "You don't know whether you'll suddenly need to rush to the bathroom, so you plan your day-to-day activities with this in mind."

Having an irritable bowel doesn't have to put you in that mindset, however. While you should see a doctor if you suspect that you have IBS, there are plenty of things you can do to lessen its symptoms.

Control your sweet tooth. Limiting the amount of sugar you eat is a key to putting the bite on IBS-triggered diarrhea. That's because sugars—especially fructose and the artificial sweetener sorbitol—aren't easily digested, which can cause the runs, says Stephen B. Hanauer, M.D., professor of medicine in the section of gastroenterology at the University of Chicago Medical Center. These sweeteners are in most sugar-free or low-calorie candy and gums as well as store-bought fruit juices. So if you like juice, make your own with a juicer.

Chill out. Being under stress makes IBS symptoms worse, and conversely, not being stressed out can help, adds Dr. Hanauer. He suggests that people under the gun manage their stress with the help of relaxation therapy techniques such as meditation, self-hypnosis, biofeedback, and regular exercise. You can also keep a "stress diary" to help you determine the source of your difficulties.

Warm up. Abdominal cramps may be relieved with a heating pad placed directly on the painful area, says Arvey I. Rogers, M.D., chief of gastroenterology at the Veterans Administration Medical Center in Miami. Just be sure to place it on the low setting to prevent burning your skin.

Watch what you drink. Coffee and other caffeinated drinks can aggravate IBS by speeding up motility, the pace at which stools move through the bowels—bad news if you're prone to diarrhea. Besides that, there's a chemical in coffee that can cause cramping, says Alex Aslan, M.D., a gastroenterologist in private practice in Fairfield, California. Meanwhile, milk may not be much better, because some people with IBS also have lactose intolerance.

Feast on fiber. A high-fiber diet tends to quiet that kvetching colon. Fiber increases stool production and reduces intestinal pressure, which can benefit those with either constipation or diarrhea (or both), says Dr. Hanauer. People with IBS are advised to eat up to 35 to 50 grams of fiber a day. Start by adding about 3 tablespoons of pure bran to your cereal each morning and eating at least four servings of fruits and vegetables each day. Grains and beans are great sources of fiber. Shoot for a cup of beans or other legumes a day. Other fiber-rich foods include whole-grain breads and cereals, pastas, and brown rice. But add fiber to your diet gradually to help avoid its gassy side effects.

Ax fat. Fatty foods can make your stomach empty more slowly, causing nausea and bloating, says Dr. Aslan. So avoid cheeses, ice cream, rich desserts, fried foods, and fatty meats such as hot dogs, sausage, and bacon.

Try the calming herb. Chamomile is another good anti-inflammatory that's also soothing to gastrointestinal tissues, says Melissa Metcalf, N.D., a naturopathic doctor in Los Angeles. She suggests taking two 400- to 500-milligram capsules three times a day for relief of symptoms.

DOUBLE CHIN

Going Neck and Neck with Aging

Mother Nature didn't do us any favors when she invented gravity. Since the day we slipped off our prom attire, it's been tugging, tugging, tugging on us, pulling body parts to places we would never have thought possible in our teens.

And of all our body parts, none is more gravity sensitive than the neck. Add a few innocent pounds, a few harmless years, and—aarrgh!—here comes a double chin.

"I must say, a double chin really seems to bother some people. It makes them feel like they're aging in a hurry," says Robert Kotler, M.D., a facial cosmetic surgeon and clinical instructor in surgery at the University of California, Los Angeles. "Every time they look in the mirror, they see it. They are conscious of it at parties or at work. And it's telling them that maybe they're not as young as they used to be."

Jaw Droppers

Three factors contribute to double chins: body fat, anatomy, and time. We tend to store fat on our necks just as easily as on other parts of our bodies, Dr. Kotler says. So if we gain a few extra pounds, there's a good chance some of it will settle under our chins.

But overweight people aren't the only ones in danger. Even those who are thin get double chins, usually because of the shape of the jaw and throat. "The less sharp the angle between the jawline and neckline, the greater the risk of a fleshy neck," says Dr. Kotler. "But the lower your Adam's apple is in your neck, the more likely you are to get a sag in your chin."

Age also increases the odds. A woman's skin starts to lose its elasticity after 35 to 40 years, a man's after 40 to 50. Even if you're fit and firm, you may still show a slight double chin simply because of looser skin, Dr. Kotler says.

From a health perspective, none of this really matters. There's nothing dangerous about a double chin unless you're seriously overweight, Dr. Kotler says. Even then, it's a symptom of obesity, not a problem by itself. "Double chins are just an unfortunate part of the aging process," Dr. Kotler says. "In the overall scheme of things, there are more important things to worry about."

Keeping Your Chin Up

Harmless or not, most people still find double chins unattractive. To help get rid of those extra folds—or at least to hide them a little—experts offer these tips.

Lose 10. Or maybe 15—pounds, that is. "The single best way to get rid of a double chin is to lose weight," Dr. Kotler says. "Lots of people come to my office wanting cosmetic surgery. But if they just take off some excess weight, the problem usually diminishes to the point where they don't need any more help."

The standard rules apply. Get regular aerobic exercise. Eat less fat. Avoid crash diets, which usually do more harm than good. And don't rely on miracle "spot-reducing" exercises for your neck. They won't remove the fat—and in some cases have caused dislocated jaws and severely strained neck muscles.

Get cropped. Long hair draws eyes to your neck—precisely what you want to avoid. Men and women should "keep it short, at or above the jawline," says Kathleen Walas, fashion and beauty director for New York City–based Avon Products and author of *Real Beauty . . . Real Women.*

For men, stay loose. Nothing exposes a double chin more than a dress shirt that is too tight around the neck. "You start to look like a stuffed sausage," says G. Bruce Boyer, a New York City fashion consultant and author of *Eminently Suitable.* Swallow your pride and buy a bigger size. Boyer also suggests shirts with bigger collars, since they help keep things in proportion. And avoid spread, round, and pin collars. They only accentuate your neck. With casual shirts, try open collars, and stay away from turtlenecks. The darker the color around the neckline, the better.

For women, drop that neckline. Open, broad necklines are more flattering for women with double chins, Walas says. Turtlenecks are a definite no-no. As for jewelry, avoid chokers and try longer necklaces. Dangling earrings—anything below the jawline—can bring attention to your neck, according to Walas.

Make up the difference. To play down a double chin, women should play up another feature. Walas suggests using blush high on the cheekbones. Or try a brighter, tasteful shade of eye shadow. If you use foundation, apply it one shade darker under your chin and blend it carefully with the foundation on your face. "That will make the rest of your face bright and attractive and your double chin much less noticeable," Walas says.

Know the skinny on surgery. Cosmetic surgery is a last resort, Dr. Kotler says. But if you have tried everything else and can't lose that extra chin—and have about $4,500 handy—you can have your neck "sculpted." The surgeon will make a small horizontal cut under your chin, then suck out the fat that has collected beneath the skin. Finally, he will make a vertical incision between the layers of the neck and jaw muscle and sew the edges together, tightening the muscle layer like a corset.

It's a relatively painless procedure that requires two Band-Aids to hide, Dr. Kotler says. Bruising is minimal, and within about 10 days you won't see anything except your old single chin. "It's a common procedure," he says. "The technique has become very refined, and the results are quite good." The operation can be performed under either general anesthesia or local anesthesia with sedation.

For an extra $500 or so, the surgeon can also add a chin implant. It's a piece of solid silicone that is slipped between your jawbone and the sheath of tissue that covers the bone. The implant gives you a more prominent jaw and further accentuates the angle between the jawline and neck, Dr. Kotler says. There is no addition to overall recovery time. Surgeons use implants in about one-fourth of all double chin procedures, Dr. Kotler says.

FATIGUE

How to Restore Your Energy

Tom is an avid jogger. But lately, his running has left him feeling drained. He felt so exhausted the other day that after less than half his normal run, he stopped and limped home.

His friend Dick regularly gets a good 8 hours of sleep, but every morning, he can barely wake up. One shower and many cups of coffee later, he still feels as weak as a kitten.

Their friend Terry is on the go all day. She's up at the crack of dawn to make breakfast and get the kids off to school. Then she runs around like a madwoman for 9 or 10 hours at work. Back at home, chores keep her busy until midnight rolls around. Waking up refreshed? It's only a distant memory.

Every now and then, every Tom, Dick, and Terry goes through a spell of fatigue. Usually, it doesn't last long. But sometimes an overwhelming bout of fatigue can last for days, weeks, months. And once fatigue hits, it can transform a person from a vibrant lover of life into a washed-up, worn-out zombie who feels 100 years old.

"Fatigue's greatest impact is on human function and activity," says Lt. Col. Kurt Kroenke, M.D., associate professor of medicine at the Uniformed Services University of the Health Sciences in Bethesda, Maryland, and an expert on fatigue. "When you don't have the strength or energy to move, even simple tasks become difficult. You become sedentary, your productivity drops, your motivation suffers. For some, this persistent weariness can be so debilitating that they can't even get out of bed."

Fatigue can take a toll on your mind as well, experts agree. Thinking becomes difficult and confused. Decisions come slowly. Even your outlook on life turns gloomy.

Eventually, fatigue can lead to poor work performance, less interaction with friends and family, and less participation in the sports and activities you enjoy.

But the good news is that with a little detective work, you can almost always get to the source of the problem and reclaim your energy and vitality.

110

What's Running You Down?

It's easy to shrug off a case of lethargy as just another sign that you're getting older or that you're coming down with something.

But for most of us, it's neither. "Most fatigue is not because of aging or a serious medical problem," says Dr. Kroenke. "More often it's a signal that the body is getting too much or too little of something, and that's making you feel run down."

Most fatigue is caused by too much work, too much stress, too much weight, too much junk food, and not enough exercise, doctors say.

"Most of us live and work in rapid, pressure-filled environments," explains Ralph LaForge, an exercise physiologist and instructor of health promotion and exercise science at the University of California, San Diego. "Much of the fatigue people experience is really because of the inability to pace themselves, to effectively stagger their workloads, or to bring a sense of order to the chaos around them."

Just dealing with the pressures of everyday life takes a lot of energy, says Thomas Miller, Ph.D., professor of psychiatry at the University of Kentucky College of Medicine in Lexington. "One of the first things we look at whenever a patient complains of fatigue is stress. Whenever anyone has a hard time coping—with family problems, relationships, job pressure—there's usually a tremendous burnout factor, physically as well as emotionally."

Fatigue also is often a signal that you're not eating right, says Peter Miller, Ph.D., executive director of the Hilton Head Health Institute, a clinic in Hilton Head, South Carolina, that develops personal health programs. "The eating habits we established when we were younger are not suited for our middle years.

"Think of the body as a car and food as the fuel," says Dr. Miller. "When you're young, you can put almost any kind of gasoline in your tank. But as you get older, the body has a harder time running on that low-octane stuff. So you need to fill up with high-test fuel and in the proper amounts."

If you're an overeater, for example, you're going to be storing more fuel than you need in the form of fat. And lugging around that excess body weight can make anyone feel sluggish. At the other extreme, undereating can also cause fatigue by depriving you of sufficient calories to propel your body through the day. That's why many people who go on "crash" or very low calorie diets often find their energy levels crashing: They're like cars running on empty.

Your activity level also has a direct effect on whether you feel fatigued, says LaForge. Lack of exercise can easily create a pattern of inactivity that is difficult to break. "A body at rest tends to remain at rest," LaForge says. "Generally, the more active and fit you are, the more stamina and energy you'll have on a day-to-day basis. Letter carriers, for example, are always on their feet. Yet they complain of fatigue much less than office workers."

On the other hand, too much exercise can have a negative effect. "Overexertion can send your energy level crashing," says LaForge. That's because when we exercise, the body produces lactic acid, a substance that accumulates in our muscles, producing weakness and body aches. When we push our bodies during workouts and don't allow our muscles time to recover, lactic acid accumulates faster than we can get rid of it. And this can leave us feeling fatigued all the time.

Other factors that can make us feel tired all the time? Smoking, so-called recreational drugs, alcohol, and inconsistent eating and sleeping patterns put enormous strain on the mind and body. Sometimes, experts agree, fatigue is simply your body's cry that your lifestyle is not one that supports a healthy body.

Get Back Your Vim and Vigor

Fatigue can be a symptom of everything from the common cold to cancer. And it's also a side effect of some of the medications used to treat serious conditions. But fatigue is rarely anything to worry about unless it's accompanied by other symptoms such as pain, swelling, or fever, or it lasts longer than a week.

If your fatigue has lasted a week or more, or you have other symptoms, see your doctor. Otherwise, here are some tips to re-energize your life.

Lighten your load. Are you one of the countless Americans who has no downtime? Do you go from work to home to your volunteer position or children's activities, leaving no time for your pleasures? Then you may be on overload, says Reed Moskovitz, M.D., founder and medical director of the stress disorders service at New York University Medical Center in New York City and author of *Your Healing Mind*. "Absolutely everyone needs true downtime to relax and recover," says Dr. Moskovitz. By downtime, he means that time when you don't have to answer to anyone, when you have no responsibilities. It's the time when you garden, read a mystery novel, go for a walk, or lose yourself in preparing a gourmet meal. The key thing: You need to cut activities that are a low priority and reclaim time for yourself—or as says Dr. Moskovitz says, stop living a human "doing" and start living as a human being.

Exercise for energy. "Even though energy is used during exercise, it also creates more energy," says William J. Evans, Ph.D., director of the nutrition, metabolism, and exercise program at the University of Arkansas for Medical Sciences in Little Rock. "The muscles and cardiovascular system are like a car engine. Regular exercise increases the efficiency and the horsepower of the engine."

Health officials say that 30 minutes of daily moderate activity is enough to gain major health benefits. You can accumulate those 30 minutes in short bursts of activity that include walking up stairs, walking short distances quickly, gardening, even dancing, says Dr. Evans.

Clear the clutter. Does a list of tasks leave you feeling zapped before you even begin? Clear away the clutter in your life bit by bit, says LaForge. Start your day with a list of four or five tasks you can definitely accomplish and work on them alone. The next day, try four or five more. What at first seemed like a mountain you couldn't climb then becomes a series of small hills you step over with ease.

Close the sleep gap. Even being an hour or so short of high-quality slumber can make you fade. "Many Americans force their bodies to run day after day on 5 to 6 hours of sleep, when they really need 7 or 8," says sleep expert Mary A. Carskadon, Ph.D., professor of psychiatry and human behavior at Brown University in Providence, Rhode Island. Shoot for a minimum of 8 hours to feel your best.

Hit the road. According to a study by Robert Thayer, Ph.D., professor of psychology at California State University, Long Beach, a brisk 10-minute walk causes a shift in mood that quickly raises energy levels and keeps them high for up to 2 hours.

And an after-meal stroll can counteract the energy drop you experience after eating a big meal, adds Dr. Peter Miller. Digesting large meals increases blood and oxygen flow to the stomach and intestines, and this draws energy away from muscles and the brain. But a walk will keep blood and oxygen circulating evenly throughout the body.

Balance your diet. A junk food diet high in sugar, fat, and processed foods gives your body few or none of the basic vitamins, minerals, and nutrients it needs to perform at normal levels. And sometimes just the slightest deficiency of any one nutrient is all it takes to send energy levels plummeting.

The answer, says Dr. Miller, is to find a balance in both the amount and the types of food that you eat. "It's important to hit all the major food groups—fruits, vegetables, grains and cereals, dairy, nuts, and meats—every day to guarantee that you're giving your body the right combination of fuel and basic nutrients to keep on running at peak levels," says Dr. Miller.

Ideally, every day you should be getting 60 percent (or more) of your calories from carbohydrate-rich foods such as pasta, bread, potatoes, and beans, 25 percent (or less) of your calories from the fat found in foods such as canola oil, olive oil, and peanut butter, and 15 percent of your calories from protein-rich foods such as chicken and fish.

Focus on the carbs. Of the three energy-supplying nutrients—carbohydrates, fat, and protein—carbohydrates pack the most fatigue-fighting punch. "Carbohydrates provide an efficient, long-lasting energy source," says Dr. Miller. To produce an abundant reservoir of carbohydrate energy, add some of these foods to your plate whenever you sit down for a meal.

Eat more frequently. Skipping meals can leave your fuel reserves dangerously low and digesting big meals can be an enormous energy drain. Unfortunately, the traditional three meals per day may contribute to the problem.

"Your body needs fuel in moderate doses throughout the day to keep performing at optimal levels," says Dr. Miller. He recommends eating four or five small meals each day. "Reducing the amount of food you eat at any one time and spreading your calorie consumption more evenly over the day make more energy available to your body throughout the day," he says.

Snack wisely. When your stomach's growling and your energy's waning, the

Do You Have Chronic Fatigue Syndrome?

Chronic fatigue syndrome (CFS) is a rare, debilitating disorder that leaves people weak, exhausted, and barely able to function for months or even decades.

The cause is still a mystery. "Because CFS usually appears after a flu or another illness, it was once thought to be caused by the Epstein-Barr virus," says Nelson Gantz, M.D., a member of the Centers for Disease Control and Prevention (CDC) Task Force on Chronic Fatigue Syndrome, and chief of medicine and the division of infectious disease at Polyclinic Medical Center in Harrisburg, Pennsylvania. "Today, we're less sure of its origins. It probably doesn't have a single cause but is a combination of viral infections, allergies, and psychological factors acting on the immune system."

There is no cure for the syndrome, says Dr. Gantz. Until one is found, people with the disease can find relief through a program of good nutrition, gentle exercise, and rest, as recommended by their personal physicians. In severe cases, nonsteroidal anti-inflammatory drugs and antidepressants are used to partially relieve symptoms, according to Dr. Gantz.

How do you know if you have CFS? The CDC task force has developed a preliminary set of criteria. To be diagnosed as having CFS, you must have suffered from persistent fatigue for at least 6 months. The fa-

---

best pick-me-ups are of the natural variety, says Dr. Miller. Fruits, raw vegetables, nuts, and unbuttered popcorn—all which are low in energy-draining fat—are some excellent energizers.

Avoid a quick fix. Sugar-loaded foods such as candy may zip up your energy level for a while, but they also cause blood sugar levels to increase and then sharply drop. Unfortunately, the result is that your energy level will dip even lower than it was before, says Dr. Miller.

Cut the caffeine. While a cup or two of coffee early in the morning has been shown to boost alertness and mental functioning, drinking large amounts day after day tends to lower energy levels. To avoid this caffeine crash, limit yourself to a couple cups of coffee, cola, or other caffeine-laden drinks and foods each day.

But drink more water. Feeling rundown is often the first sign of dehydra-

tigue must not have existed previously, must persist despite bed rest, and must cut your daily activity level in half for at least 6 months.

Also, the fatigue must not be related to the existence of any other disease, infection, malignancy, or condition that may produce similar symptoms, or to the use of any drugs, medications, or chemicals.

You must also have had 8 of the following 11 symptoms for at least 6 months:

1. Mild fever or chills
2. Sore throat
3. Painful lymph nodes (glands on the sides of your neck)
4. Unexplained general muscle weakness
5. Muscle discomfort or pain
6. Fatigue of 24 hours or more after levels of exercise that used to be easily tolerated
7. Unusual headaches
8. Aches and pains (without swelling or redness) that travel from joint to joint
9. Any of these complaints: forgetfulness, excessive irritability, confusion, difficulty thinking, inability to concentrate, depression
10. Difficulty sleeping
11. Extremely swift development of these symptoms, from within a few hours to a few days

tion, says Dr. Miller. Drinking at least eight glasses of water every day—more if you're active or trying to lose weight—will prevent this type of fatigue.

Avoid booze and pills. Regular use of alcohol, sleeping pills, and tranquilizers will make anybody act like a zombie, says Dr. Kroenke. And believe it or not, stimulants and pep pills can take you from way, way up to way, way down after their immediate effects have worn off.

Check your medicine cabinet. Antihistamines and alcohol, both which are found in a wide variety of over-the-counter and prescription cold medications, can make you feel groggy, says Dr. Kroenke. Ask your doctor or pharmacist if she can recommend a nonfatiguing alternative.

Explore alternative approaches. Many people fight fatigue by going beyond the traditional limits of Western science, says LaForge. Meditation, yoga, and massage are just a few of the nontraditional options that practitioners say will energize, refresh, and revive both body and mind.

Studies at Harvard Medical School show that taking a deep breath, exhaling, then sitting quietly for 20 minutes as you focus on a word that reflects your personal faith—*God, Allah, Krishna*, or *shalom*, for example—will relax and re-energize both mind and body.

Check the Yellow Pages of your local telephone book for organizations that teach these techniques. In many cases, you'll also find them at your local YMCA.

Ask your doctor about supplements. In addition to a balanced diet, a multivitamin/mineral supplement should ensure that you're getting all the vitamins and minerals that you need, says Dr. Kroenke. Talk to your doctor about which one is right for you.

FOOT PROBLEMS

Sidestepping the Ache

The trouble started long ago and innocently enough, with Mom and Dad cheering and steering you as you fumbled your way past the coffee table and La-Z-Boy chair on your maiden trek across the living room floor. You were mobile. Going places. And the world was at your feet—quite literally.

But that thrill of victory as a toddler learning to walk paved the way for today's agony of the feet.

"The moment you begin to walk, you begin the process of wear and tear that could lead to future foot problems," says Glenn Gastwirth, D.P.M., deputy executive director of the American Podiatric Medical Association.

Often, foot problems are simply issues of neglect. Since they're located 5 feet or so from our faces, we often don't give our feet the respect they're due. We wear shoes that are too tight just because we like the style or color. We walk for hours in stiff dress shoes that leave our feet blistered and burning. We wear old, poorly supporting sneakers that should have been retired years ago because, well, they fit like an old soft shoe. The abuse is rampant.

Foot problems especially are an issue for women who wear high-heeled shoes. Those heels that give legs shape also put incredible pressure on the feet. According to a 15-year study by Michael J. Coughlin, M.D., an orthopedic surgeon in private practice in Boise, Idaho, 80 percent of foot surgery patients are women, and most of the problems stem from their shoes.

"High heels can be terrible for your feet," says Philip Sanfilippo, D.P.M., a podiatrist in private practice in San Francisco. "They can cause your feet to slide forward, making you prone to bunions and other problems. And many women develop shortening of their Achilles tendons from wearing heels for too long. After time, this may result in tightness of the tendon and the inability to wear flat shoes or to walk barefoot without pain." Also, pointy-toed shoes can cause neuromas, pinched nerves surrounded by fibrous tissue that can become very painful.

But woman or man, foot pain is more than a nuisance. It can make you hurt all over and feel old before your time. "Bad feet can throw your posture out of whack, setting you up for possible knee pain, hip pain, back pain, and neck pain," says Marc A. Brenner, D.P.M., a doctor of podiatric medicine in private practice in Glendale, New York.

Tight Isn't Right

Beyond the shoes themselves, part of the reason so many people are bothered with foot problems as they age is because of middle-age spread—of the feet. "What happens is that as we age, our feet become longer and wider, a process called splaying," says Dr. Sanfilippo. "This occurs as the ligaments in our feet begin to collapse and the arches fall because of gravity and wear and tear. This flattens out our feet.

"Unfortunately, many people aren't aware of this process—which can occur in your thirties or forties—and they continue to wear the same size shoes they've always worn. And that causes the problem."

Pregnancy can make this splaying occur earlier and be more severe. "When a woman is pregnant, she releases hormones that prepare the connective tissue around the birth canal for delivery," says Dr. Gastwirth. "What this does is weaken some of the connective tissue in other parts of the body. So if you're not wearing supportive shoes or you're doing a lot of barefoot walking during pregnancy, this splaying of the foot may be even more pronounced."

The end result in all cases: Many of us end up wearing shoes that are much too tight, which is a primary cause of corns, calluses, blisters, and other foot problems. In fact, Dr. Coughlin's study estimates that we spend $2 billion on conditions caused by tight shoes.

And if that weren't shocking enough, a study by the American Podiatric Medical Association found that nearly half of all women and one in five men knowingly buy and wear shoes that are too tight strictly for appearance's sake.

Getting Your Feet to Toe the Line

Shoes aren't the only reason for foot pain. Besides causing the feet to splay, the natural aging process also wears away the fat pads on the balls of our feet, which cushion our steps and absorb shock. "It's like the padding of a carpet. When it's installed, it's nice and cushy. But after 20 years, that padding can get pretty worn," says Dr. Gastwirth.

Another common problem is the loss of moisture in the skin of your feet, which frequently occurs after age 30 and can result in itchy feet and make you more susceptible to athlete's foot and other types of fungus. Some people, especially smokers and those with Raynaud's disease, have circulatory problems that take a toll on the feet, causing a loss of sensation, particularly in cold weather. Says Suzanne M. Levine, D.P.M., adjunct clinical instructor at New York College of Podiatric Medicine in New York City and author of *My Feet Are Killing Me*, "Any foot older than 25 is an aging foot."

But suffering isn't inevitable. With a little know-how, you can dance around foot problems and breathe new life into tired tootsies.

Foot and Heel Pain: Support Yourself

There are several causes of those "unexplained" pains in your foot or heel, and most are the result of long-term use of your feet. They include fallen arches, Achilles tendon stiffness, plantar fasciitis, which is an inflammation in the bottom of the foot, and heel spurs, which are tiny growths of bone that may form from the constant pulling of ligaments through jumping, walking, or running. "Usually, these problems result from overuse of your feet," says Richard Braver, D.P.M., sports podiatric physician for teams at Seton Hall University in South Orange, New Jersey, Fairleigh Dickinson University in Rutherford, New Jersey, and Montclair State College in Upper Montclair, New Jersey. No matter what the cause, here are the solutions.

Get some support. There's no getting around the deterioration of your feet's fat pads, but you can do something about the pain it causes on the soles of your feet. "Wearing high-quality, supportive, cushioning insoles in your shoes can certainly ease some of your discomfort," says Dr. Sanfilippo. These insoles are available at drugstores and sporting goods shops. If the pain is centered on your heel, a heel cup, also sold in these stores, can help prevent excess heel movement and ease pain. But perhaps more important than insoles and heel cups is wearing supportive shoes.

Stretch out your calf. For heel pain, many people find relief by stretching the heel cord, or Achilles tendon, on the back of the foot, says Gilbert Wright, M.D., an orthopedic surgeon in private practice in Sacramento, California. Stand about 3 feet from a wall and place your hands on the wall. Lean toward the wall, bringing one leg forward and bending your arms at the elbows. Your back leg should remain straight, with the heel on the floor, so you feel a gentle stretch.

Roll away pain. For heel spurs and plantar fasciitis, try massaging the bottom of your foot. "Roll your foot from heel to toe over a rolling pin, a golf ball, or even a soup can," advises Dr. Braver. "This eases pain by stretching out the ligaments."

Heat feet in the morning. "If you feel stiffness in your foot when you wake up, heat it to stimulate blood flow," says Dr. Braver. He recommends placing a warm compress or hot water bottle on the bottom of your foot for about 20 minutes.

Ice them in the evening. Suzanne M. Tanner, M.D., assistant professor in the department of orthopedics at the University of Colorado Sports Medicine Center in Denver, suggests placing an ice pack on your foot for 20 minutes, removing it for 20 minutes, and then reapplying it for 20 minutes. Be sure to wrap the ice in a towel to prevent ice burns or frostbite.

Neuromas: The Big Squeeze

This is almost exclusively a woman's problem because of tight and narrow shoe styles. "What happens is that the shoe pushes your foot in tighter and pinches a nerve," says Dr. Braver. "But then tissue grows around this pinched nerve, causing a great deal of pain." Neuromas usually occur between the third and fourth toes or along the sole of your foot. In extreme cases, surgery may be required. But before the pain gets that far, here's what Dr. Braver suggests.

Pad it. "Anything that can be done to support the arch will help women with neuromas," says Dr. Braver. "One of the best things you can do is get an arch support pad, available at drugstores, and place it in your shoe. This reduces pressure to the nerve."

Give it the big chill. A nightly application of an ice pack reduces swelling and numbs pain, adds Dr. Braver. Remember to wrap a towel around the ice pack and follow the 20 minutes on, 20 minutes off routine (described in the previous section on foot and heel pain).

Try physical therapy. "Basic massage won't help, but electrical nerve stimulation and therapies that reduce swelling can," says Dr. Braver. You'll need the help of a physical therapist for this. Steroid injections by a doctor can also ease pain.

Corns and Calluses: Things That Go Bump

Corns are lumps of built-up dead skin that form on the bony areas of your feet, such as the toes. They're caused by friction, usually the result of wearing shoes that are too tight. Calluses are essentially corns on nonbony places. Both can make you feel as though you're walking on pebbles. Unless you have severe, constant pain, in which case you'll need a doctor's care, you can usually remedy these problems by yourself. Here's how.

If it doesn't fit, don't wear it. "If you have good-fitting shoes, you usually won't have corns and calluses," says Jan P. Silfverskiold, M.D., an orthopedic surgeon in private practice in Wheat Ridge, Colorado, who specializes in foot problems.

To make sure your footwear fits, have both your feet measured for length and width each time you shop for shoes, advises Dr. Gastwirth. Be aware that the shape of your foot influences the best style of shoe to purchase. In general, the best styles for the corn-prone include sandals and running and walking shoes, which have roomy toeboxes. If you're a woman and you must wear heels, "buy shoes with wide, stable heels that don't exceed 2 inches and look for comfort-type pumps that provide greater cushion for shock absorption," suggests Dr. Gastwirth.

Apply a moisturizer. Since corns and calluses result from excessive friction, it's best to keep skin soft and well moisturized. Dr. Levine recommends that you apply a skin moisturizer to your feet immediately after your bath or shower. If your skin is already hardened with corns and calluses, scrape it with an emery board or a pumice stone anywhere from once a day to twice a week, adds Dr. Silfverskiold.

Be careful with the remover. Over-the-counter corn and callus removers (such as Dr. Scholl's) contain salicylic acid, which will erode lumpy lesions on your feet. But take care: These medications should be applied only to the affected area, since they can burn healthy skin, Dr. Levine says. Also, don't use products containing salicylic acid if you have diabetes or poor circulation, cautions Dr. Levine. There are nonmedicated cushions available (such as Dr. Scholl's Advanced Pain Relief Corn Cushions) that you can use to protect your corns.

Blisters and Bunions: Bubbles and Bone

Blisters are painful bubblelike rips in the skin that usually fill with fluid because of excessive friction. Bunions are bumps of bone and thickened skin on the side of your foot just below the base of your big or little toe. They can be accompanied by splaying of the foot and drifting of the big toe toward the little toe. Tight shoes, arthritis, and heredity can all lead to bunions. As with corns and calluses, wearing properly fitting supportive shoes can prevent blisters and bunions. But if you already have either problem, here's how to fix it.

Pamper or pop 'em. Insoles, moleskin, or even little balls of cotton stuffed between your toes can alleviate the immediate agony of blisters and prevent them from recurring. When blisters become too large for pads, however, pop them by pushing the fluid to one end of the "bubble" and pricking that area with a needle that's been sterilized with a flame or rubbing alcohol. After draining the liquid, repeat the procedure 12 hours later, and then again 12 hours after that, to ensure that you've removed all the liquid, advises Rodney Basler, M.D., a dermatologist and assistant professor of internal medicine at the University of Nebraska at Omaha. Don't pull off the skin, but if it has been torn off, wash the sore with hydrogen peroxide or soap and water and apply an antibiotic ointment.

Try a splint. Bunion pain can be relieved with a toe-straightening splint that's available at most pharmacies without a prescription. The most common version is a rubber plug that "pulls" the big toe away from the second toe, easing pain. While moleskin pads are often used by bunion sufferers, they're not as effective as these splints.

Athlete's Foot: Calming the Itch

This fungus, which leaves feet scaly, itchy, cracked, and reddened, can be picked up just about anywhere—especially in warm, moist areas such as locker room floors (hence the name). Once you get it, athlete's foot is hard to get rid of because it thrives in your shoes. Over-the-counter medications are the preferred course of action. Lotions are better than creams, since creams can trap moisture. Still, the best way to deal with athlete's foot is to avoid it. Here's how.

Sock it to 'em. When you take off your socks, rub one up and down the web of each toe, advises Dr. Basler. This helps keep feet desert-dry. If sock rubbing isn't your style, you can use a hair dryer set on the low setting to dry those trouble areas. And if you have a problem with sweating after your feet have been dried, you can roll some antiperspirant on your feet after showering, he adds.

Be a shoe swapper. Try wearing different pairs of shoes as often as possible, says Dr. Basler. This gives your shoes, which are full of moisture after a day of wear, the time they need to dry out. If you don't have many pairs of shoes, spray them with Lysol at the end of the day to help disinfect them and prevent athlete's foot.

Get cooking with baking soda. There are plenty of over-the-counter powders to prevent athlete's foot, but baking soda does essentially the same thing for a lot less money, says Dr. Levine. Just sprinkle it on daily to absorb excess moisture.

Ingrown Toenails: Pain That Digs In

All it takes is a teeny bit of nail to cause big-time pain. Once again, tight shoes can contribute to this problem by forcing the nail downward. If your nail is ingrown to the point that you're in constant agony, you may need a doctor to remove it. But here's how to avoid that anguish and keep nails trouble-free.

Cut nails straight across. Leave the half-moons for cloudy nights. The best way to cure an ingrown nail and prevent a new one from forming is to cut the nail straight across, not slightly curved or in a half-moon shape as most people do, says William Van Pelt, D.P.M., a Houston podiatrist and former president of the American Academy of Podiatric Sports Medicine. And don't cut it too short; it should be just over the crease of your nail fold. Be sure to soak your feet in warm water beforehand in order to make the cutting easier.

Take your piggies to market. There are several over-the-counter products that can soften an ingrown nail and the skin around it, thereby relieving pain. Dr. Levine recommends Dr. Scholl's ingrown toenail reliever and Outgro solution as two common brands. Make sure you follow the instructions carefully. Don't use these products if you have diabetes or circulation problems because they contain strong acids that could be dangerous to people who have lost sensation in their feet.

Nail Fungus: Avoidance Is Best

Nail fungus doesn't hurt. It won't harm your health. In fact, people won't even notice those thick, raggedy-looking toenails if you keep your shoes on. But take off your shoes for a day at the beach—well, that's another story.

Some experts believe that nail fungus is often caused by an immune system problem and aggravated by moisture. So keeping your feet clean and dry is essential for keeping nail fungus at bay. There is at least one antifungal treatment available by prescription, but even then the treatment process is lengthy and involves a doctor's care, especially if your feet tend to be sweaty. Here's how to avoid getting it in the first place.

Loosen up. "One way to prevent nail fungus is to make sure your shoes are big enough that toes have room to breathe," says Dr. Braver. "Runners, dancers, and other athletes often get nail fungus because they get microtrauma to their toes from their toes hitting the front of the shoes. If you can, wear looser shoes."

Apply an antiperspirant. Sweating makes matters worse, so prevent a potential problem by treating your feet like underarms—apply a daily dose of roll-on deodorant, says Dr. Braver. "There is a prescription product called Drysol made especially for this purpose. It's like using a much stronger underarm antiperspirant."

Plantar Warts: A Powerful Punch

Like other warts, these ¼-inch nasties that form on the soles of your feet are caused by a virus, which is probably picked up walking barefoot. The problem with plantar warts, however, is that the pressure of walking flattens them until they are covered by calluses. When the calluses harden, you feel the plantar's punch, which is similar to walking on a pebble.

"About 13 percent of all plantar warts disappear on their own, with no treatment," says Dr. Braver. "However, several strains of the wart virus have been known to spread rapidly." He advises aggressive treatment to get rid of the warts before this happens. Try these measures.

Eat your vegetables. "There is substantial evidence that vitamin A helps protect against warts," says Dr. Braver. While vitamin A in supplement form can be toxic, you can get this added protection by eating more yellow or orange vegetables and fruits, such as carrots, squash, sweet potatoes, cantaloupe, apricots, and nectarines, as well as green leafy vegetables such as spinach.

Go commercial. Using an over-the-counter wart or corn remover (such as Occlusal) can rid you of plantar warts, says Dr. Braver. These products are available at drugstores without a prescription.

Stop going barefoot. The best way to avoid plantar warts is to wear shoes or sandals, says Dr. Braver. "It's important to keep the soles of your feet covered, especially when you're around pools and other moist areas that are attractive to the virus." If a family member has a plantar wart, prevent it from spreading by keeping floors and showers clean and disinfected.

See a doctor. If you have tried the above measures for 6 weeks and notice little improvement, or if the problems are getting worse, see your podiatrist for care. Professional treatment may include freezing or burning the warts and traditional or laser surgical removal methods.

GOUT

Beating the Arthritis That Prefers Men

If the word *gout* brings to mind the image of an old, scowling, overfed, Charles Laughton–type cursing the world as his bandaged foot teeters precariously on a stool, you have a fairly good picture of the condition and its effect.

For one thing, gout is predominantly a male condition. For another, it can be a hellish experience. "Gout has been described as a man's answer to labor pains," says Jeffrey R. Lisse, M.D., director of the division of rheumatology and associate professor of medicine at the University of Texas Medical Branch at Galveston. "The difference is that women eventually come out of labor; gout can linger."

Gout is a form of arthritis that strikes out of thin air. It can affect any joint but often begins by producing a deep, excruciating pain that leaves the big toe swollen, tender, and red-hot.

Gout can make you feel old and crotchety. It can also be crippling. One Pearl Harbor–style sneak attack can put you out of commission for days and make getting around difficult for even longer. If the attacks become frequent, you can lose some of the function in the joint. And if the condition is allowed to progress untreated, it can disable a joint totally.

Even though gout is more common as we age, you don't have to be old to be shot down in flames. While most men experience their first attacks in the forties, bouts can occur much earlier. For years, it was thought to be the exclusive domain of royalty and the idle rich (who were paying the price for a life of excess). Today, we know that gout crosses all class and social lines. "The sedentary middle-age guy who eats and drinks in abundance while his weight and blood pressure go up is a primary target for gout," says David Pisetsky, M.D., Ph.D., co-director of the Duke University Arthritis Center in Durham, North Carolina, and medical adviser to the Arthritis Foundation.

The Cause Is Crystal Clear

Your throbbing toe may come on like a bolt out of the blue, but chances are it was years in the making. Normally, your body produces a chemical called uric acid that's excreted through the urine. Some men produce extremely high levels of this waste product or have trouble urinating it out. It has to go somewhere, and that somewhere can be the skin, the kidneys (where it can form stones), or other parts of the body, usually with little fanfare.

But when this excess uric acid beelines for your joints, watch out. "When uric acid collects in the joints, it forms long, needlelike crystals," says Christopher M. Wise, M.D., associate professor of internal medicine at the Virginia Commonwealth University Medical College of Virginia in Richmond. "These crystals irritate the joint and trigger an extremely violent response."

One reason for astronomical uric acid levels is diet. Certain foods—particularly rich and fatty ones—contain high amounts of purines, chemical substances that turn into uric acid in the blood. But you can't place all the blame on culinary excesses. Often it is an inherited tendency. It can also be related to certain conditions, such as kidney disease. And many medications can produce high uric acid levels.

Give Gout the Kick

Fortunately, there's a lot you can do to deal with gout and make sure it doesn't come back.

Raise your raging joint. During an attack, keep the affected joint elevated and at rest, says Dr. Lisse. Prop it up with some pillows so that it rests several inches above your torso, and try to move it as little as possible. This will drain fluids away from the joint and reduce the inflammation.

Chill out. Applying ice packs for 20 minutes at a time, several times a day, will lessen the pain and inflammation, says Dr. Lisse.

Reach for ibuprofen. When you need fast relief for the pain and swelling, the best over-the-counter product you can use is ibuprofen, says Dr. Pisetsky. The inflammation is the primary cause of the pain, and ibuprofen is a reliable pain-relieving anti-inflammatory. Aspirin, normally an effective pain reliever and anti-inflammatory, can actually raise uric acid levels, making the pain and inflammation worse.

Wet your whistle. Gout-producing uric acid is more likely to crystallize in your joints if you are dehydrated, says Dr. Lisse. Make sure you drink plenty of water every day. It will help the body flush out excess uric acid in your urine.

Lock up your liquor cabinet. Alcohol in the bloodstream causes uric acid levels to go through the roof and inhibits the body's ability to excrete these chemicals, says Dr. Wise. If you are a heavy or frequent drinker, you should either go on the wagon or reduce your consumption significantly. If your uric acid levels are already high, one or two nights of debauchery could be enough to send levels into the danger zone.

Hold the Anchovies

Living high on the hog? Love to eat rich, fancy foods? Your expensive tastes may be not only socking it to your wallet but also stabbing you where it really hurts: your aching joints. "Some rich foods are sky-high in purines, compounds that your body turns into uric acid. And a uric acid overdose can trigger a gout attack," says Christopher M. Wise, associate professor of internal medicine at the Virginia Commonwealth University Medical College of Virginia in Richmond.

"Diet alone will probably not bring on a gout attack. But it's still worthwhile, if you're prone to gout, to limit your intake of high-purine foods," says Dr. Wise.

Here are foods to watch for.

Foods with Extremely High Purine Levels
(probably best to avoid)

Anchovies	Kidneys
Beer	Liver
Brain	Mussels
Fish roe	Sardines
Gravies	Sweetbreads
Heart	Wine
Herring	Yeast

Foods with Moderately High Purine Levels
(limit to one daily serving)

Dry beans and peas	Seafood
Meats	Shellfish
Poultry	

Slim down. Overweight people run a greater risk of having higher uric acid levels and getting gout, says Dr. Wise.

Avoid crash diets. In general, losing weight is good. But if you lose too much weight too soon, or if you become malnourished, you can actually encourage gout, says Dr. Lisse.

Control your blood pressure—naturally. Because people with gout tend to have high blood pressure, doctors often recommend lowering your blood pressure to prevent future attacks, says Dr. Pisetsky. Unfortunately, certain drugs prescribed to lower blood pressure, such as diuretics, can actually raise uric acid levels. Along with treatment from your doctor, try other proven ways to control high blood pressure, such as losing weight, exercising, and watching your intake of sodium, fats, and cholesterol.

Take Some Natural Steps

Along with medical remedies, there are a number of herbal and nutritional supplements that are good allies, say alternative medicine experts. Many can help improve the kidney, the liver, and the blood, according to Luc Maes, D.C., N.D., a chiropractor and naturopathic doctor in Santa Barbara, California. Others can help fight inflammation. Here are several to consider.

Fight the flame with EPA. Fish-oil supplements are particularly rich in an omega-3 fatty acid called eicosapentaenoic acid (EPA), which discourages inflammation, says Priscilla Evans, N.D., a naturopathic doctor at the Community Wholistic Health Center in Chapel Hill, North Carolina. EPA is also available from flaxseed oil.

Supplements can't do the whole job, Dr. Evans emphasizes. "It's very important to cut back on vegetable oils and saturated fats that promote inflammation. Just adding fish oil is not enough if you're still eating a lot of red meat and fat."

Dr. Maes suggests taking 500 milligrams of fish oil three times a day with meals. You should also take 400 to 1,200 international units of vitamin E a day, she says. It works along with the EPA to act as an anti-inflammatory and also serves as an antioxidant.

Benefit from bromelain. An enzyme with an appetite, bromelain, which comes from pineapple, is nature's anti-inflammatory medicine. "Bromelain inhibits those proteins that are promoting inflammation in the body. It kind of digests the products of inflammation," says Dr. Evans. She recommends 500 milligrams of bromelain three times a day between meals to help reduce inflammation during acute gout attacks. For milder cases of gout, you'll probably want to start out with a smaller dose, since bromelain sometimes causes a burning feeling in the gut. If the gout lingers more than 4 to 5 days, cut back the bromelain to 125 to 250 milligrams three times a day, advises Dr. Evans.

Block it with berries. In the 1950s, researchers discovered that cherries could decrease uric acid levels and prevent a gout attack. Of course, you'd have to eat a lot of cherries—a half-pound a day—to make a dent in gout. For the same results, you can take a bioflavonoid supplement or 2,000 milligrams of berry extract a day, says Dr. Maes. The best are those that have a combination of all the bioflavonoids or the extracts of several different berries, he says.

Settle on nettle. Nettle, a natural antihistamine that has long been used by old-time herbalists to treat inflammation of the joints, also works as a diuretic to help lower uric acid levels. "Nettle works as a blood cleanser and detoxifying agent," says Dr. Maes. To get the full benefit, take 300 to 600 milligrams of a freeze-dried extract daily, he advises. Nettle may be used long-term, but Dr. Maes recommends not using it for more than 2 to 3 months at a time. Avoid tinctures of nettle. They contain alcohol and may aggravate gout.

Get Thee to a Doctor

If you awake one morning in sheer agony, like your big toe is being stabbed with a rusty knife, you'll probably want to get medical help. Your doctor can pre- scribe medications to stop the inflammation, says Dr. Wise. Popular choices are a drug called colchicine and nonsteroidal anti-inflammatory drugs such as asin- domethacin (Idameth) and prescription-strength ibuprofen.

If your attacks are frequent or unusually severe, your doctor may prescribe medications to reduce the amount of uric acid in your system and to reverse the deposit of crystals in the joints, says Dr. Wise. Drugs such as allopurinol (Zylo- prim) and probenecid (Benemid) are very effective at preventing gout attacks, but they must be taken regularly.

GRAY HAIR

Rethinking Your True Colors

You roll out of bed, move slowly to the bathroom, and turn on the light. You lean toward the mirror for a close, close look.

How many more gray hairs will there be today?

Besides wrinkles and sagging skin, few things say "aging" louder than gray hair. While some of us love the look and wear it well, a whole lot of us don't. And there's a multimillion dollar industry out there catering to our needs to keep our changing true colors a secret.

"If you're going gray, I guarantee you're not happy about it," says Philip Kingsley, a hair care specialist based in New York City. "I have seen tens of thousands of people over the years, and none of them wants gray hair. It can really make people feel old before their time."

The Roots of Your Family Tree

Most of us have about 100,000 hairs on our heads. Before we go gray, every one of those hairs contains the pigment melanin, which gives hair its color. But for reasons doctors don't understand, the pigment cells near the roots of each hair start to shut down as we get older. So when a blonde, brown, or red hair falls out, it's often replaced by a gray one. A white one, actually—though we call it gray because that's what it looks like in contrast to the hair that still has color.

If you're looking for someone to blame, start with Mom, Dad, Aunt Judith, or Great-grandpa Joe. "There's a very strong hereditary link with gray hair," says Diana Bihova, M.D., clinical assistant professor of dermatology at New York University Medical Center in New York City. "If your family goes gray early, it's very likely you will, too."

Whatever you do, don't chalk it up to stress. Playing parent, boss, worker bee, cook, chauffeur, gardener, handyman, or some combination all at once won't give you gray hair—unless the stress is so bad that you deplete your store of some B vitamins. (And the evidence remains sketchy on this explanation.)

129

Overexposure to the sun might also cause hair to gray early, Dr. Bihova says. The theory is that ultraviolet rays cause pigment cells on your scalp to work overtime, just as they do on your arms or legs when you get a tan. If they work too hard and burn out early, Dr. Bihova says, the result could be gray hair. Again, there's no concrete evidence of this. But Dr. Bihova still suggests wearing a hat or using hair care products that contain sunscreen. "Let's just say it can't hurt," she says.

The average Caucasian adult starts developing gray hair at age 34, while the typical African-American adult gets about a 10-year reprieve. Dr. Bihova says most people start graying at the sides, then on the crown, and finally the back of the neck. The process can go in fits and starts, with more gray hair growing in some years and less in others.

Eventually, the rule of 50 kicks in. That means by age 50, 50 percent of adults will be 50 percent gray, Dr. Bihova explains.

Follicle Fallacies: The Myths of Gray

There are a million tales out there about gray hair—and precious few good, hard facts. While doctors might not know just yet what causes gray, they do know a few things that won't.

Gray Hair Myth #1: You can go gray instantly because of a shocking event. It's physically impossible—existing hair does not turn gray. Diana Bihova, M.D., clinical assistant professor of dermatology at New York University Medical Center in New York City, says you get gray only when a regular hair falls out and is replaced by a gray one in the same follicle.

Gray Hair Myth #2: Your hair can return to its normal color after it has gone gray. Sorry, but no. When a hair follicle starts producing gray hair, it doesn't change back. There are a few exceptions, Dr. Bihova says. Your hair could temporarily go gray if you have an endocrine gland disorder, are malnourished, suffer an injury or a disease of the nervous system, or have an autoimmune disorder. Even then, hair may not come back in its original color, she says.

Gray Hair Myth #3: If you pull one gray hair, two more will grow out. Nope. You go gray follicle by follicle. If you pull out a gray hair, it will be replaced by a gray hair in the same follicle. "You can't stop the process," Dr. Bihova says. "But pulling white hairs isn't going to speed it up, either."

Generally, the hair on your head starts to change first, followed some time later by the hair on your legs, under your arms and in your eyebrows, and, finally, in your pubic area. But again, everyone's different.

The good news in all this is that there's usually nothing physically wrong with getting gray hair—it doesn't mean you're aging faster than friends who haven't had a single gray strand yet. Studies show that people who go gray at an early age are usually not suffering from anything but a case of unwelcome family genetics.

The bad news is that graying is irreversible.

For Many of Us, It's to Dye For

So gray hair is on the way, like it or not. That leaves you with two choices. You can accept it as an inescapable, even desirable, part of maturing. Or you can put it on hold for a while, using some form of hair dye.

"Some people grow to be quite comfortable with gray hair," Kingsley says. "The most important point to remember about gray hair, or hair in general, is that you have to be comfortable with it. If it makes you feel wise or dignified, that's fine."

Here's some advice from the experts on how to handle that gray.

Be yourself. Harrison Ford, Vanessa Redgrave, Judy Collins, George W. Bush. None of these people looks worried about going gray—and who wants to argue with them? Your initial reaction to gray hair might be shock. But before you color your hair, take stock of the situation. Does it really make you look old? Or does it add a little maturity? A little warmth? A little realness?

Crop it. If you do decide to stay gray, Kingsley suggests keeping your hair cut short. "It's really simple," Kingsley says. "If you don't want gray hair or you're not sure about it, then short styles leave less gray to show."

Condition it. As time passes, your hair and scalp may get drier. To keep your gray looking healthy, Kingsley suggests using a conditioner each time you shampoo. And he suggests letting your hair air-dry once in a while, instead of using a blow dryer.

When You're Dyeing for a Change

What if you've tried the gray look for a little while, and you don't like it? Then certainly try a dye—only do it right. Here are some options the experts recommend

Bring on the highlights. Highlighting, in which scattered strands of hair are dyed, can blend away some of the gray. Choose a color that's a couple of shades lighter than your natural hair.

Lighter dyes also help you avoid unsightly gray roots. When your hair grows out, the gray won't show as much.

Go all the way. The experts call this process color, and it means that all your hair will be dyed one shade. If you opt for this, stay away from the darkest shades, which tend to make your hair look flat and unnatural. "Black colors don't really work well," Kingsley says. "All the hair is colored exactly the same, and you can instantly see that it's dyed."

There's also some question about whether dark hair dyes can cause cancer. Some studies have linked use of such dyes to increased risk of bone cancer and lymphoma.

The bottom line? "There isn't one yet," says Sheila Hoar Zahm, Ph.D., an epidemiologist at the National Cancer Institute in Rockville, Maryland. "The risk of getting cancer from hair dye isn't as high as getting lung cancer from smoking. But we definitely need to study the relationship further."

Pass on progressive dyes. Kingsley says you should be wary of so-called progressive dyes that promise to slowly hide your gray hair. He says these products can give your hair an unnatural, yellowish green tint. They can also dry out your hair, making it unmanageable and brittle.

And once you start using them, it's hard to switch over to a regular dye. "That can turn your hair all sorts of colors that you would never want hair to be," Kingsley says.

Semipermanent dyes that wash out over several weeks offer somewhat better color but are not as good as permanent dyes. If you want to try a slow route to darker hair, Kingsley suggests doing it with increasingly darker permanent dyes.

HAIR LOSS

Winning over Thinning

Most of us think of hair loss as a "man's problem"—after all, the most common term is "male pattern baldness," isn't it? But women experience their share of hair loss, too. In fact, 20 million American women are transforming from Goldilocks to fallen locks right now.

Man or woman, if you're losing your hair, the major cause is poor inheritance: You just got the wrong genes when the assets were passed down from mom's side of the family.

Hair loss begins between the ages of 25 and 40. For men, hair starts disappearing on the crown and at the hairline. Women are more likely to lose hair evenly over the entire scalp. Where a woman once had five hairs, she may now have only two. She may also develop a widow's peak, with a slightly receding hairline and more noticeable hair loss around her temples.

The Other Loss Cause

Not all hair loss is inevitable, however, nor is the decline entirely controlled by genes. Stress, hormone changes, fad and crash diets, anemia, childbirth, and vitamin and mineral deficiencies also can lead to fast fallout. Other culprits: conditions such as arthritis and lupus, and drugs, including birth control pills, anabolic steroids, beta-blocker blood pressure drugs, and drugs derived from vitamin A.

Moreover, you're likely to lose hair faster if your hair follicles become inflamed or if you get skin disorders that affect your scalp.

"I've had patients who have lost all their hair because of major stresses in their lives," says Hope Fay, N.D., a naturopathic doctor in Seattle. "When you're under stress from illness or work, sometimes the circulation in the scalp is so constricted that the hair follicles lose blood supply, which causes them to die and fall out." Dr. Fay is quick to add, however, that if people lose their hair under these circumstances, it often grows right back in when they're no longer under extreme stress.

To help the hair return when the loss isn't a matter of inherited baldness, you can try a number of tactics. The solution usually lies with improving your diet and making lifestyle changes to relieve stress, says Dr. Fay. In addition, you can supplement your diet with nutrients that aid in hair growth, she says.

In other words, you have to feed your head using strategies like these.

Mine your minerals. Deficiencies of selenium and zinc generally lead to hair loss, researchers have observed. Normally, we get all we need of these trace minerals from the soil in which our food is grown. It doesn't always work that way, however, says Elizabeth Wotton, N.D., a naturopathic doctor at Compass Family Health Center in Plymouth, Massachusetts. "Unfortunately, in some areas of the United States, some trace minerals just aren't in the soil in high enough quantities," she observes. "You could be eating what you think is a good diet but still be lacking."

If that's your problem, there's a quick fix. Take a trace mineral supplement that includes 200 micrograms of selenium, 20 milligrams of zinc, and a wide variety of other trace minerals. You can also try taking 30 milligrams of zinc daily and see if you stop losing hair or even start to grow it back, says Dr. Wotton. If your hair loss is from a zinc deficiency, you could see regrowth in as little as a week. You should talk to a doctor before taking this amount of zinc, however.

Get the nettle you need. While you're at the store, you might also look at some herbs that could help. One is nettle. "It's really high in mineral content and can make your hair much healthier," Dr. Fay says. Nettle can be found in a tincture or capsules. In either form, simply follow the dosage directions on the bottle. For 480-milligram capsules, for example, the typical dose is one capsule twice a day. A typical tincture dose is 15 to 20 drops in ¼ cup of water or juice twice a day.

Regulate your hormones. In the first few months after their children are born, some women may begin to lose hair because of hormonal changes. Hormone upsets aren't limited to new mothers, however. Stress, menopause, and illness can also bring on changes.

To ease hormonal transitions, Dr. Wotton suggests women should eat more foods containing phytoestrogens, plant compounds that mimic the biological activities of female hormones. These foods include legumes and soy products, such as tofu.

Dr. Wotton also suggests supplementing your diet with a few important minerals and vitamins. She recommends 150 milligrams of magnesium twice a day, 400 to 800 international units of vitamin E daily, and a daily vitamin B-complex supplement that contains 100 milligrams of B_6 and 50 micrograms of biotin.

In addition, you might consider supplementing with essential fatty acids from flaxseed oil or evening primrose oil, says Dr. Fay. These kinds of fats form the biological backbone of many hormone molecules. The oils are rich sources of omega-3 and omega-6 fatty acids, good fats that are important for healthy skin and hair.

Dr. Fay suggests taking 1,000 milligrams of evening primrose oil three times a day or one teaspoon of flaxseed oil once or twice a day. You can take the flaxseed oil by the spoonful or put it on salads and other foods.

Growing It Back—Sometimes

If you've just noticed that your hair has started to thin, remember this: Minoxidil—the hair loss cure that comes in a topical prescription formula—works for men and women.

"Women can achieve significant results with the use of minoxidil," says Dominic A. Brandy, M.D., medical director of Dominic A. Brandy, M.D., and Associates, a permanent hair restoration practice in Pittsburgh. "In fact, in some of my patients, the results seem to be better than with men."

Minoxidil is the active chemical ingredient in the topical medication sold under the brand name Rogaine. Clinical tests have shown that Rogaine can help people return some fullness to their hair. But there are limits to Rogaine's effectiveness.

Dr. Brandy says Rogaine won't grow hair at the frontal hairline or in areas that are completely bald. At best, he says, it will slightly thicken existing hair and return a fuller look to your locks.

"But in most cases, it simply retards the progression of baldness," Dr. Brandy says. "That's what I tell most people to expect. Anything more is a bonus."

One more thing to think about: Rogaine is expensive. Treatments typically cost $500 to $700 per year, and you have to use Rogaine forever. If you stop, you'll lose everything you had gained within 6 months.

Researchers are evaluating these alternative treatments. Some may not be available yet.

Aromatase. People with thinning hair appear to be deficient in this enzyme—which, when present in normal levels, causes follicles to grow hair. Marty Sawaya, M.D., Ph.D., assistant professor of dermatology at the University of Florida Health Sciences Center in Gainesville, and other researchers are working to refine a method of restoring natural aromatase levels.

Tricomin solution. Karen Hedine, vice president of business development for the drug's maker, ProCyte of Kirkland, Washington, says this drug appears to work by stimulating the growth of new follicles in the scalp and by preventing existing follicles from becoming dormant.

Diazoxide. Like Rogaine, this drug appears to work by dilating blood vessels in the scalp.

Electrical stimulation. Tests involving low-current doses of electricity to men's scalps have shown promise in Canadian tests. Researchers predict treatments could be available in the United States soon.

Shortcuts to Thicker Hair

Whether hair thinning or hair loss is temporary or permanent, there are some things you can do to disguise the problem.

Do the wave. The fastest way to hide thinning hair is with a curly perm, says David Cannell, Ph.D., corporate vice president of technology with the Redken Product Laboratory in Canoga Park, California.

"With a wavy pattern, individual hairs push against each other," Dr. Cannell says. "The overall effect is that they push up and out, making your hair look fuller."

Dr. Cannell also advises women to avoid hairstyles that require small curlers or tightly pulled hair. The more pressure you put on your hair, the more likely it is to pull out.

Get in condition. Avoid oily hair dressings and other products that advertise "creamy-rich" results. Dr. Cannell says these tend to weigh down and flatten hair, which can make your hair look thin.

He suggests trying a lighter, leave-in conditioner that may add a microscopic amount of thickness to individual hairs.

Give yourself a pat on the head. After showering, dry your hair carefully. Pat it lightly with a towel instead of rubbing.

Comb with care. Dr. Cannell says to be gentle with brushes and combs. Never brush your hair when it's wet (pulling on a tangle is always a no-no). Try using a comb with widely spaced teeth instead.

And forget the 100-stroke gospel your great aunt used to preach. Dr. Cannell says you should brush your hair only as long as it takes to get it styled the way you want it.

Lighten up. Choose a new, lighter hair color. Shades that closely match your skin tone are best, Dr. Cannell says, since they blend with your scalp.

"The worst thing you can do is dye your hair jet-black," Dr. Cannell says. "That really shows your scalp, which is the last thing you want to do."

Keep your hands off. Drop nervous habits such as tugging on your hair or curling it with your fingers. You may be pulling on it more than you realize, since you're conscious of how it looks.

"Even when a hair is ready to fall out, it will stick around for quite a while—if you leave it be," Dr. Cannell says. "The more you manipulate it, the faster it will go."

HEARING LOSS

Fending Off the Sounds of Silence

Until a hundred years or so ago, the loudest noise that people were likely to hear would be the roar of a waterfall, the sound of musket fire, or maybe a church bell rung too loud and too often by an overly zealous parishioner.

All that changed with the Industrial Age. When locomotives, jackhammers, and, later, rock and roll amplifiers came along, the soundtrack of life increased far beyond anything nature had to offer.

The result? Hearing loss.

Hearing loss is not only a significant problem for people today, it's one that's striking earlier and earlier in life.

"Hearing loss is occurring at younger ages and is more prevalent than is generally thought," says J. Gail Neely, M.D., professor and director of otology, neurotology, and base of skull surgery at Washington University School of Medicine in St. Louis.

Overall, about 23 million Americans have significant hearing impairment, and nearly 7 million of those people are under age 45, according to the American Speech-Language-Hearing Association. In a survey of 2,731 people with hearing impairment, nearly 57 percent said they first noticed the problem before age 40, says Laurel E. Glass, M.D., Ph.D., professor emeritus and former director of the Center on Deafness at the University of California, San Francisco, School of Medicine.

The toll of that hearing loss is enormous, doctors say. It can lead to social isolation, limit your job prospects, complicate your sex life, rob you of your self-esteem, and make you feel as if life's parade is passing you by.

Hear Ye, Hear Ye

Before looking at why people have developed hearing problems, it's important to understand how your ears work. When your best friend tells you the

The 5-Minute Hearing Test

Suddenly, everyone around you mumbles, mutters, or whispers. Could it be that you have a hearing problem? To find out, take this quiz prepared by the American Academy of Otolaryngology-Head and Neck Surgery. Your choices are almost always (A), half the time (H), occasionally (O), and never (N).

1. I have a problem hearing over the phone.
2. I have trouble following conversation when two or more people are talking at the same time.
3. People complain that I turn the TV volume too high.
4. I have to strain to understand conversations.
5. I miss hearing some common sounds, such as the phone or doorbell ringing.
6. I have trouble hearing conversations in a noisy background, such as at a party.
7. I get confused about where sounds come from.
8. I misunderstand some words in a sentence and need to ask people to repeat themselves.
9. I especially have trouble understanding the speech of women and children.
10. I have worked in noisy environments (on assembly lines, with jackhammers, near jet engines, and so on).

punchline to her latest joke, the sound of her voice enters your ear canal and strikes the eardrum, a cone-shaped elastic membrane stretched across the end of the canal. As the eardrum vibrates, it causes tiny bones in the middle ear to move back and forth. These movements trigger small waves of fluid in the inner ear that ripple through a snail-shaped organ called the cochlea. Inside the cochlea, 30,000 hairlike cells transmit impulses to the auditory nerve, which carries the sounds to the brain. There they are interpreted as the funniest joke you've ever heard, and you laugh.

Some hearing loss is a natural part of aging, says Debra Busacco, Ph.D., audiologist and coordinator of the Lifelong Learning Institute at Gallaudet University in Washington, D.C., the world's only liberal arts university for the deaf. The eardrum stiffens with age, thereby reducing its ability to vibrate. Age-related changes to the bones in the middle ear, such as the degeneration of joints and cal-

11. I hear fine—if people just speak clearly.
12. People get annoyed because I misunderstand what they say.
13. I misunderstand what others are saying and make inappropriate responses.
14. I avoid social activities because I cannot hear well and fear I'll reply improperly.

To be answered by a family member or friend:

15. Do you think this person has a hearing loss?

Scoring
Give yourself three points for each time you answered "almost always," two points for every "half the time," one point for every "occasionally," and no points for every "never."

0 to 5. Your hearing is fine.

6 to 9. The academy suggests that you see an ear, nose, and throat specialist.

10 and above. The academy strongly recommends that you see an ear, nose, and throat specialist.

cium deposits in those joints, cause the middle ear system to become stiffer, resulting in less effective transmission of sound. Over time, irreplaceable hair cells in the inner ear are damaged by a combination of aging, noise exposure, medication, decreased blood supply to the ear, and infection. And once they're damaged, the auditory nerve becomes less efficient. But most of those changes don't occur until you're at least 60 years of age.

If symptoms of hearing loss appear at an earlier age, the most common cause is excessive noise exposure, says Susan Rezen, Ph.D., professor of audiology at Worcester State College in Massachusetts and author of *Coping with Hearing Loss*.

Sudden loud noises close to the ear, such as firecrackers or gunshots, can cause immediate hearing loss. But usually, noise-induced hearing loss happens gradually, over years. In general, the longer you expose yourself to sounds louder than 85 decibels, whether it's a rock concert or a leaf blower, the more likely you are to destroy cilia in the inner ear and damage your hearing, Dr. Rezen says. "The effects of noise exposure are long term," says Dr. Rezen. "When people are continually exposed, their ears wear out faster, and the effects of aging show up earlier."

How Loud Is Loud?

Decibels are how hearing experts measure sound intensity (sound pressure), beginning with the softest sound a person can hear in a laboratory setting, which is 0 decibels. Using this system, 20 decibels is 10 times more intense than 0, 40 decibels is 100 times more intense, 60 decibels is 1,000 times more intense, and so on.

So how loud is 85 decibels? It's about the same amount of noise as a vacuum cleaner, a blender, or a power lawn mower. In contrast, a normal conversation is about 65 decibels. Noise levels at some rock concerts come close to exceeding 140 decibels, a level that can cause rapid and irreparable hearing damage in some sensitive ears. Even symphony orchestras can generate sounds louder than 110 decibels, which can cause ear discomfort and pain in some people.

In fact, just one 2-hour rock concert can potentially age your hearing by nearly 2½ years if you don't wear ear protection, according to calculations by Daniel Johnson, Ph.D., an engineer who tests hearing protectors for the military at Kirtland Air Force Base in Albuquerque, New Mexico.

Another example: Say you're 30 years old and you work 8 hours a day without hearing protection near machinery that produces noise averaging 95 decibels. By age 40 you could have the high-frequency hearing loss of a 70-year-old.

High-frequency hearing loss affects your ability to hear sounds such as the consonants *sh*, *ch*, *t*, *f*, *h*, and *s*, which are frequently used in conversation.

"If you miss hearing those high-frequency sounds, the remaining part of a word won't make sense to you," Dr. Neely says. "You literally won't know if people around you are talking about fish or tin cans. That can be very confusing and frustrating."

Defending Your Ears

Although most of us will suffer some hearing loss because of aging, you can keep your hearing sharp well into your golden years if you protect your ears from noise now. "Imagine that your hearing is a big barrel of sand. Either you can empty it out gradually with a teaspoon, so it will last a long time, or you can use a shovel and run out of it a lot sooner," says Flash Gordon, M.D., a primary care physician in San Rafael, California, and cofounder of Hearing Education and Awareness for Rockers (HEAR), a San Francisco–based nonprofit organization that encourages high-decibel musicians and fans to turn down the volume and wear earplugs.

Here are some ways to prevent hearing loss.

Turn it down. You probably can't do much about traffic noise, jackhammers, and many other sources of excessive sound. But you can turn down the volume on your stereo, says Stephen Painton, Ph.D., an audiologist at the University of Oklahoma Health Sciences Center in Oklahoma City. Some sound systems can produce noise equal to the loudest rock concerts. Here's a way to tell if your stereo is too loud. Turn it on, then walk outside your home, and close the door. If you can hear the music, it's too loud. The same rule applies to your car radio. And if you use headphones or a personal stereo, the person standing next to you shouldn't be able to hear the sound.

If you have to shout, get out. If you have to raise your voice to be heard by someone standing a foot or two away from you, that's a clear warning that the noise level may be dangerous, and you should get away from it as soon as possible or wear ear protection, says John House, M.D., associate clinical professor of oto-laryngology at the University of Southern California in Los Angeles.

Keep plugs handy. Stuffing cotton or pieces of shredded paper napkin into your ears does virtually nothing to minimize damage to your hearing. Instead, get in the habit of carrying earplugs with you, Dr. Busacco says. Most earplugs are small and can easily be carried in your purse or pocket. That way, she says, you'll be prepared for unexpected noise, such as an unusually loud movie. The foam rubber types are good because they are inexpensive and available over the counter at most drugstores, and they can be quickly rolled up and placed in your ears. Look for the noise reduction rating on the side of the box, Dr. Painton says. This will tell you how many decibels of sound the earplugs will muffle. Buy plugs that have a rating of at least 15. Those plugs will reduce noise by 15 decibels and slash the chances that your hearing will be damaged. If you want better protection, an audiologist can design a pair of custom-made plugs for about $80 that reduce noise by about 35 decibels, Dr. Busacco says.

Take timeouts. The longer you expose yourself to loud sounds without a break, the more likely you are to cause permanent damage to your hearing, even if you're wearing earplugs. So give your ears a 5- or 10-minute break from noise every 30 minutes, Dr. Gordon says. "It's like putting your head underwater for 20 minutes. You can do it if you hold your breath for a minute at a time, then take a 10-second break. But if you'd try to do it in two 10-minute segments, you'd be dead. If you give your ears an occasional break, they can rest and recover from the excessive work that loud noise makes them do."

Spread out the noise. Placing several loud appliances or power tools near each other will compound your noise problem. So if your TV set is in the same room as your dishwasher, for example, you might be tempted to turn up the TV volume excessively when you do a load of dishes. Instead, move the television into a quieter room, says Lt. Col. Richard Danielson, Ph.D., supervisor of audiology in the Army Audiology and Speech Center at Walter Reed Army Medical Center in Washington, D.C.

Swab the deck, not your ears. Attempting to clean wax out of your ears with a cotton swab, matchstick, or anything else smaller than the Love Boat does

When the Ringing Won't Quit

At 31, Elizabeth Meyer was finding her way in life. She was taking marimba lessons and theater classes and looking forward to a career as a musician. Then the morning after an African music concert in Portland, Oregon, she noticed a ringing in her ears; over the next few weeks, she also developed an intense sensitivity to sound.

Soon she could speak on the telephone only if she held a pillow between her ear and the receiver. Before she gave up going to the movies, she was wearing two pairs of earplugs and industrial-strength earmuffs like airport baggage handlers wear. She couldn't travel for more than 15 minutes in a bus because the noise and the ringing in her ears overwhelmed her.

"Overnight, I felt like I'd aged 30 years," says Meyer. "I literally felt like I was 60. It has gotten a bit better, but the first year I spent just trying to stop myself from jumping up and banging my head against the wall every 30 seconds. At first I went through a suicidal period. Finally, I realized that although my condition might not improve, my ability to cope with it certainly would."

Meyer is one of the 3.5 million American women who endure chronic tinnitus, an annoying ringing, humming, or buzzing in the ears that can be a symptom of everything from excessive earwax to high blood pressure to heart disease. One in three women who has tinnitus, like Meyer, also develops hyperacusis, which is an extreme sensitivity to sounds. Both tinnitus and hyperacusis can also be signs of noise-induced hearing loss caused by damage to the cilia, hair cells in the inner ear that help conduct sound to the auditory nerve in the brain, says Christopher Linstrom, M.D., director of otology and neurotology at the New York Eye and Ear Infirmary in New York City.

more harm than good, says Dr. House. A small amount of earwax is actually good for you. It repels water and helps keep dust away from your sensitive eardrum. Sticking small objects in your ear pushes the wax farther into your ear and can cause infection. To handle earwax in your outer ear, wipe the ear with a warm, wet washcloth every day. For earwax in the inner ear canal, "the best thing to do is leave it alone," Dr. House says. If it becomes bothersome, see your physician or get an over-the-counter earwax removal kit that contains drops that will soften the wax and allow it to flow naturally out of your ear.

Hyperacusis, for instance, causes individual hair cells, each of which is normally stimulated only by certain frequencies, to react to the same range of sounds. As a result, more and more hair cells vibrate in unison, and that can make the quietest noises seem loud and jarring. When this damage occurs, sounds that are quite tolerable to many people can be painful to you, says Lt. Col. Richard Danielson, Ph.D., supervisor of audiology in the Army Audiology and Speech Center at Walter Reed Army Medical Center in Washington, D.C.

In some cases, tinnitus can be treated with drugs or surgery, particularly if it's caused by excessive fluid in the middle ear, high blood pressure, a partially blocked artery in the neck, or allergies. But in most instances, there is no cure for either tinnitus or hyperacusis, Dr. Linstrom says.

Once tinnitus or hyperacusis is diagnosed, you should avoid loud noises and wear earplugs to prevent more hearing damage that can make these conditions worse. Masking devices that produce pleasant sounds such as raindrops or ocean waves can help people with tinnitus drown out the ringing, Dr. Linstrom says. Caffeine and nicotine aggravate both conditions, so quit smoking and avoid coffee, tea, and chocolate, he says. Some medications such as aspirin, antibiotics, and anti-cancer drugs can also cause tinnitus and hearing sensitivity. A hearing aid might help, because the better you hear, the less noticeable the ringing may be, says John House, M.D., associate clinical professor of otolaryngology at the University of Southern California in Los Angeles.

If you have questions about these hearing problems, see your physician or write to the American Tinnitus Association, P.O. Box 5, Portland, OR 97207.

Muzzle your medication. Taking six to eight aspirin a day can cause ringing in your ears and temporary hearing loss, Dr. Gordon says. Antibiotics such as gentamicin (G-Mycin), streptomycin, and tobramycin (Nebcin) can also damage your hearing, says Barry E. Hirsch, M.D., a neurotologist at the University of Pittsburgh School of Medicine. If you are taking any drug and develop hearing problems, ask your doctor if the medication could be causing it.

Stop smoking. Smoking reduces blood flow to the ears and may interfere with the natural healing of small blood vessels that occurs after exposure to loud noise, Dr. House says. In a study of 2,348 workers exposed to noise at an aerospace factory, researchers at the University of Southern California School of Medicine found that smokers had greater hearing loss than nonsmokers. So if you smoke, quit.

Cut the coffee. Like nicotine, caffeine cuts blood flow to the ears, increasing your chances of hearing loss, says Dr. House. Drink no more than two 8-ounce cups of coffee or tea a day. If possible, drink decaffeinated brews.

Balance your diet. The same fatty and cholesterol-laden foods that are bad for your heart also endanger your ears, according to Dr. House. High blood pressure and atherosclerosis, a buildup of plaque on artery walls, not only cause heart disease but also can reduce blood flow to the ears and gradually strangle your hearing, Dr. House says. So cut the fat with a balanced daily diet that includes at least five servings of fruits and vegetables, six servings of breads and grains, and no more than one 3-ounce serving of lean red meat, poultry, or fish.

Exercise. Walk, run, swim, or do any other aerobic exercise for 20 minutes a day, three times a week, Dr. House suggests. It will stimulate blood circulation, lower your blood pressure, and help keep your ears in peak condition.

Making the Best of It

The average person waits 5 to 7 years after first noticing a hearing problem to seek help for it. Those can be years of unnecessary social isolation and frustration, Dr. Busacco says, because the earlier you seek help, the sooner your hearing problem can be diagnosed and treated.

"People are a lot more self-conscious about their hearing than they are about their vision," Dr. Hirsch says. "It's often an issue of vanity. Wearing a hearing aid somehow implies aging, while wearing glasses doesn't."

If you suspect that you have a hearing problem, particularly if you have ringing in your ears or develop a sudden sensitivity to loud noises that didn't bother you in the past, see your doctor or a physician who specializes in diseases of the ear, nose, and throat. Some hearing problems such as Ménière's disease, a disorder that causes ringing in the ears and dizziness, can be treated with prescription medication or surgery. Other conditions, such as perforated eardrums and otosclerosis, may be corrected with surgery.

Even if the loss can't be fully corrected, powerful but inconspicuous hearing aids—some small enough to fit inside the ear canal—are available to help you get back in touch with the world. An audiologist, a professional trained to fit hearing aids, can help you choose one that fits your needs.

Here are other ways to cope with a hearing loss.

Don't be shy about it. If you have difficulty hearing or understanding people, tell them, says Philip Zazove, M.D., assistant professor of family medicine at the University of Michigan Medical School in Ann Arbor who has had profound hearing loss since birth. Simply saying "I don't hear as well as I used to," "Could you repeat that?" and "Talk a little slower" can prevent a lot of misunderstandings, frustration, and anger, he says.

When to See a Doctor

If you feel that you've had a sudden, unexplainable hearing loss accompanied by ringing in your ear (especially on one side), see your doctor, says Jennifer Derebery, M.D., otologist at the House Ear Clinic at the University of Southern California School of Medicine in Los Angeles. The problem could be anything from an infection to a tumor, but only the experts can tell for sure.

In fact, whether the hearing loss is sudden or slow-building, experts say you should see a doctor before taking any other action. Don't just run out and get a hearing aid. Depending on the source of the problem, some hearing losses can be fixed without a hearing aid, says Dr. Derebery. But you won't know that for sure unless you're checked out by a doctor.

Light up your sex life. Hearing loss can cause havoc in the bedroom. Those whispered sweet nothings you used to enjoy so much when you were making love are often the first casualty. Leave in your hearing aid if there is any possibility of sex, or ask your partner to leave on the light so that you can see well enough to lip-read, Dr. Rezen suggests. Talk about what you want sexually before you go into the bedroom. If necessary, develop your own secret code, such as "Two taps on the back means kiss me." "If you don't plan, you may lose the opportunity altogether," she says.

Find a quiet spot. If you really want to talk to an interesting person at a party, pull her away from the middle of the room and into a secluded corner. Not only is that more intimate, you can concentrate on what she's saying and don't have to compete with laughter, music, and other background noise that just makes it that much harder to hear, Dr. Zazove says. At home, consider turning off the television, radio, or other noisy appliances before you try to listen to someone.

Laugh it off. A good sense of humor is vital if you have a hearing problem, says Dr. Painton. So what if you misunderstand a word or two and say something inappropriate? Enjoy the moment and join the laughter.

Do your homework. If you're attending an important business meeting or conference, get there early and try to nab a front row seat facing the person who you think will do most of the talking, Dr. Zazove says. Also try to get a written summary of the topic or agenda, so you'll be prepared for words or phrases that might come up. That way, if you do miss a few words, you'll have a better chance of filling them in accurately.

Maintain eye contact. Seeing a person can actually help you understand what he's saying. You'll pick up visual cues and body language. And that can help you fill in the blanks of what you don't hear, says Dr. Glass.

HEART ATTACK

Don't Ignore the Possibility

Every so often you hear about someone cut down in the prime of life by a heart attack. So you wonder, "Can it happen to me?"

It's an unsettling question—one that makes you feel like an older person worried about vitality and mortality. In most cases, though, heart attacks spare the young. Only 12 percent of heart attacks occur in men ages 44 and under and for women the percentage is even less. Thanks to the natural protection of the hormone estrogen, just over one-half of 1 percent of heart attacks occur in women ages 44 and under.

Though heart attacks may be uncommon, it doesn't mean you shouldn't be concerned about having one. After all, as you grow older your risk does rise and the things you do now could reduce your later chances of having an attack.

When Luck Runs Out

A heart attack occurs when a sudden clot blocks or reduces blood flow in a coronary artery. The symptoms may include crushing chest pain, heavy sweating, and shortness of breath. But there are other warning signs, too: pain in the back, jaw, or neck; nausea or lightheadedness.

Men are more likely to feel the classic chest pain and heavy sweating. Women are somewhat more likely to feel short of breath or nauseous, or have back or jaw pain.

One-third of these heart attacks are fatal. Four in five heart attack deaths occur in those ages 65 and older.

As you grow older, your heart and the blood vessels that nourish it begin to show and feel their age, even without the dramatic intrusion of a heart attack. The heart gradually starts to pump a little less efficiently, and the walls of the arteries become a little stiffer and less flexible.

But a heart attack is something different. In just minutes or hours, it can take a devastating toll upon your body, as though you were adding 20 or 30 years to your age overnight. As the supply of blood to your heart is impaired, the heart cells can become severely injured. The longer this blood flow is interfered with, the greater the chance of irreversible damage, producing cell death and the demise of part of the heart muscle.

But there's good news, too. Most heart attacks are preventable, no matter what your age, if you adopt lifestyle habits that can slow the buildup of fatty deposits in your coronary arteries.

Fight the Good Fight

So where do you begin? Here are some crucial strategies to keep in mind.

Know yourself. "It's important to know where you stand," advises Richard H. Helfant, M.D., vice chairman of medicine and director of the cardiology training program at the University of California, Irvine, Medical Center and author of *Women, Take Heart.* That means being aware of the risk factors that may increase your chances of having heart problems. If close relatives have had heart attacks at early ages—less than 55—you need to be extra cautious. If you're a woman going through menopause, be aware that your natural protection from estrogen will decrease because estrogen dwindles after menopause. Also, woman or man, if you have conditions that increase your risk that you can change—high blood pressure, an elevated blood cholesterol level, diabetes, or a cigarette habit—you need to control them before they attack your heart. Talk to your doctor about how to do that.

Toe the line. No one is asking you to be a fanatic. You don't have to swear off red meat or work out at the gym until you can't see straight. But if you live a reasonably careful, energetic lifestyle, you can keep your heart beating with the vigor of a much younger person, and with less worry about the Big One.

Get active. If you're one of those people who feels more comfortable with a TV remote control in your hand than with a tennis racquet, it's time for a change of heart. Regular exercise, such as brisk walking for just 30 to 45 minutes three times a week or some laps in the pool, can turn that pump in your chest into a mean machine.

"Exercise is beneficial for your heart in a number of ways," says Stephen Havas, M.D., associate professor of epidemiology and preventive medicine at the University of Maryland School of Medicine in Baltimore. "It can boost your HDL (high-density lipoprotein) cholesterol, which is the protective component of your blood cholesterol level. It also can modestly decrease your blood pressure and help you control your weight." It can help keep your heart fit and conditioned, too, just as it gets the other muscles in your body into shape.

Eat right. It's not a magic bullet, but proper diet can be the heart and soul of any personalized cardiac care program. According to Fredric J. Pashkow, M.D., medical director of the Cardiac Health Improvement and Rehabilitation Program at the Cleveland Clinic Foundation in Cleveland and author of *The Woman's Heart Book*, research shows that the best way to keep your heart out of danger is to slash the fat and cholesterol in your diet. That means when it comes to menu planning, choose fish more often than steak, skim milk more frequently than whole milk, egg whites rather than whole eggs, and low-fat frozen yogurt instead of ice cream. Keep your daily dietary fat intake to 25 percent or less of total calories.

Consider hormones, if you're a woman. Estrogen replacement therapy can cut your risk of heart attack by as much as one-half to one-third, according to Dr. Helfant.

But you must talk over your options with your doctor. "There's a potential downside to hormonal therapy," says Dr. Helfant, "such as an increased risk of endometrial cancer and perhaps breast cancer, too." If you have a family history of endometrial or breast cancer or other risk factors, you and your doctor may decide that hormonal therapy isn't for you.

After You've Been Struck

Prevention may sound good, but what if you've already endured the terrifying experience of a heart attack? Well, count your blessings that you survived it—and then make a commitment to some health habits that might keep you from going through it a second time and that might put you on the fast track to a zestful, healthful life. If you've bought into the belief that a heart attack will permanently impair your mobility, activity level, job function, or sex life, it's time to dispel those myths. Despite your heart attack, your best years can still be ahead of you.

With lifestyle changes, you should be able to reduce your risk of having another heart attack, says Dr. Helfant. "These changes will also allow you to take control of your health and live a purposeful, meaningful life while protecting yourself to the maximum degree possible."

So what kind of action should you take? The recommendations may sound familiar, but here's the specific impact they can have when a heart attack is part of your medical history.

Eat healthfully. After something as major as a heart attack, you might think the damage that has been done to your heart makes simple measures such as healthier eating about as helpful as applying a Band-Aid to your chest. But when researchers at the National Heart, Lung and Blood Institute conducted an analysis of studies of heart attack survivors, they found that people could significantly decrease their chances of having another heart attack by reducing their high blood cholesterol readings. Various studies have shown that declines in blood cholesterol levels of 10 percent cut the risk of having a second heart attack by between 12 and 19 percent. A key to lowering blood cholesterol is cutting back on saturated fat (the kind found in animal products and tropical oils) and dietary cholesterol (found in most animal products).

Move it. In many programs for heart attack recovery, physical activity is the center of attention, often beginning at very modest levels even while patients are still hospitalized. Most cardiac rehabilitation programs recommend exercising for 15 to 30 minutes at least three times a week.

"People who have done no exercise in the past would certainly be better off doing even a little bit now," says Peter Wood, Ph.D., professor of medicine emeritus and associate director of the Stanford University Center for Research in Disease Prevention in Palo Alto, California. By gradually increasing the amount of physical activity you do—with your doctor's guidance—your heart will reap even more benefits, Dr. Wood says.

Take aspirin. In this age of high-powered, high-priced medications, can a simple aspirin make you the picture of health? An American Heart Association team of researchers analyzed six studies in which patients were given aspirin after heart attacks. This inexpensive white pill reduced the death rate from heart disease between 5 and 42 percent and cut the rate of subsequent nonfatal heart attacks between 12 and 57 percent.

One other piece of good news: You needn't go overboard on aspirin dosages. "A baby aspirin a day is all that's necessary," says Dr. Helfant. Nevertheless, some people should probably stay away from aspirin completely, despite its potential benefits. "If you have a bleeding disorder or an ulcer, for example, taking aspirin is not a good idea," says Julie Buring, Sc.D., principal investigator of the Women's Health Study and associate professor of ambulatory care and prevention at Harvard Medical School in Boston. She suggests talking with your doctor before taking aspirin.

HEART DISEASE

The Sooner You Act, the Better

Imagine cutting your risk of heart disease to zero—in other words having the healthy, normal cardiovascular system you probably had in your youth.

Impossible? Not for most of us. With reams of data collected during decades of research, scientists have a pretty good idea why some people get heart disease and some don't. It boils down to things such as poor diet and lack of exercise.

As it turns out, almost every one of the factors that can lead to heart disease is within your control. And curbing your chances of a heart attack or related problems is simply a matter of following three steps.

"Know, monitor, and change controllable risk factors," says William P. Castelli, M.D., former director to the famed Framingham Heart Study and retired medical director of the Framingham Cardiovascular Institute in Massachusetts. "If all Americans did this, heart disease would be eradicated, just as polio was."

Committing to Change

Heart disease doesn't happen overnight. Most heart disease results from a narrowing of the coronary arteries, known as atherosclerosis, over decades. What makes arteries narrow? Largely, it's the way we Americans live our lives. In some other countries, where lifestyles are simpler, arteries are healthy and wide open even in the very elderly.

The encouraging news is pretty straightforward: You can slow the progression of heart disease, and in some cases even reverse it, without drugs or surgery. Best of all, you don't have to go to extremes or have a will of steel to do so. "Moderate changes go a long way," advises Richard H. Helfant, M.D., vice chairman of medicine and director of the cardiology training program at the University of California, Irvine, Medical Center and author of *Women, Take Heart.* "You don't have to be a fanatic or be perfect to make a difference in your health."

150

Here are some strategies that can keep your heart pumping as though it inherited an extra decade or two of life.

Give up the cigarettes—now. When you smoke, your blood vessels constrict, which places extra strain on your heart, your heart beats more rapidly, and your blood pressure jumps. The result is as brutal as it comes: According to the American Heart Association, cigarettes directly cause nearly one-fifth of all deaths from heart disease.

If you're a woman who smokes and takes oral contraceptives, you're asking for even more trouble. Together, those two make you up to 39 times more likely to have a heart attack than a woman who uses neither.

Cut your cholesterol. You need some cholesterol for essential body functions to take place. But the fact is that your own liver produces all the cholesterol your body requires. When you add to that total by eating foods that are high in saturated fats, such as meats, milk, eggs, and butter, you fill your bloodstream with cholesterol, especially low-density lipoprotein, the "bad" cholesterol. LDL eventually collects on the walls of your arteries, hardening into a dense, fatty layer called plaque that can narrow or block your blood vessels. The result? Heart attack city.

If your total blood cholesterol readings get to 240 milligrams per deciliter of blood (mg/dl) or above, you will double your chances of heart disease. What you need to shoot for is a total cholesterol level below 150 mg/dl. The key: Cut your total consumption of fat to no more than 25 percent of your daily calories, and limit your saturated fat consumption to 7 percent of your daily calories.

Making this change not only will put you on a heart-healthy track, it could even reverse atherosclerosis. When Dean Ornish, M.D., president and director of the Preventive Medicine Research Institute in Sausalito, California, shifted patients to a comprehensive program that included a very low-fat diet, moderate exercise, no smoking, and stress management training, the results were astonishing. After 1 year, 82 percent of the people significantly reduced the fatty deposits that had clogged their coronary arteries.

But don't think that to prevent heart disease you need to adopt a deprivation diet. "No one ever got a heart attack from a steak or a piece of pie," says Dr. Helfant. "We're talking about an overall change in lifestyle and not worrying about an occasional slip."

Tip the triglyceride scale. As if cholesterol weren't enough to worry about, you and your doctor should keep tabs on your triglycerides, too. They are a type of fat in the bloodstream, and though they appear to play a role in heart disease, their exact role in that process is still not as clear as the link between cholesterol and heart problems.

Many experts say that a triglyceride level above 150 mg/dl should serve as a warning flag. What's one of the best ways to temper your triglycerides? Regular exercise, says Peter Wood, Ph.D., professor of medicine emeritus and associate director of the Stanford University Center for Research in Disease Prevention in Palo Alto, California.

Maintain your best weight. In a country that seems obsessed with slogans like "Thin is in," a lot of us could never be mistaken for being undernourished. About 34 million Americans are a bit more than pleasantly plump (approximately 20 percent or more over their desirable weights). Putting on those extra pounds is a little like playing Russian roulette with your heart. Data from the Framingham heart study, the longest-running research project to assess the risk factors for heart disease, found that people who are more than 30 percent over their desirable weight double their chances of heart disease.

So whether or not you consider flab to be unattractive, it's clearly hazardous to your heart. "If you're obese, the heart has to work harder to move nutrients to the additional cells in your body," says James Martin, M.D., family physician with the Institute for Urban Family Health at Beth Israel Medical Center in New York City. That extra strain on the heart can be particularly worrisome if you already have other risk factors that can contribute to heart disease, such as high cholesterol or high blood pressure. Set some goals for shedding extra pounds by relying more on low-fat foods and getting more exercise.

Sweat a little. Sure, it's tempting to toss out the exercise shoes, cancel your health club membership, and spend every weekend entrenched like Gibraltar in front of the television or camped out on the beach with a best-selling novel. If

---

If the Worst Happens

Sometimes even the most conscientious efforts at prevention just aren't enough. If you start to feel the warning signs of a heart attack—such as pressure or squeezing sensations in the chest, pain shooting into the shoulders, arms or neck, or shortness of breath and nausea—you need to respond rapidly.

As the American Heart Association warns, "Delay can be deadly!"

Clot-dissolving drugs called thrombolytics are administered in the emergency room and can restore blood flow, thus minimizing damage to the heart muscle.

But time is crucial. "The later you come in to the emergency room, the less likely a thrombolytic is going to be effective," says Gerald Pohost, M.D., director of the Division of Cardiovascular Disease at the University of Alabama School of Medicine in Birmingham. "The first 2 hours are the best time, but as time passes, the success of these drugs diminishes."

that's your idea of Shangri-La, you're not alone—but you are paying a price. In fact, almost 60 percent of Americans don't get any exercise, a lifestyle choice that greatly increases their risk of heart attack.

Exercise can do more than just get you some fresh air and make you feel more invigorated. "It strengthens the heart muscle," says Dr. Wood. "With regular exercise, the heart becomes a more efficient pump. As a result, the heart rate becomes slower for a given amount of effort." Each beat is more efficient, he says, and so the heart doesn't need to work as hard as it would if you were out of shape.

Exercise is particularly important because it boosts a good type of cholesterol called high-density lipoprotein (HDL). HDL can diminish some of the damage that LDL cholesterol causes. You don't need to push yourself to exhaustion to reap the benefits of exercise. Even just walking at a faster pace will improve your HDL level.

Deflate your blood pressure. High blood pressure is called the silent killer, quietly doing sinister work that puts so much extra strain on the heart and arteries that it can ultimately provoke a heart attack (not to mention a stroke or kidney failure).

But by pulling the plug on your high blood pressure—which you can do by reducing sodium in your diet, losing weight, exercising, and (if necessary) taking one of many available medications—you can give your heart a breather. Here are some comforting statistics: For each one-point decline you can achieve in your diastolic blood pressure (the bottom number), you can cut your risk of a heart attack by 2 to 3 percent. And with proper therapy, it's not uncommon for people with high blood pressure to lower their diastolic readings by 20 points or more.

Consider aspirin. It may not be the Fountain of Youth, but the drug that can keep your heart vital may be as close as the medicine cabinet in your bathroom. Aspirin, the tiny white pill that has been relied on a zillion times to zap headaches and other mild pain problems, appears to be a heart-saver as well.

In the Nurses' Health Study at Harvard University, women who took from one to six aspirin tablets per week over a 6-year period had about a 32 percent decreased chance of having a first heart attack compared with women who took no aspirin. Women over age 50 seemed to get the most protection. But particularly if you're prone to bleeding problems, consult your doctor before self-prescribing aspirin, since it's a medication that discourages blood clotting in your body.

Feast on fish. There's a healthful kind of fat called omega-3 fatty acids. Found in most fish and also in flaxseed, omega-3's can help prevent clots from forming in the bloodstream. In addition, they help lower potentially dangerous triglycerides. Studies show that eating fish once or twice a week can help keep your arteries clear and your heart working well. Looking for a good fish? Consider salmon, because it contains high levels of omega-3's.

Sip a little health. It's a tradition in many countries to raise a glass of wine and give a toast to good health. As it turns out, what's in that glass can make the toasts come true. Studies have shown that drinking moderate amounts of alcohol raises levels of beneficial HDL cholesterol. Plus, alcohol acts like motor oil in the

---

Are You an Apple or a Pear?

In the fruit basket, pears tend to age somewhat faster than apples. But when it comes to your heart—and "pear" and "apple" are describing different body shapes—the pear definitely ages slower.

People who tend to put on weight around their midsections (apples) are at higher risk of heart attack (as well as of diabetes, stroke, and high blood pressure) than those who gain weight around their hips (pears).

Why is a jelly belly so malicious? One theory is that abdominal fat is more easily converted to cholesterol.

No matter what the cause turns out to be, make an effort to trim the size of your own "apple" by losing a few of those extra pounds. Here's a guideline for you to keep in mind: To cut your risk, your waist measurement should not be more than 80 percent of your hip measurement if you're a woman, and 90 percent if you're a man.

---

blood. It makes platelets, the tiny disks that aid in clotting, a little more slippery, so they're less likely to stick together and cause heart-damaging clots in the bloodstream. All alcohol can help boost HDL cholesterol and reduce the tendency of blood to clot. But red wine is particularly good because it also contains heart-healthy flavonoids.

To get the benefits of alcohol without the problems, doctors advise drinking in moderation. For men, this means having no more than two drinks a day. Women, who are more susceptible to alcohol's effects, should limit themselves to one drink a day. (A drink is defined as 12 ounces of beer, 5 ounces of wine, or 1½ ounces of liquor.)

The Value of Vitamins and Minerals

While the steps mentioned above are key ingredients in the fight against heart disease, doctors are beginning to realize that there are other potent weapons you can bring to bear. Specifically, vitamins and minerals. Here are some of the best they've discovered.

Vitamin E: The cholesterol neutralizer. Several studies indicate that vitamin E may help prevent LDL cholesterol from creating the plaque that clogs arteries. In the Health Professionals Follow-Up Study of almost 40,000 men, conducted by researchers at Harvard School of Public Health, men who took at least 100 international units of vitamin E a day for at least 2 years reduced their risk of heart disease by 37 percent. A companion study of more than 87,000 nurses between the ages of 34 and 59 found similar results. Even people who have undergone angioplasty, a procedure to open blocked arteries, or who had bypass surgery, appear to benefit from taking vitamin E daily.

Although some doctors involved in vitamin E research do not recommend vitamin E supplements, others feel that 100 to 200 international units of vitamin E a day might prove beneficial.

Beta-carotene: A potent protector. Beta-carotene, the nutrient that gives yellow, orange, and red vegetables their color, is a champion on the dinner plate when it comes to fighting heart disease. In study after study it's been shown to cut heart attack risk and protect people who have risk factors that predispose them to heart disease, such as smoking and high cholesterol.

To protect yourself against heart disease, researchers across the board resoundingly recommend you eat five or more servings of fruits and vegetables a day, including some servings rich in beta-carotene. Foods high in beta-carotene include carrots, cantaloupe, kale, leafy greens, peaches, sweet potatoes, and tomatoes.

Vitamin C: An antioxidant attack ship. Vitamin C seems to work in concert with vitamin E and beta-carotene to improve your heart health. In one study, University of California, Los Angeles, researchers checked the amounts of vitamin C taken by more than 11,000 men and women between the ages of 25 and 74. They found that people who got more than 50 milligrams of vitamin C a day, in addition to a multivitamin/mineral supplement, reduced their risk of death from cardiovascular disease by 28 percent.

The exact amount of vitamin C you need to achieve good heart health is still unknown, but many cardiologists are recommending taking somewhere in the range of 250 to 500 milligrams a day.

There are also key minerals that may be able to reduce your risk. Researchers have found that low levels of at least two elements—selenium and zinc, generally found in meats, seafood, cereals, and vegetables—seem to increase your risk of heart disease. In a study in Denmark of nearly 3,000 men between the ages of 53 and 74, researchers found that those with the lowest levels of selenium in their diets increased their risk of heart disease by 55 percent. What's more, the researchers suspected that close to 19 percent of the heart attacks among men in the study might in fact have been caused by low levels of this nutrient. The Daily Value for selenium is 70 micrograms. Most researchers agree, however, that you can take up to 100 micrograms daily without harm.

Zinc might also play a role in preventing heart disease, researchers say. Laboratory studies at the University of Kentucky in Lexington indicate that zinc may be necessary to safeguard the heart's arterial walls from the damage triggered by high blood pressure, high cholesterol, and tobacco smoke. The Daily Value for zinc is 15 milligrams a day.

HIGH BLOOD PRESSURE

The Silent Thief of Youth

There's a hidden aging problem out there, one that's far more dangerous than varicose veins, farsightedness, or gray hair. High blood pressure, also called hypertension, is directly linked to the deaths of more than 32,000 Americans each year—and it contributes to the deaths of untold thousands more.

It can make you 12 times more likely to suffer strokes, 6 times more likely to suffer heart attacks, and 5 times more likely to die of congestive heart failure. It's also a major risk factor for kidney failure.

And even though it affects more than 64 million Americans, nearly half of those who have high blood pressure aren't aware of it.

"There really aren't any noticeable outward signs. But if you have high blood pressure, it is doing damage," says Patrick Mulrow, M.D., chairman of the department of medicine at the Medical College of Ohio at Toledo and chairman of the American Heart Association's Council for High Blood Pressure Research.

The saddest part? "We could save lives if people discovered they have high blood pressure and then took measures to control it," Dr. Mulrow says.

Pressure Builders

Doctors take two measures when they check your blood pressure. The first is called the systolic reading. It indicates how hard your heart pumps to push blood through your arteries. The second measure, called the diastolic reading, shows how much resistance your arteries put up to the blood flow. A reading of about 120/80 is considered healthy.

Your blood pressure varies widely throughout the day. Generally, it will rise when you're exercising and drop when you're asleep. But when your baseline, or resting, reading creeps up to 140/90, you have borderline high blood pressure. That means your heart is working too hard to pump blood, either because your arteries have narrowed or stiffened with plaque or because you have too much blood in your system because of water retention or other problems. The result of

Try to Remember

If you have to be reminded to control your blood pressure, then maybe it's already too high. That's because high blood pressure may weaken your memory.

A study of 100 adults found that people with higher blood pressure scored lower in a process called short-term memory retrieval. That means it took longer for them to remember whether a number shown to them had been part of an original set of numbers that they had seen earlier.

No one's sure why high blood pressure fogs your memory. It may be related to the way blood circulates in the brain or to a reduction in the amount of oxygen that reaches the brain. "Whatever the mechanism, this is just another reason to keep your blood pressure under healthy control," says David J. Madden, Ph.D., professor in the department of psychiatry at Duke University Medical Center in Durham, North Carolina.

the extra stress can be heart disease or dangerous blood clots that can cause stroke or heart attack.

In 90 to 95 percent of cases, Dr. Mulrow says, the exact cause of high blood pressure is unknown. But researchers have identified a number of risk factors that may increase your risk of developing high blood pressure. Family history is one. If several members of your immediate family have high blood pressure, you're more likely to develop it. African Americans and members of other minority groups are at higher risk than Caucasians. Obesity is another major factor. Studies show that 60 percent of people with high blood pressure are overweight.

The Sodium-Stress Link

The amount of sodium in the foods you eat is one of the biggest contributors to high blood pressure, experts say. Sodium makes you retain water, Dr. Mulrow says, which increases the volume of blood in your body and makes your heart work harder to pump it. There's also evidence that sodium in some way damages the linings of blood vessels, making scarring and clogged arteries more likely.

The vast majority of your sodium intake is from the salt in food. After analyzing dozens of studies on sodium and high blood pressure, one British research team found that cutting salt by 3,000 milligrams per day—that's a little less than a teaspoon's worth—could prevent 26 percent of all strokes and 15 percent of heart attacks caused by blood clots.

Some people are more sensitive than others to the effects of salt or, more specifically, of sodium, says Robert DiBianco, M.D., director of cardiology research at the Washington Adventist Hospital in Takoma Park, Maryland. "Maybe you can eat a lot of salt, process, and get rid of it quickly and not have to worry about it," he says. But maybe not. There's no reliable test for salt sensitivity. If you are overweight, don't get a lot of exercise, or have a family history of high blood pressure or diabetes, Dr. DiBianco says you're probably more at risk and need to limit your salt intake.

Psychological factors can also play a role in high blood pressure. A 2-year study of 1,123 American adults found that severe anxiety and worry make middle-age men twice as likely to develop high blood pressure. Another study of 129 college students at the University of British Columbia in Vancouver showed that women who felt they got little social support from friends, family members, or co-workers had slightly higher systolic readings.

Job stress may lead to high blood pressure, too. Then there's alcohol. Scientists have long known that excess drinking can contribute to high blood pressure. But a study from the Research Institute on Alcoholism in Buffalo, New York, shows that how often you drink may be as important as how much you drink. Researchers looked at 1,635 residents of Erie County, New York, and found that people who drank every day had systolic readings 6.6 points higher and diastolic readings 4.7 points higher than people who drank only once a week. But the study found no significant relationship between blood pressure and the total amount of alcohol consumed.

Easing the Pressure

Lots of prescription drugs help reduce high blood pressure. Diuretics flush excess fluids from the body. Beta-blockers reduce the heart rate and the heart's total output of blood. Vasodilators widen arteries and allow easier blood flow. Sympathetic nerve inhibitors also prevent blood vessels from constricting.

But drugs should be a last resort. They can cause fatigue and inhibit your sex life, among other problems. The trick is to avoid high blood pressure in the first place—and the tips below will get you started. Even if you already have mild high blood pressure, the advice could reduce your dependence on drugs and maybe even let you control things naturally.

Have it tested. There's only one way to know for sure if you have high blood pressure: Have your doctor check your blood pressure. Once a year should be sufficient, unless your doctor orders more tests. If you show a borderline high reading, the doctor may order several retests over a couple of weeks or months.

Lighten up. If you're overweight, even moderate weight loss may help lower your blood pressure, says Marvin Moser, M.D., clinical professor of medicine at Yale University School of Medicine in New Haven, Connecticut, and senior adviser to the National High Blood Pressure Education Program. In some cases, he says, weight loss of 10 to 15 pounds may be enough to lower slightly elevated blood pressure to normal and help you avoid medication.

Move it. Exercise, combined with a low-fat diet, is the best way to lose weight and keep your arteries clog-free. Research shows that people who don't exercise are 35 to 50 percent more likely to develop high blood pressure. And the American College of Sports Medicine says that regular aerobic training can reduce systolic and diastolic blood pressure by as much as 10 points.

You don't have to be a marathon runner to reap the benefits, either. In fact, some studies have found that lower-intensity workouts such as walking are as good or better at lowering blood pressure than running or other heavy-duty aerobic activities. Many experts recommend working out at least three times a week for 20 minutes a pop.

Shake it off. Remember that not everyone is sensitive to the effects of sodium. But until doctors can reliably tell who is or isn't, it's a good idea to limit your intake. "It certainly isn't going to hurt anyone to cut down on salt and probably will be of real value if you're successful," Dr. DiBianco says.

Cut salt from your diet wherever you can. Most of us are eating about 2½ times more than we should. Swearing off the table shaker will have some effect. But research shows that three-fourths of all the salt we eat comes from processed foods such as cheese, soup, bread, baked goods, and snacks.

"You have to read labels," Dr. Mulrow says. Check for sodium content and shoot for a daily total of about 2,400 milligrams. When shopping, look for labels that say "low sodium." That means they contain no more than 140 milligrams of sodium per serving. Be careful when you eat out, too. You'll be surprised how fast sodium can add up. A hamburger from your favorite fast-food restaurant, for instance, may give you almost half a day's total.

DASH to the produce aisle. DASH stands for Dietary Approaches to Stop Hypertension, and it is the name of a large scientific experiment that tested whether a healthy way of eating could lower blood pressure. The study found that people could significantly reduce high blood pressure by consuming 8 to 10 daily servings of fruit and vegetables and about 3 daily servings of low-fat dairy products, and limiting the total fat in their diets to 25 percent of calories.

"Following the DASH combination might be an effective nutritional approach to preventing high blood pressure, " says Lawrence J. Appel, M.D., a DASH investigator and associate professor of medicine, epidemiology, and international health at the Johns Hopkins University Medical Institutions in Baltimore.

Pile on the potassium. Studies have shown that eating 3,500 milligrams of potassium can help counteract sodium and keep blood volume—and blood pressure—down. And it's easy to get enough. A baked potato packs 838 milligrams of potassium all by itself, and 1 cup of spinach has 800 milligrams. Other potassium-packed foods include bananas, orange juice, corn, cabbage, and broccoli. Check with your doctor before taking potassium supplements. Too much may aggravate kidney problems.

Meet your magnesium needs. Researchers seem to have found a link between low magnesium intake and high blood pressure. But just how much magnesium you need to combat high blood pressure remains unclear. For now, Dr.

How Low Can You Go?

When it comes to blood pressure, the lower the better.

"It doesn't really matter how low your reading is, even if it's something very, very low, like 85 systolic. As long as you're not feeling any ill effects from it, that's just fine. In fact, you should feel good knowing you're in a low-risk group," says Robert DiBianco, M.D., director of cardiology research at the Washington Adventist Hospital in Takoma Park, Maryland.

The landmark Framingham Heart Study, which took a decades-long look at the health of more than 5,200 residents of Framingham, Massachusetts, found that people with systolic blood pressure readings below 120 mm Hg (millimeters of mercury) had the least chance of suffering heart attacks. The risk rose steadily with increased pressure. People with the highest readings, 170 mm Hg or above, were more than three times more likely to die of heart attacks than those at or below 120 mm Hg.

Still, there are a couple of problems to watch for with low blood pressure. As people age, they're more likely to suffer from a form of temporary low blood pressure called orthostatic hypotension—the sensation you get when you hop out of bed and suddenly feel weak, like the room is spinning or the lights are dimmed. "If you have ever fainted from that, or if it happens more than very, very rarely, you should see a doctor," Dr. DiBianco says. The problem could be caused by mild dehydration, a reaction to medication, fever, illness, or heat exhaustion, he says.

For some people, especially the elderly and people with diabetes or heart disease and possibly those being treated for high blood pressure, readings that fall too low may be a particular risk. If you fit in one of these groups, consult your doctor, Dr. DiBianco says.

DiBianco says, your best bet is to get the Recommended Dietary Allowance (RDA) of about 280 milligrams.

Unfortunately, America's intake of magnesium has been dropping for a century, since we started processing foods and robbing them of their trace elements. Good sources of magnesium include nuts, spinach, lima beans, peas, and seafood. But don't overdo it by taking supplements; Dr. Mulrow says too much magnesium can give you a nasty case of diarrhea.

Keep up your calcium. The link between calcium intake and blood pressure is controversial. Some studies show that extra calcium can lower blood pressure, while others show that it has no effect.

But experts aren't yet convinced that large doses of calcium are going to help. Dr. Mulrow says getting the RDA of 800 milligrams per day—three 8-ounce glasses of skim milk provide more than enough—and keeping your other risk factors under control is the best advice for now. Other calcium sources include low-fat cheeses, canned salmon, and other canned fish with bones. If you want to take calcium supplements, see your doctor, since too much calcium can cause other problems, such as kidney stones.

Fill up with fiber. A Swedish study of 32 people with mild high blood pressure found that taking a 7-gram tablet of fiber each day helps lower diastolic blood pressure by five points. No one is sure why; perhaps it's because of weight loss from people being fuller and eating less or because they eat less sodium. Whatever the reason, 7 extra grams of fiber is easy to find. There's almost that much in a bowl of high-fiber cereal.

Drink in moderation. "A little alcohol isn't going to hurt," Dr. Mulrow says. "But drinking every day, and drinking to excess, could mean trouble." If you're fighting high blood pressure, 3 ounces of alcohol a week seems to be about the limit. A 12-year study of 1,643 women, with a mean age of 47, showed that both systolic and diastolic pressure readings begin to rise steadily after that. That means three 12-ounce beers, three 5-ounce glasses of wine, or three cocktails containing 1½ ounces of hard liquor a week.

Stop smoking. Smoking markedly increases your risk of developing a stroke or damaging blood vessels from high blood pressure, says Dr. Mulrow. When you smoke, it encourages your body to deposit cholesterol within your coronary arteries. This decreases the size of your vessels and forces your heart to work harder. "Anyone with high blood pressure should stop smoking immediately," advises Dr. Mulrow.

Shrug off stress. When you are stressed, your body pumps out hormones that make your blood vessels contract and your heart race, a combination of reactions that can launch your blood pressure into the high-risk regions. One of the best ways to defeat stress is to spend time every day focusing on your breathing, says Patricia Liehr, R.N., Ph.D., associate professor of nursing at the University of Texas, Houston School of Nursing and a stress-management consultant.

"When you are stressed, your breathing becomes very shallow and that becomes a pattern." If you breathe deeply, however, you can reset your nervous system at a calmer level. Spend 5 minutes every morning and evening just taking slow deep breaths, she advises. "Just pay attention to the breath going in and out. If other thoughts enter your mind, simply turn your attention to the breathing," she says.

IMPOTENCE

Living Well Reduces Your Risk

For most men, the very word *impotence* suggests a whole range of emotions that they'd rather deny, situations they'd prefer to forget, and issues they'd rather not face.

But face them they should, because often the underlying factors that lead to impotence can be prevented or cured. Address those problems and there's no reason you can't maintain a healthy sex life into your forties, fifties, sixties, and beyond.

An estimated 10 to 15 million American men regularly suffer from impotence, defined as the inability to achieve and maintain an erection long enough to have satisfactory sexual intercourse. Of those men, 75 to 85 percent are under the age of 65.

For men over 50, the most common cause of impotence is clogged arteries in the penis. The most frequent cause of the clogs: a buildup of cholesterol and fatty deposits inside artery walls. For men under 50, stress, depression, anger, fatigue, and performance anxiety are the most common triggers for impotence.

Men also can become impotent as an offshoot of medical conditions such as diabetes, thyroid problems, stroke, heart disease, and multiple sclerosis. And sometimes, erection problems are a reaction to blood pressure medications, tranquilizers, antidepressant drugs, or antihistamines. Then there's alcohol consumption and smoking, both of which can compound the problem of achieving an erection.

Clearly, there are a number of things that can lead to impotence. The good news? Just growing older isn't one of them.

"Theoretically, there is no reason for your potency to change as you age," says Joseph Khoury, M.D., a urologist in private practice in Bethesda, Maryland, who knows men in their eighties who still have sex three times a week. The one thing they have in common: They took care of themselves better than most men.

162

A Maintenance Manual for Potency

Like keeping a smooth-running sports car in tip-top shape, the key to a healthy life is maintenance. Here are some maintenance ideas that could prevent impotence, as suggested by a Boston University Medical Center study on male sexuality.

Work out, eat right. Low levels of high-density lipoproteins, the "good" cholesterol, seem to be linked to sexual dysfunction. In the Massachusetts study, men being treated for heart disease, diabetes, and high blood pressure were up to four times more likely to become completely impotent in later life than men without those problems. "These are problems that regular exercise and a healthy diet can really combat," says Kenneth Goldberg, M.D., founder and director of the Male Health Institute in Irving, Texas.

Check the meds. If you're taking medication for other health problems, these drugs might be affecting your sex life. Impotence is much more common among men who are taking medications, especially for blood pressure, heart disease, and diabetes. "Talk to your doctor about drug substitutions," says Dr. Goldberg. Some medications may have no substitute, but if your doctor can recommend a drug that won't impair your sex life, you may want to try it.

Drop some weight. Since being overweight is a factor that raises your risk of all the impotence-related diseases, shedding pounds is an important preventative measure. And the components of a weight-loss program—a healthy diet and regular exercise—can help preserve blood flow, a big factor for good sex. "Most of the problems noted in the study were vascular in nature—that is, impaired blood flow contributed to impotence," says Irwin Goldstein, M.D., professor of urology at the Boston University School of Medicine and co-director of the New England Reproductive Center-Medical Center in Boston. So avoid fatty, cholesterol-boosting foods. It may not only keep you from expanding your waistline but may also help prevent blockages in the arteries in the penis.

De-stress for sex. The mind may be one of the most important factors for preventing impotence. In the Massachusetts Male Aging Study, depression, anger, and submissiveness were strongly linked to increased sexual difficulties. Among men who reported feeling the most angry, 35 percent were unable to maintain an erection and have intercourse at least some of the time, and nearly 20 percent were completely unable to achieve an erection.

"This may suggest that dealing with stress is important," says Dr. Goldberg. When we get excited or stressed-out, our nerves release a form of adrenaline that has been shown to stop an erection in its tracks. "Stress reduction, through relaxation, exercise, or both, is a must," he says.

Stop smoking. You already know what smoking does to the lungs and heart, but the Massachusetts Male Aging Study makes the erection connection. Fifty-six percent of the smokers in the study were completely impotent, compared to 21 percent of nonsmokers. "Tobacco can also cause circulatory problems, reducing blood supply to your penis and destroying tissue flexibility," says Dr. Goldberg.

Recharge your batteries. The more erections you have, the more you are likely to have them. Erections supply your penis with the stuff it needs most, oxygen-rich blood. Research suggests that if a man's penis doesn't get enough oxygen through circulation, permanent damage to blood vessels or penile muscles may occur. "This is not the sole reason men become impotent, though. So men shouldn't feel that not having frequent erections will ultimately lead them to becoming impotent," says Dr. Goldberg. "But there is increasing evidence that having more of them helps—you might call it the 'use it or lose it' syndrome."

Alternative Cures

While Viagra has become the chemical cure for impotence, alternative medicine practitioners believe that nutritional supplements—taken as part of a program that includes exercise and a healthy diet—also can help restore the ability to achieve erections. They say that a combination of nutritional supplements could speed your progress toward sexual health and that certain herbs are potent enough to dramatically increase blood flow to the penis and boost your sex drive, says Thomas Kruzel, N.D., a naturopathic doctor in Portland, Oregon. Additionally, some vitamins and minerals provide the building blocks for sexual health.

Keep in mind, though, that since impotence could be a side effect of prescription drugs or a symptom of other health problems, you should see a doctor to evaluate your overall condition before you take any nutritional supplement. After that stop, you may want to consider these herbs and vitamins.

Charge your sex life with yohimbine. For centuries, people have used yohimbe, the bark from a West African tree, to boost sex drive. It is said to increase blood flow to the penis, which makes it possible to attain and sustain an erection. But the natural form of yohimbe can cause nasty side effects including anxiety, increased heart rate, and hallucinations. For this reason, herbalists suggest taking a prescription form of the herb, called yohimbine (Yocon, Yohimex).

Yohimbine is powerful yet has milder side effects than yohimbe. One may even be pleasing: Men who use it report having a pleasant tingling sensation along their spines and in the genitals. This said, you shouldn't take yohimbine if you have certain health conditions or with certain foods and drugs. Be sure to discuss possible interactions and side effects with your doctor.

Improve circulation with gingko. Ginkgo, a medicinal plant with a long tradition, is mainly used to improve blood circulation to the brain. It may also aid mental alertness and memory and even relieve depression. Because it can improve blood flow throughout arteries and veins, it's been successfully used to treat many men whose impotence is caused by poor blood circulation, says Dr. Kruzel.

In one study, 60 men with impotence who didn't respond to injection treatments with a prescription medication were given 60 milligrams of ginkgo daily for 12 to 18 months. The first signs of improvement in blood circulation occurred after 6 to 8 weeks. When the men were evaluated again after a 6-month period, 50 percent of those who took the ginkgo reported that they had regained potency.

"You can try 60 to 240 milligrams a day, but don't go any higher than that," says James A. Duke, Ph.D., botanical consultant, former ethnobotanist with the U.S. Department of Agriculture who specializes in medicinal plants, and author of *The Green Pharmacy*. High amounts of ginkgo may cause side effects.

Restore energy with ginseng. Asian ginseng, also called panax, Korean, or Chinese ginseng, tops the list of herbs used to restore vitality, boost energy, reduce fatigue, and improve physical performance. It protects the body from the negative effects of stress. Traditionally, it's been used as an aphrodisiac, and research seems to back up its reputation, showing that it can increase blood flow to the penis, says Dr. Kruzel.

The amount of ginseng you should take for impotence depends on the species you buy and how much of the active ingredients is in the product. Dr. Kruzel recommends that most of his patients take 500 milligrams daily, but he says that it's best to consult your doctor for the optimum dose.

Choose the building block for sexual health. The most important nutrient for overall sexual health is zinc. This trace mineral is vital for a number of functions. It enhances the production of testosterone, the male hormone that's required for sexual development and potency. It also influences sperm motility—that is, the speed and mobility of sperm—which can be a factor in fertility.

Certain forms of zinc are better absorbed than others. Zinc picolinate, zinc citrate, and zinc monomethionine are the most absorbable. If you're experiencing impotence, Dr. Kruzel says that you can take 15 to 30 milligrams of zinc daily, but he advises that you talk to your doctor if you're considering taking more than 20 milligrams. If you don't see results after 4 to 6 weeks, Dr. Kruzel recommends that you see your doctor for a re-evaluation.

He also recommends taking a high-potency multivitamin and mineral supplement in addition to the zinc to help keep your urinary tract in good working order and to lay the foundation for sexual health. "Vitamins C and E are also found in high concentrations in the prostate gland, so they can help speed your recovery from impotence," says Dr. Kruzel. He recommends 2,000 to 4,000 milligrams of vitamin C with meals and 400 to 800 international units of vitamin E daily.

While it's annoying, an occasional inability to get or maintain an erection shouldn't worry you too much, doctors say.

"As you age, it takes longer to get an erection and more physical and psychological stimulation to maintain it," says Roger Crenshaw, M.D., a psychiatrist and sex therapist in private practice in La Jolla, California. "It's the guy who notices that his erection is fluctuating and worries about it who will become psychologically impotent, because he isn't accepting that his body is aging."

INJURIES
AND ACCIDENTS

They're Easy to Avoid

$\mathbf{T}$he ice pack is doing its job. The pain has receded, the swelling is down, and your knee—except for an interesting configuration of cuts and colors—looks the way it's supposed to.

But it's going to be a few days before you're up and around. And right now, confined to a chair, feeling stiff and sore, you know that the next time you rush for that return at the net, you won't try the full-out body stretch that Venus Williams uses on TV.

Nothing is more likely to make you feel like your body is 110 years old than an injury that lands you on your back or confines you to a chair. And whether the injury is caused by a car accident, a fall, or a tricky move in a game of volleyball, nearly all of us are at risk at one time or another. For people between the ages of 25 and 44, when a problem occurs, it is most likely to be a strained or torn muscle from a sports injury.

The Sports Connection

Sports injuries result in 6,000 deaths a year. Nonfatal injuries in recreational activities such as baseball and softball, basketball, football, and bicycling put more than 2 million people in the emergency room every year. Add to that the mammoth numbers of strains and sprains that are treated in locker rooms, plus injuries suffered in dozens of other sports, and you can understand why the National Safety Council estimates that the total number of sports injuries exceeds 3 million each year.

People between the ages of 25 and 64 account for more than 74 percent of all emergency room visits for scuba-diving injuries, 68 percent for squash, racquetball, and paddleball injuries, 51 percent for horseback-riding injuries, 45 percent for fishing injuries, 44 percent for tennis injuries, 42 percent for volleyball injuries, and 40 percent for weight-lifting injuries.

Why are so many people in this age group getting hurt? "By age 25, people have become 'weekend athletes,'" explains Stephen J. Nicholas, M.D., associate team physician for the New York Jets and associate director of the Nicholas Institute of Sports Medicine and Athletic Injuries at Lenox Hill Hospital in New York City. "They're getting more involved with work, and social demands begin to take precedence over physical well-being.

"It's like putting your body in a cast and taking it out only on weekends," says Dr. Nicholas. "The muscles get short, weak, and stiff. And they're no longer able to function at their optimal levels."

Unfortunately, most of us still think we're in peak condition, says Dr. Nicholas. So when we play tennis on the weekend, we push our bodies the way we used to when we were playing several times a week.

The result? The muscles fatigue, cramp, strain, then pull to the point where they can actually tear, says Dr. Nicholas.

How to Reduce Your Risk

It's difficult to rein yourself in when you're going for that extra mile or point, Dr. Nicholas adds. But here's how you can help your body keep up—and reduce your risk of injury.

Take a high school exam. If you're over age 25 and participating in weekend sports, schedule a physical exam with a family physician who does the local high school's team physicals, suggests Rosemary Agostini, M.D., a staff physician at the Virginia Mason Sports Clinic and clinical associate professor at the University of Washington, both in Seattle.

Ask him to give you the same type of physical that he gives the local football or basketball team, including a review of any previous sports injuries. Combined with a "weekend warrior" approach to sports, old injuries have a way of coming back to haunt you—sometimes on a chronic basis, says Dr. Agostini. A physician can evaluate the likelihood of that happening and make specific suggestions to avoid reinjury.

Balance your diet. You can't build muscle or improve performance without eating a balanced diet, explains Dr. Agostini. A lack of calcium to build strong bones, a lack of iron to build red blood cells, or a lack of protein to build and maintain muscle can not only sabotage your performance but set you up for injury as well.

Ask the doctor who does your physical to recommend a local sports nutritionist. Then work with her to develop an eating program that suits your particular needs.

Turn in your shoes every 500 miles. Shoes need to provide good support and shock absorption to prevent injuries, says Dr. Agostini. Replace them every 6 months or 500 miles, whichever comes first. And check your shoe size before you buy. Feet widen and change as we age.

Keep moving. "You'll be able to minimize injuries if you go on a regular exercise program—one that involves 30 or 40 minutes every day or at least three or four times a week," says Dr. Nicholas. The point is that your body not be allowed 5 or 6 days in a row in which to stiffen up.

Stretch. Begin your exercise program with at least 25 minutes of stretching every time you work out, Dr. Nicholas says. The muscles in the back and front of your thighs—the hamstrings and quadriceps—plus those in the lower back are the most important to loosen up.

"They usually don't get any stretching during the day unless you specifically set out to do it," says Dr. Nicholas. "Yet one of the most common causes of lower back pain is a hamstring tightness that causes a pelvic tilt.

"If you can maintain your hamstrings in a loosened fashion," he adds, "you might minimize not only the number of hamstring pulls or lower extremity injuries you get but also the amount of lower back pain you develop in the future."

Make your body work. After you stretch, do any aerobic exercise—walking, running, jumping—that accelerates your heart rate and keeps you breathing hard—hard, not panting—for 20 minutes, says Dr. Nicholas.

Lift. Strengthen your muscles by lifting at least a minimal amount of weight, says Dr. Nicholas. Get an athletic trainer to review your doctor's exam and recommendations and then to prescribe the specific weights and number of repetitions you should do. And don't forget to stretch before your workout.

When You Make a Mistake

No matter how carefully you keep your body in shape, every once in a while you're going to pull or strain something when you twist the wrong way, intensify your exercise program, or simply fall over your own two feet.

So here's what Dr. Nicholas advises you to do about a pulled or strained ligament, tendon, or muscle.

Apply RICE. RICE may be the sports world's most important acronym. It means Rest, Ice, Compression, and Elevation. And that's exactly what you should do for any new injury, says Dr. Nicholas. The idea is to minimize the amount of inflammation that occurs. It's inflammation that produces the swelling that causes the pain, which can then limit your movement.

"Put ice on the injury for 3 or 4 days," Dr. Nicholas says. "Apply it for 20 minutes of every hour you're awake." Wrap an elastic bandage around the injured area afterward, then elevate the injured muscle.

Take ibuprofen. "I also tell people to take Advil if they don't have any stomach problems," says Dr. Nicholas. That also reduces inflammation. Just follow package directions.

Use wet heat. Once you have RICE'd yourself for 3 or 4 days, it's time to work on getting your normal function back and preventing the injured area from becoming a chronic problem, says Dr. Nicholas.

The difficulty is that after 3 or 4 days, dried blood from torn or traumatized muscle fibers is sitting at the injured site.

"We need to get it out of the area," says Dr. Nicholas. "So we start what we call the wet heat program. We wrap a warm, wet towel around the injured area, put plastic—the kind of plastic bag you get at the dry cleaner's—around the towel to provide insulation, then put a heating pad on top.

"We leave it that way for about an hour and a half, three times a day, being careful not to burn the skin," he adds. "It will liquefy the dried blood in the injured area, bring the blood to the surface, and help the body absorb it.

"It also helps with the healing process by loosening up the muscles."

Re-stretch the injured muscle. Once a muscle has been injured, both it and the surrounding muscles have contracted into shorter lengths, says Dr. Nicholas. So before you can resume your normal workouts, you have to re-stretch the muscles until they achieve their normal resting lengths. Ask an athletic trainer which stretches are best for your particular injury.

"If you don't achieve that resting length, you're more subject to chronic pulls that can occur again and again," says Dr. Nicholas.

Falling Down on the Job

Sports injuries may be costly in terms of time, pain, and aggravation, but falls are more likely to kill.

While falls that occur in the home are most likely to involve older folks with failing eyesight or wearing floppy footwear, falls by men and women between the ages of 25 and 44 are more likely to occur on the job, says researcher John Britt, R.N., state injury prevention program coordinator at Harborview Hospital in Seattle.

People fall when they're moving from one height to another on everything from stairs and stages to ladders and girders, according to safety experts at the Occupational Safety and Health Administration (OSHA) in Washington, D.C. Railings may stop unexpectedly before the last step, movable sets may not be clamped into place on stages, safety ropes may be torn or frayed on ladders, tools may inadvertently be left on girders.

Want to make sure you're not the next one to go bottoms up at work? Here's how Britt says you can reduce your risk.

Find the fall guy. Every company has someone whose job it is to make detailed reports of accidents to insurance companies, safety committees, and workers' compensation, says Britt. Find that person. Then ask when and where every injury took place during the past 12 months. Then make sure you don't fall into the same traps that others did.

Make the invisible visible. People tend to pay attention to the little things and ignore huge ones, says OSHA. They see the tiny X-Acto blade that might slice their fingers in the art room but not the pool of ink on the floor that can cause them to slip.

Walk into any room at your workplace, stand in a corner, and look for anything that can trip you up or hurt you in any other way. Then either report the hazard to management or take care of it yourself.

Leave the high heels at home. If your company suggests you wear flats, nonskid soles, boots, or other special footwear designed to keep you from falling down on the job, do it.

Be a Road Scholar

Many of the men and women who survive the 10 million or so traffic accidents in the United States each year can no longer expect friends and co-workers to automatically extend their sympathies.

Instead, says Britt, their accident recitals are just as likely to be met with the question, "Were you wearing your seat belt?" or "Did you stop by the bar before you drove home?"

"There's been a subtle shift in public opinion about motor vehicle accidents in the past couple of years," Britt explains. People used to feel sorry for accident victims. But today there's more of a sense that accidents are preventable.

What can you do? Here are three safety strategies that Britt feels will help you prevent—or survive—motor vehicle accidents.

Don't drink. Safety studies indicate that between 40 and 50 percent of all fatal accidents involve drunk drivers, says Britt. Alcohol is most likely to be involved in fatal crashes with adult male drivers between the ages of 20 and 55. And the more violent the crash, the more likely a drunk was at the wheel. So don't drink before you drive.

Stay alert on Fridays and Saturdays. One-third of all fatal crashes occur between 6:00 P.M. and 6:00 A.M. on Fridays and Saturdays, researchers report. So stay particularly alert during those times.

Use lap/shoulder belts. Many people simply won't wear safety belts in the mistaken belief that they have less chance of injury if they're "free" to get out of the car quickly. Unfortunately, these are the people who are least likely to get out of their vehicles at all. A study by the National Highway Traffic Safety Administration indicates that when they're worn carefully, lap/shoulder belts reduce the odds of occupant death in a crash by 45 percent.

LOW IMMUNITY

Fortifying the Troops

A co-worker sneezes and a cloud of viruses fills the air. Pick up a pen or a pair of socks and you're exposed to thousands, possibly millions of bacteria. Walk barefoot across the lawn and you're picking up fungi, parasites, and still more bacteria.

A dangerous world? It would be if you didn't have your immune system to protect you.

"Our bodies are constantly bombarded with bacteria, viruses, and other organisms trying to gain entry," says Thomas Petro, Ph.D., associate professor of microbiology and immunology at the University of Nebraska Medical Center in Lincoln. "The immune system is the one defense we have against this takeover."

It's truly a battle for survival. A single inch of freshly washed skin may be home to more than 1 million bacteria. Without strong immunity, microbes in and on your body would quickly multiply to unimaginable numbers. Yet every minute of every day, your immune system keeps these microscopic marauders in check.

To a large extent, your ability to maintain a healthy immune system as you grow older depends directly on good nutrition, researchers believe. Research has shown, for example, that in parts of the world where healthy, nutritious food is in short supply, people frequently have weak immune systems, and they are much more prone to developing infections.

Similarly, in this country nutrition may play a role in the health of older Americans. "We know that in many older folks, immune response is compromised," says Adria Sherman, Ph.D., professor and chair of the department of nutritional Sciences at Rutgers University in New Brunswick, New Jersey. "It's not clear whether this is an inevitable characteristic of aging, a physiological process, years of nutritional depletion, poor eating habits, or increased needs. But in my opinion, it's probably some combination of all of these."

Having a low level of even a single nutrient may cause the immune system to pay the price. In one small study, for example, researchers at Tufts University

School of Nutrition in Medford, Massachusetts, put eight people on diets that were very low in vitamin B_6. Within 3 weeks, their levels of disease-fighting white blood cells plummeted. Then, when the people were allowed to eat foods high in vitamin B_6 once again, their immune systems quickly regained strength.

"Food is powerful medicine," says Keith Block, M.D., medical director of the Cancer Institute at Edgewater Hospital in Chicago.

A Diet for Defense

The most powerful protection you can give your immune system is to eat a well-balanced diet containing a variety of fruits, vegetables, whole grains, seeds and nuts, and seafood, says Michelle S. Santos, Ph.D., a research associate at the Jean Mayer USDA Human Nutrition Research Center on Aging at Tufts University in Boston. These foods are high in vitamins, minerals, and other nutrients that can help keep your immune system healthy.

Beyond that general advice, here are the specific nutrients researchers say may boost your immunity.

Vitamin A. This vitamin seems to top the A-list of nutrients that are vital for a strong immune system. Vitamin A deficiency causes damage to the naturally protective mucous membrane barrier of the respiratory tract, and it's thought that bacteria and viruses take advantage of that damage. After a flu virus attacks, for example, the lining of a normal throat will repair itself. Not so in those who are vitamin A-deficient.

"Instead, you might get that once-healthy cell replaced by an abnormal cell," says Charles B. Stephensen, Ph.D., associate professor in the department of international health at the University of Alabama in Birmingham. "That may predispose you to having a more severe episode of an infection or having another infection on top of a viral infection."

The Daily Value (DV) for vitamin A is 5,000 international units. You can get your fill by eating green, leafy vegetables, drinking fortified milk, or, if necessary, taking a supplement.

Beta-carotene. Beta-carotene is the pigment that helps turn carrots, cantaloupe, sweet potatoes, and other fruits and vegetables orange or yellow. But researchers are discovering that this nutrient does a lot more than add color to your favorite produce. In fact, studies have shown that beta-carotene does quite a bit of immune-boosting work of its own.

Researchers in one study found that the number of T-helper cells in male volunteers jumped 30 percent after the men took 180 milligrams (almost 299,000 international units) of beta-carotene a day for 2 weeks. (T-helper cells are important components of the immune system.)

There is no DV for beta-carotene, but nutrition experts generally recommend getting 8,300 to 10,000 international units a day from a combination of foods and a vitamin supplement.

B_6. Research shows that people who don't get enough vitamin B_6 in their diets are likely to have a depressed immune system. You can boost your vitamin B_6 intake by eating chickpeas, prune juice, turkey, potatoes, and bananas. A banana provides 33 percent of your DV of B_6, while an 8-ounce glass of prune juice provides 28 percent.

Vitamin C. The body uses vitamin C to make interferon, a protein that helps destroy viruses in the body. Plus, vitamin C may increase levels of a compound called glutathione, which has also been shown to keep the immune system strong.

In one large study, researchers at the University of Helsinki in Finland reviewed 21 smaller studies that looked at how well vitamin C was able to beat colds. They found that people getting 1,000 milligrams of vitamin C a day were able to shorten the duration of their illnesses and reduce their symptoms by 23 percent.

The DV for vitamin C is 60 milligrams, but many researchers say that 200 milligrams is probably the minimum amount you need to maximize immunity. It's easy to get this much vitamin C in your diet. Half a cantaloupe, for example, has 113 milligrams of vitamin C, while a half-cup of brussels sprouts has 48 milligrams, 80 percent of the DV. Of course, you can also get a lot of vitamin C in citrus fruits, broccoli, rutabagas, radishes, and rose hips tea.

Vitamin E. This vitamin has also gotten a lot of attention for its role in boosting immunity. The body uses vitamin E to produce a powerful immune protein called interleukin-2, which has been shown to tackle everything from bacteria and viruses to cancer cells. In one study, researchers at the Jean Mayer research center at Tufts found that people taking large amounts (800 international units) of vitamin E a day were able to increase their levels of interleukin-2 by 69 percent.

How much vitamin E is enough to create this immune-boosting effect? Experts generally recommend getting 400 to 800 international units a day. There's simply no way to get such large amounts of vitamin E from foods alone, which is why some doctors recommend taking vitamin E supplements.

Reduce Fat, Raise Immunity

Just as eating the right foods can help the immune system stay strong, eating the wrong ones—specifically, those that are high in fat—put it at a disadvantage. "A high-fat diet speeds up the aging of the immune system, although we don't know why," says Dr. Petro. "But we do know that it results in the production of more cell-damaging free radicals."

Studies have shown, in fact, that people who cut back on fat in their diets have a rapid increase in natural killer cell activity, which is a sign of immune-system strength. In one study, researchers at the University of Massachusetts Medical School in Worcester put men on low-fat diets for 3 months. For every 1 percent the men were able to reduce the amounts of fat in their diets, the activity of their natural killer cells went up nearly 1 percent.

It isn't necessary to go on an extremely low-fat diet to boost immunity, Dr. Petro adds. For most people, getting no more than 30 percent of calories from fat—and preferably getting between 20 and 25 percent—is probably ideal.

A lot has been written about strategies for cutting fat, but in fact it's quite simple. Eat fewer processed foods, such as those that come in cans, packets, and boxes. With the exception of canned fruits, beans, and vegetables, many processed foods are often high in fat. Eat more fresh fruits and vegetables, beans, whole-grain breads, and cereals. In addition, switching from whole-fat dairy products to skim milk and low-fat yogurt and cheese and eating less red meat will help bring your fat levels into the safety zone.

MEMORY PROBLEMS

Forget This Myth of Aging

Boy, is this going to be a day. At 10:00 A.M., you have to see Barb about the Bonner project. At 11:00 A.M., it's Bob and the Bagelman account. This afternoon, the boss has booked a briefing with Bonny in Boston about the Bledsoe bookkeeping blowup.

And so you call Barb at 10:00 A.M. to talk about Bonner. But Barry butts in with a bulletin about the Browning building. By then you have to rush to call Bob about the Bledsoe books—or was that Bonny with the Bagelman account? Belinda with Borghoff? Oh, brother. How bad can it get?

A few years ago, you probably could have kept it all straight. But you're having more trouble remembering things now, like birthdays, clients' names, phone numbers. Wait. Isn't forgetfulness a sign that age is creeping up on you?

"There's no doubt, when you forget things, it makes you feel like your mind is slipping away on you," says Douglas Herrmann, Ph.D., a memory researcher at the National Center for Health Statistics in Washington, D.C., and author of *Super Memory*.

But Dr. Herrmann says there's plenty of room for optimism. You may need to pay a little more attention to your memory, but it's probably still fully functional. "In all likelihood, you're not losing your memory," he says. "With a little focus and a little work, your memory will be just as good as it was in your teens and twenties—maybe even better."

Still a Gray Area

Experts still don't really know how we store and recall information. One theory holds that people may keep memories in holographic, three-dimensional form, using networks of neurons and electrochemical reactions to gain access to the system. Researchers do know that you can reach the same memory through a number of different paths. Smells can trigger a memory, as can a familiar sight, word, or phrase.

Be Predictable

Always losing your keys? Designate a spot for them in your house or office. If you put your keys—or glasses or other things—in the same place every day, you'll always know where they are, says Douglas Herrmann, Ph.D., a memory researcher at the National Center for Health Statistics in Washington, D.C., and author of *Super Memory*.

Most scientists break down memory into three parts. First is the working memory, also called the scratch-pad memory. Dr. Herrmann says people use this to recall phone numbers or other information they need for a very short period of time—usually about a minute. Then it's usually just forgotten.

The midrange, or intermediate, memory keeps all the information you've consciously and unconsciously absorbed within the past few hours or days. Eventually, you either forget that stuff because it's not important (what did you have for breakfast 3 days ago?) or transfer it to long-term memory. There you store permanent recollections, such as important addresses and names, Mom's apple pie recipe, and memories of childhood Christmas mornings.

For years, studies kept showing that scratch-pad and midrange memories start declining relatively early in life—even in your forties. But the research was flawed, Dr. Herrmann says. New evidence shows that you probably won't suffer serious memory loss until well into your sixties or seventies, he says.

So why are you forgetting things more than you used to? Stress could be the culprit. "Your ability to concentrate and make decisions, along with short-term memory, may be one of the first areas of mental functioning hit by stress," says Paul J. Rosch, M.D., president of the American Institute of Stress in Yonkers, New York. And try not to worry about forgetting things; Dr. Herrmann says anxiety about memory makes it even harder to remember.

Then there's just plain old sensory overload. When life pulls you five ways at once, Dr. Herrmann says, you're less likely to concentrate on details. "And the less you pay attention, the less you're going to remember," he says.

For most people, memory loss never becomes a serious problem. But some diseases, most notably Alzheimer's, lead to direct memory trouble. If you forget significant appointments at work, can't recall the names of family members or good friends, or become severely disoriented or confused, see a doctor, warns Francis Pirozzolo, M.D., a neuropsychologist at Baylor College of Medicine in Houston.

Hold That Thought

Your brain is not a computer. You can't just run to the store and buy more memory; you have to learn to use what you have.

Fortunately, you already have plenty of storage space. Here's how to take better advantage of it.

Jog your mind. Regular exercise may give you a memory boost. In one study, people who took a 9-week water aerobics class scored better on general memory tests than a similar nonexercising group. "The aerobic exercise may have increased oxygen efficiency to the brain," says the study's coauthor, Richard Gordin, Ph.D., professor in the department of health, physical education, and recreation at Utah State University in Logan.

Dr. Gordin stresses that the results are preliminary. But other studies are coming up with similar findings. And then there are the added benefits of lower risk for heart disease and stroke and all the other helpful side effects of exercise.

Pay attention. This is the most basic—and most forgotten—memory aid. Don't expect to memorize a client's product line while you're talking to another client long distance. Don't expect to remember a person's name if you're thinking about what you're going to have for lunch when you make your introductions.

"It's simple," Dr. Herrmann says. "Focus, focus, focus. If it doesn't register in your brain initially, you have no chance of remembering it." So when there's key information to recall, drop what you're doing and spend a couple of minutes concentrating. Then move to the next task at hand.

Sleep on it. A good night's rest will do wonders for your memory. Research shows that people who are awakened during dream sleep fail to process memories from the day before and thus forget more. Dr. Herrmann also says that regular sleep allows your entire body to recharge, making you more alert and more

Byte Off What You Can Chew

Computers remember information in small pieces, or bytes. That's the best way for you to do it, too, according to Francis Pirozzolo, M.D., a neuropsychologist at the Baylor College of Medicine in Houston.

The process is called chunking. Since your mind remembers items in groups of five to nine, break down lists into segments of that size. It's much easier to remember five groups of 5 items than it is to remember a list of 25 items, Dr. Pirozzolo says. And if you can group similar things together—fruits on one list, paper products on another—you'll do even better.

attentive to detail. "And avoid sleeping pills," he says. "You don't get the same quality sleep, and you're less likely to remember things during the following day."

One more hint: If you're studying or working into the night, go to sleep as soon as you're done. Going out afterward for a drink or a cup of coffee, or staying up to watch the news, makes it harder to remember the information the next day.

Be selective. We have invented telephone books, address books, computer files, pencils, pens, and those little yellow sticky pads—all to help us remember things. So use them. "Why spend time trying to memorize giant shopping lists when you can just write them down?" Dr. Pirozzolo asks. "If you are a busy person with lots to remember, making lists frees up your memory to recall more important items."

Boost your brain with B. The B vitamins are perhaps the most essential nutrients for helping to keep your mind sharp. Your body uses B vitamins to turn food into mental energy and to manufacture and repair your brain tissue. "Deficiencies in thiamin, niacin, and vitamins B_6 and B_{12} can all cause mental dysfunction," says Vernon Mark, M.D., author of *Reversing Memory Loss*. "In fact, pellagra, a niacin deficiency, used to be a leading cause for admissions into state mental hospitals," he explains.

The easiest way to make sure you get enough brain-boosting B vitamins is to eat foods containing enriched grains. One cup of enriched spaghetti, for example, has 0.3 milligram of thiamin, 20 percent of the Daily Value (DV), and 2 milligrams of niacin, 10 percent of the DV. Meat is also a good source of these nutrients. Three ounces of pork tenderloin, for example, provide 0.8 milligram of thiamin, 53 percent of the DV. For niacin, 3 ounces of chicken breast deliver 12 milligrams, 60 percent of the DV.

It's not as easy to get additional amounts of vitamins B_6 and B_{12}, because it's harder for the body to absorb them as you get older. So, it's a good idea to try to

Be a Slow Learner

You'll remember information longer if you absorb it gradually rather than all at once, according to Harry P. Bahrick, Ph.D., professor of psychology at Ohio Wesleyan University in Delaware, Ohio. In an 8-year study, he found that people who practiced their Spanish vocabulary once a month remembered four times more words than people who practiced daily. Dr. Bahrick says the principle works for physical skills, too. "If I was learning how to golf, I'd practice an hour a week for 7 weeks rather than an hour a day for 7 days," he says.

GLAD You Can Remember

You have to buy *g*as, pick up the *l*aundry, get some *a*pples, and make a bank *d*eposit. To remember the list, try forming a word using the first letter of each item—in this case, GLAD. It's called mnemonics, according to Francis Pirozzolo, M.D., a neuropsychologist at the Baylor College of Medicine in Houston. If you convert information into a familiar form, such as a simple word, you're more likely to remember it, he says.

get more than the DV of both of these nutrients. Vitamin B_6 is abundant in baked potatoes, bananas, chickpeas, and turkey. One baked potato provides 0.4 milligram of vitamin B_6, 20 percent of the DV, and one banana provides 0.7 milligram, 35 percent of the DV. For vitamin B_{12}, meat and shellfish are good choices. Three ounces of lean ground beef will provide 2 micrograms of vitamin B_{12}, about a third of the DV. Clams are an incredible source, with 20 steamed clams providing 89 micrograms, 1,483 percent of the DV.

Mind your minerals. There's nothing better for your memory than a balanced, healthy diet with lots of fruits and vegetables, Dr. Herrmann says. There's also some evidence that keeping up your intake of zinc and boron can revive your memory, according to James G. Penland, Ph.D., research psychologist with the U.S. Department of Agriculture's Grand Forks Human Nutrition Research Center in North Dakota. One study showed that women on low-zinc diets scored lower on short-term memory than they did when they got their Daily Value of 12 milligrams. A half-dozen steamed oysters gives you a whopping 76.4 milligrams of zinc. Other good sources include wheat germ, lean meats, and pumpkin and squash seeds.

The same held true for boron, which your body needs in trace amounts. People who ate high-boron diets of about 3 milligrams per day scored higher on tests of attention and memory. That's the same amount you'll find in three apples. Other good boron sources include prunes, dates, raisins, and peanuts.

Dr. Penland points out that these studies show that you're better off with recommended levels of boron and zinc than you are at low levels. But that doesn't mean taking high doses of the two will improve memory further; proving that will take more study.

Can the coffee. Caffeine is a proven memory killer, Dr. Herrmann says. More than one cup during the workday is probably going to overstimulate you and make it harder to concentrate. "It's an out-and-out myth that coffee helps you re-

Tune Out

Are you sometimes forced to remember information amid the chaos at home or work? Practice will help. Turn on the television loudly and then try to concentrate on something else for a few minutes, such as reading a book or memorizing a phone number. This will help you overcome the background noise and pay attention, says Douglas Herrmann, Ph.D., a memory researcher at the National Center for Health Statistics in Washington, D.C., and author of *Super Memory*. You could also try watching two televisions at the same time. That forces you to pay attention only to important information and helps you hone your concentration.

member. It may keep you awake, but by wrecking your sleep you'll remember even less," Dr. Herrmann says.

Smoking causes the same problem with overstimulation, Dr. Herrmann says. And alcohol, even one drink, reduces the ability of individual brain cells to process and store information. Long-term drinking also kills brain cells, Dr. Herrmann says.

Ignore miracle cures. Lots of pills and powders advertise themselves as "miracle memory boosters." They don't work, according to Thomas H. Crook, Ph.D., a clinical psychologist and president of Memory Assessment Clinics, based in Bethesda, Maryland. There has been promising research into memory enhancement drugs, but Dr. Crook says nothing on the market today will help. "They're really just nutritional supplements masquerading as cures," he says.

MENOPAUSAL CHANGES

Reinventing the Change of Life

Though it's a sure signal your body is aging, for many women, menopause is a time of great exuberance. Unfettered by monthly periods or concerns about pregnancy, it's natural to feel a sudden rush of freedom—as though the rest of your life truly is your own.

"There's no more creative force in the world than the menopausal woman with zest," said anthropologist Margaret Mead, who did some of her most exciting work when she was well past her fifties.

Still, the body does undergo a number of physical changes during menopause that can take the zest from the best. Hot flashes, mood swings, and insomnia are just a few of the symptoms many women experience around this time.

For years, women (and their doctors) assumed that the discomfort of menopause was an inevitable part of the process. As it turns out, however, many of the problems of menopause can be controlled or even eliminated simply by improving your nutrition and making other lifestyle changes.

Understanding Menopause

Literally speaking, menopause refers to a woman's last period. Technically, a woman must not have menstruated for an entire year to be menopausal. The average age for menopause in the United States is 51, although women can go through it earlier. About 1 percent of women experience menopause before they reach age 40.

Women who have their ovaries removed during a hysterectomy become menopausal virtually overnight, says Joan Borton, a licensed mental health counselor in Rockport, Massachusetts, and author of *Drawing from the Women's Well: Reflections on the Life Passage of Menopause*. They often feel as if they were propelled into menopause without any preparation. Women who have undergone chemotherapy can also go into early menopause.

In natural menopause, a woman's final period is surrounded by a number of years in which other physical changes occur. This is what is known as perimenopause. It generally begins several years before menstruation ends, says Brian Walsh, M.D., director of the Menopause Clinic at Brigham and Women's Hospital in Boston. During this time, women can experience a whole range of physical changes, including hot flashes, night sweats, sleep difficulties, vaginal dryness, skin changes, hair loss, mood swings, depression, and weight gain. Hot flashes, which are often the symptom of most concern to women who are approaching menopause, affect approximately 75 to 85 percent of women.

All these changes, and the loss of the periods themselves, are triggered by decreasing levels of estrogen and progesterone, two of several hormones produced by the ovaries. As a woman ages, her ovaries do, too; they shrink in size, stop releasing eggs, and produce less hormones.

Your Risks down the Road

When estrogen levels dip, cholesterol rises, which is why women have a higher risk of heart disease after they have passed menopause. Before age 65, one in nine women will experience a heart attack, according to the American Heart Association. After 65, that rate skyrockets to one in three.

Estrogen decline also affects bone strength and quality, placing you at increased risk for osteoporosis, a disease in which bones become brittle and fragile. Osteoporosis results in an estimated 1.5 million fractures per year. One-third of all women over age 65 experience spinal fractures, and one in three women in their nineties fracture their hips (compared with one in six men). Overall, between 25 and 44 percent of women experience fractures after menopause because of the disease.

Planning Ahead

You can't avoid menopause. But there are some things you can do now, before you get there, that can make the whole experience a little easier for you. Menopause doesn't have to be a trying time, and it doesn't have to make you look and feel older. Here's what you can do.

Get a move on it. Exercise is one of the best things women can do ahead of time to fare better during their menopausal years, says Dr. Walsh. Exercise places stress on bone, increasing its density and strength. Women's bones lose density after menopause—at the rate of about 4 to 6 percent in the first 4 to 5 years. So the stronger they are to start off with, the better. Weight-bearing activities such as walking and running are best, experts say. Exercise also helps keep your cholesterol levels down, offering protection against heart disease.

Cut the fat. Get on a nutritious diet low in saturated fat, says Dr. Walsh. This will help reduce cholesterol and the risk of heart disease, he says, both of which go up after menopause. Experts recommend that you keep your fat intake to 25 percent or less of the total calories you consume.

Keep an eye on PMS. If you have premenstrual syndrome, or PMS, keep a log of your symptoms and pay attention to any changes. Sometimes PMS symptoms become far more intense as women enter menopause, and they can serve as a signal for you that you are becoming menopausal, says Ellen Klutznick, Psy.D., a psychologist in private practice in San Francisco who specializes in women's health issues. Some possible changes you might notice are PMS symptoms that last longer than usual and a feeling that your mind is fuzzy, she says. If you notice changes, tell your doctor. She can perform a simple blood test called the FSH test, which measures the amount of FSH, or follicle-stimulating hormone. Before menopause, your body produces enough FSH to help follicles develop and trigger ovulation. At menopause, however, you have fewer follicles, and it takes more FSH to get one to mature and ovulate. So your body pumps out more of the hormone than it used to. If your test shows a high FSH level—say, above 40—that means you are officially in menopause.

Quit smoking. If you stop smoking at a younger age, that can help you experience a gentler menopause, says Dr. Walsh. Smokers are more likely than nonsmokers to have menopausal symptoms, he says. Smokers also have a tendency toward lower bone mass, putting them at greater risk for osteoporosis. Smoking can cause you to experience menopause earlier, experts say. They think it's because nicotine may somehow contribute to the drop in estrogen. So stopping smoking now could delay menopause a bit.

Get your calcium now. While the decrease in bone mass accelerates at menopause, it begins around age 35. After 35, women lose 1 percent of their bone mass per year. So be sure to consume enough calcium. The current Daily Value for adults is 800 milligrams of calcium, but some experts suggest 1,000 milligrams a day for premenopausal women and 1,500 milligrams for postmenopausal women.

Unfortunately, most women consume only about 500 milligrams a day through diet. You can come closer to the protective amounts by adding low-fat dairy products and canned fish with bones (such as salmon) to your daily diet. For example, one serving of low-fat milk gives you 300 milligrams of calcium, and one serving of low-fat yogurt contains 415 milligrams. Three ounces of canned sockeye salmon contains 203 milligrams of calcium, and ½ cup of raw tofu contains 258 milligrams.

Another way to increase your calcium intake is through supplements. The amount that you should take and the type of tablet you use—calcium carbonate, calcium lactate, or calcium citrate—will depend on your individual health needs, so consult your doctor.

Know your cholesterol levels. Get your cholesterol levels checked, says Dr. Walsh. Menopause can cause levels of HDL (high-density lipoprotein) cholesterol, the "good" kind, to decrease and levels of LDL (low-density lipoprotein) cholesterol, the "bad" kind, to rise. So the better your cholesterol profile before menopause, the greater your chances of keeping it low once you hit menopause. Experts say that the best measurement to use is the ratio of total cholesterol to HDL cholesterol. A ratio of less than 3.5 is considered low, between 3.5 and 6.9, moderate, and over 7, high.

Hormone Replacement Therapy— the Natural Way

In conventional hormone replacement therapy (HRT), the estrogen that's given to menopausal women is often collected from the urine of a pregnant horse. That fact alone might prompt you to go another route. You might want to try natural hormones that are manufactured from soybeans and wild yam in the laboratory and are identical to the estrogen and progesterone in the body, says Lauri Aesoph, N.D., a health-care consultant in South Dakota who specializes in helping doctors and their patients find safe and effective ways to integrate natural therapies.

Plant-derived hormones have actually been around and in use for a long time. When compared to HRT, the hormones used in natural hormone replacement (NHR) offer similar relief from symptoms, says Dr. Aesoph. She notes as well that the number and severity of side effects is often lower than with the natural hormones.

When a woman uses NHR as opposed to conventional HRT, she usually takes two or three types of estrogen. These are the same two or three types that a woman's body makes on its own.

Natural hormones are not as strong as those used in HRT, so the dosages prescribed will be stronger. Dr. Aesoph advises that you work closely with your doctor for the first few months, making adjustments as necessary until you find the dose that's right for you. Hormones taken by mouth lose some of their effectiveness because they pass through the digestive system, says Dr. Aesoph. A special type of progesterone, called oral micronized progesterone, solves this problem. Prometrium (a natural oral progesterone pill) is one brand. Some doctors also use natural estrogen or progesterone drops placed under the tongue, which is another way to bypass the digestive tract.

"Many women tolerate and like natural hormones better," says Dr. Aesoph. "So they stick with them, which is just one way that these hormones can be more effective than conventional therapy."

When the Time Comes

If you think you may be entering menopause, or if you're there already, here are some things you can do.

Get support. "The most valuable thing is gathering together with other women," says Borton. By talking with other women, either one-on-one or in support groups, you can learn about various symptoms and gather information about doctors and health care professionals whom other women go to, like, and recommend, she says. "Talking with other women and sharing experiences helps women feel supported and not so isolated," agrees Dr. Klutznick. One option is to join a support group. Call your local hospital to find out about groups in your area. Or talk to other women.

Find the right doctor. Menopause will bring lots of physical changes and lots of questions, particularly about hormone replacement therapy (HRT). HRT is recommended to help replace missing estrogen and keep bones strong. But it is also controversial, mainly because it may increase your risk of certain cancers. "The key is to get a doctor who will work with you—one who will honor your decision," says Borton. Ask your friends about their doctors. And don't be afraid to shop around until you find a doctor you like.

Choose a mentor. Find a woman 10 to 15 years older than you who has been through menopause and whom you admire and respect, says Borton. "Spend time with older women, exploring with them what it is that holds meaning in their lives," she says. "Numbers of us feel that doing this has helped us cross the threshold into seeing ourselves as older women and embrace it in a way that feels really wonderful." In addition to identifying or finding women who can serve as mentors in your day-to-day life, look for older women in the public eye whom you can follow and learn from, she says.

Try some tofu. Soy products such as tofu and tempeh contain large amounts of phytoestrogens, plant compounds that act very much like natural estrogen. Since many of the problems of menopause are caused by low levels of estrogen, it makes sense that replacing some of the estrogen will make you healthier. In fact, research has shown that eating more soy foods can help bring down cholesterol levels and the risk of heart disease.

Fight hot flashes with food. Here, too, the phytoestrogens in soy can help. In Asian countries, where soy foods predominate, only about 16 percent of the women have a problem with hot flashes. Compare that to 75 percent of women in this country. And it's not only soybeans that help. Black beans and ground flaxseed are other good sources of phytoestrogens. You don't have to eat a lot of phytoestrogen-rich foods to get the benefits. Just 2 ounces of tofu or tempeh a day can help prevent hot flashes. Or you could have a bowl of miso soup, which is flavored with a salty condiment made from soybeans and salt.

Keep it cool. If you're bothered by hot flashes and food treatments aren't doing the trick, it can help to dress in layers and to keep the environment cool, experts say. Some women suck on ice cubes and drink cold liquids or visualize themselves walking in the snow or swimming in a clear lake. Hot liquids and spicy foods can trigger hot flashes, so keep those to a minimum.

Stay lubricated. The decrease in estrogen that women experience with menopause can cause vaginal dryness. The elasticity and size of the vagina changes, and the walls become thinner and lose their ability to become moist. This can make sex painful or even undesirable, says Dr. Klutznick. Surveys indicate that this happens in 8 to 25 percent of postmenopausal women. While premenopausal women can generally lubricate in 6 to 20 seconds when aroused, it can take 1 to 3 minutes for a postmenopausal woman.

Women can stay lubricated by using water-based vaginal lubricants such as K-Y jelly, Replens, and Astroglide, which are available over the counter, says Dr. Klutznick. Steer clear of oil-based lubricants such as petroleum jelly; studies indicate that they don't dissolve as easily in the vagina and can therefore trigger vaginal infections. HRT can also help alleviate the problem, says Dr. Klutznick.

Stay sexually active. Studies indicate that women who stay sexually active experience fewer vaginal changes than those who don't. Sexual activity promotes circulation in the vaginal area, which helps it stay moist. For women without partners, masturbation helps promote circulation and moistness in the vagina, she says.

METABOLISM CHANGES

A Different Kind of Energy Crisis

Remember when you could diet for a few days and drop an easy 10 pounds? Well, nowadays it's not so easy. Oh, sure, you're eating less than you did back in your twenties and making a habit of passing on dessert and that midafternoon candy bar. But for some reason, you're a few sizes larger. And the pounds are piling on.

Here's what's happening: Your metabolism—how your body converts food into energy and then burns that energy as calories—is slowing down. This is a natural process that begins at about age 30. From then on, your body burns energy about 2 to 4 percent slower every 10 years. So fewer calories are burned, and more are stored as fat. You can see that if you do nothing to counter this trend, you'll become heavier and less energetic. And you'll put yourself at greater risk for serious health problems such as high blood pressure and heart disease. Hardly a recipe for a youthful life.

For women, some of what's happening is beyond control. Women naturally burn calories slower than men do. And women's bodies also have a higher fat content than men's, with the percentage of body fat inevitably increasing with time.

But man or woman, "metabolism changes are a direct response to changes in body composition," says Robert Kushner, M.D., director of the Nutrition and Weight Control Clinic at the University of Chicago. "As we age, we tend to lose muscle and gain fat. Since muscle burns a lot of energy, our energy needs diminish as we lose muscle, and our metabolism slows."

Unfortunately, most of us develop habits that tend to intensify the problem. Yes, we lose some muscle as we age, but "the major cause of this muscle loss is inactivity," says Eric T. Poehlman, Ph.D., associate professor of medicine at the University of Maryland at Baltimore Department of Medicine. "The more inactive we become with age, the less lean muscle we have. The less lean muscle we have,

The Male Advantage

Did you ever wonder why men can eat twice as much as women and hardly gain a pound? Call it biological sexism: The average man burns calories more efficiently than the average woman—and over the same amount of time and with the same amount of physical activity, he'll lose more weight than you will.

Men burn calories faster for two reasons. One, they are usually heavier and are burning more calories all the time. Two, they have a greater proportion of fat-burning muscle. As a result, the average basal metabolic rate in women is 5 to 10 percent lower than in men.

Men are also more likely to put on fat around the belly, which happens to be the easiest location to lose fat. But thanks to estrogen, women tend to carry fat in the thighs, hips, and buttocks—those hard-to-slim-down spots. This further slows down metabolism.

Estrogen plays another role in metabolism, because it also influences a woman's appetite. Researchers have observed that food intake drops at the time of ovulation, when estrogen levels are at their peak, then increases in the second half of the menstrual cycle.

the more inactive we become. Over the years, the two feed on each other, and our metabolism plummets."

How do you break out of this trap? Unless you have thyroid disease, which can play havoc with how your body burns energy, you can get your metabolism cranked up again by making some lifestyle changes. But first, here's what's going on inside.

Overfueled and Underactive

Add up all the energy needed to power the activities in a resting body—everything from breathing and digestion to the activity of nerve cells during thinking—and you have your basal metabolic rate, the minimum energy requirement you need to stay alive. For most women, this is about 1,000 to 1,200 calories per day; for most men, around 1,800 calories per day.

Your total calorie needs per day consist of your basil metabolic rate, plus the calories you need to power your additional activities—everything from playing jacks with your kid to jumping jacks in aerobics.

This means, of course, that two people may have the same basal metabolic rate but burn very different amounts of calories every day. For example, a very active 125-pound woman can easily burn 2,200 calories a day, while a sedentary 125-pound type can barely burn 1,750.

Which takes us to the punchline of this brief lesson in calories—the metabolic formula for not gaining weight. Calories in must equal calories out. The calories that aren't "out" are stored in your body as fat. But if you burn more calories than you take in, stored fat is burned, and you lose weight.

So the way to not gain weight as you get older is simple: Cut back on calories. Pretend you like rice cakes. You know the routine. But there's a small problem. Your body doesn't know you're on a diet; it thinks you're starving to death. So instead of burning fat, your metabolism goes into famine mode, trying to preserve your fat stores.

"Very low calorie dieting can decrease your basal metabolic rate by 15 to 30 percent, making weight loss even more difficult," says Dr. Kushner. A very low calorie diet is one that consists of fewer than 600 calories a day. Because your body is trying to save you by keeping your fat level intact, it chooses another source of fuel: muscle. You've heard the phrase "Diets don't work." Now you know why.

Your metabolic rate doesn't return to normal after you stop dieting, because your body thinks another famine might be around the corner. Dieting actually prevents long-term, permanent weight loss.

And dieters typically add one more insult to metabolic injury: They cut calories without paying much attention to what kind of calories they're cutting. One gram of fat contains twice the calories of one gram of carbohydrates—and carbohydrates have the added benefit of burning faster than fats. So instead of cutting back on calories across the board, you'd be better off not cutting calories and maintaining a low-fat, high-carbohydrate diet that emphasizes fruits, vegetables, pasta, and grains. "The fat you eat is much more likely to become the fat you carry," says Dr. Kushner.

Exercise: Your Metabolism's Best Friend

Okay, dieting isn't the answer. So what can you do when your age causes your body's metabolism to shift into a lower, slower gear?

Exercise.

Aerobic exercise—walking, riding a stationary bike, aerobic dancing, any activity that boosts your heart rate for 20 minutes or more—is the best way to burn calories. And the benefits of exercise just keep going and going. Exercise sets your metabolism at a higher rate, so calories are incinerated for hours after you've stopped.

But the best way to boost your metabolism is to participate in an aerobic activity and a regular period of a strength-training exercise, such as weight lifting. "The major reason one person burns 1 calorie per minute and another burns 1.5 is that the second person has more muscle mass, and muscle is an extremely energy-hungry tissue," says Dr. Poehlman. "Strength-building exercises such as

What's Your Calorie DV?

If you knew exactly how many calories your body burns in the course of a day—your Daily Value (DV)—you'd know how many calories you need to eat to maintain or lose weight. Here's a handy formula for balancing your energy equation.

First, multiply your weight by 10. This is your basal metabolic rate, the minimum number of calories that you need to keep your system running.

Next, determine your activity level from the table below and multiply your basal metabolic rate by the appropriate percentage. This gives you the additional calories you require for the day.

Sedentary activity refers to the time you spend sitting around the house watching television, reading your favorite magazine, or talking on the phone. Light activity includes things such as housework, cooking, and a stroll around the block after dinner. Moderate activity includes swimming or walking at a brisk pace while able to talk without gasping for breath. Strenuous activity includes heart-pounding exercise such as running or aerobics.

weight lifting will add muscle mass at any age. And the more you do such exercises, the better for your metabolism."

To prove that point, Dr. Poehlman and his associates measured the basal metabolic rates of 96 people: 36 did aerobic activity, 18 did weight lifting, and 42 did nothing. The aerobic group had a 13 percent higher metabolic rate than the sedentary group; the strength group's metabolic rate was 18 percent higher than the sedentary group's.

This study, says Dr. Poehlman, shows that either aerobic exercise or strength training may provide a metabolic boost.

Maximize Your Metabolism

Convinced that exercise is the best way to beat the middle-age bulge? Here's what you can do to rev your engine.

Step up the pace. An easy way to burn more calories in the same amount of time is to put a little more speed into your current aerobic workout. Suppose you're a walker who covers a mile in about 15 minutes (about 4 miles per hour), burning roughly 365 calories per hour (or about 90 calories per mile). If you bump

Activity Level	Percentage
Sedentary	30–50
Light	55–65
Moderate	65–70
Strenuous	75–100

Add these two numbers together, and you have your total calorie needs for the day. If you're a 120-pound woman whose daily activity level is on the low end of the strenuous scale, you would need 2,100 calories.

$$120 \times 10 = 1,200$$
$$1,200 \times 0.75 = 900$$
$$1,200 + 900 = 2,100$$

This figure is only an estimate, however. Your metabolism can be measured much more accurately by an exercise physiologist or a physician specializing in weight loss and metabolism.

up your speed to a 12-minute mile (5 miles per hour), your calorie burn increases to about 585 for the same hour. That's a bonus of 27 calories a mile. That extra calorie burn each day can translate to a weight loss of about 15 pounds in less than a year.

Go longer. If you're already working out at your top speed, don't go any faster, but try to go longer. "Just like a car, your body will burn more fuel—in this case, fat—the longer it is engaged in an activity," says Dr. Kushner.

Work your arms and legs. Exercises that vigorously use both arms and legs are better fat burners than those that involve only your legs. "Cross-country skiing rates highest in lab tests for burning the most calories per minute because you're using your legs, upper body, and even your torso," says Wayne Westcott, Ph.D., strength-training consultant for the International Association of Fitness Professionals. Stationary rowers and bikes with moving hand levers also rate high.

Start your day with breakfast. Experts say your body burns calories at a slower rate as you sleep. Breakfast acts as your metabolism's wakeup call, kicking it into the calorie-burning mode. If you don't eat something in the morning, you may ultimately burn fewer calories during the day. And it's more likely that when you do eat, you'll grab the first high-fat snack you see.

Spread out your meals. Eating small meals throughout the day instead of your standard three squares may be better for fat burning. After you eat, your body releases the hormone insulin, which causes your body to store fat. The larger the meal, the more insulin your body releases. But smaller, more frequent meals keep insulin levels lower and more stable. The less insulin you have in your blood, the more fat you burn, and the less you store.

Don't skip meals. Skipping meals and then eating one big meal at night can be a triple whammy, says Dr. Kushner. First, it puts you into a slow burn mode during the day. Second, the big meal provides an energy overload: The body can metabolize only so much food at one time, so the excess is likely to become fat. Third, most of the metabolizing will take place while you sleep—when your metabolic rate is at its lowest.

Exercise after you eat. A moderate workout right after a meal gives you a fat-burning bonus. A brisk 3-mile walk on an empty stomach burns about 300 calories. But walking on a full stomach will burn about 345 calories. That's because eating gives your metabolism a boost; add exercise, and your metabolism gets a double boost and burns even more calories.

Spice up your life. Keeping an eye on your metabolism doesn't mean you have to give up tasty foods. In fact, hot, spicy foods such as mustard and chili may even shift your metabolism into high gear for a short period. In a study by British researchers, spicy food was shown to increase basal metabolic rate by an average of 25 percent.

Stay away from stimulants. Caffeine, alcohol, and other stimulants may raise your metabolic rate, but once they're out of your system, your metabolism crashes back to normal or below. The wise move, says Dr. Poehlman, is to avoid any artificial means of raising your metabolism unless it's prescribed by a doctor.

Have your thyroid checked. An underactive thyroid causes the body to burn energy at a slower rate than normal, and an overactive thyroid has the opposite effect. More women than men have thyroid disease. So if you suspect yours is out of whack, have it checked by your doctor. If a thyroid hormone deficiency exists, it can often be regulated with prescription drugs.

MIDLIFE CRISIS

It Doesn't Happen to Everybody

For years you've balanced career and family with the grace of a dancer. You waltzed around worries and pirouetted past problems. But now this choreography seems out of touch with your life.

You suddenly feel old, uncertain, and vulnerable: "Who am I?" "Why am I here?" "Where am I going with my life?"

You're questioning career choices, re-evaluating commitments to friends and family, worrying about fading looks, and mourning the passage of youth.

Welcome to a midlife crisis—that uncomfortable time when you no longer feel secure about your life as it is, and you can't look backward without regret or look forward without foreboding.

"There are three wakeup calls in midlife. First, you realize that you're not going to live forever. Second, you realize you're never going to be president of the company, or if you are president of the company, you're not enjoying it as much as you thought you would. Finally, you realize your family life doesn't look like *Ozzie and Harriet*," says Ross Goldstein, Ph.D., a San Francisco psychologist and author of *Fortysomething: Claiming the Power and Passion of Your Midlife Years*. "That's the drumbeat of midlife, and the question is, what do you do about it?"

How you cope with those realizations can literally make you feel older or younger than your years, says Leonard Felder, Ph.D., a psychologist in Los Angeles and author of *A Fresh Start: How to Let Go of Emotional Baggage and Enjoy Your Life Again*.

"Some people become more discouraged because they realize that they've set some goals they're having trouble following through on or made choices they're not comfortable living with," Dr. Felder explains. "But many who go through a midlife crisis get motivated to do what they've always wanted to, and that gives them more energy and a greater sense of being alive."

Beyond the Myths

Although most of us will experience some degree of anxiety and upheaval between the ages of 30 and 60, the average woman doesn't suddenly dash to a fat farm, have plastic surgery, take up belly dancing, buy a fur coat, or have an affair with her tennis instructor. And the middle-age man doesn't suddenly dye his hair, buy a fire-engine red sports car, change careers, and start cheating on his wife.

Instead of a complete overhaul, midlife for most people is like a minor tuneup, says Gilbert Brim, Ph.D., a social psychologist and director of the John D. and Catherine T. MacArthur Foundation Research Network on Successful Midlife Development, headquartered in Vero Beach, Florida.

So instead of starting over, a typical person may make a subtle change, such as taking up volunteer work, beginning a fitness program to tone up an aging body, or getting finances in order for the first time, Dr. Goldstein says.

"Most people look at midlife challenges as an opportunity," Dr. Brim says. "They tell us things like, 'Yeah, I got fired, but that wasn't a crisis. It was a chance to get a better job' or 'Yes, my mother died, and I miss her, but it was a release of a burden.'"

In fact, only about 10 percent of people go through what we view as a midlife crisis, Dr. Brim says in his book *Ambition: How We Manage Success and Failure throughout Our Lives*. And researchers suspect as few as half of them suffer severe psychological symptoms such as confusion, anxiety, suicidal thoughts, substance abuse, and doubts about family choices and career. Most of those who do have problems during middle age also had difficulty handling stress and trauma at other times in their lives.

"If you had chronic troubles in your relationships or on the job earlier in your life, you're more likely to have trouble dealing with midlife events," Dr. Brim says.

Some psychologists even see similarities between adolescence and midlife. "At both times, everything gets tossed in the air, and you find yourself rebelling against the phase of your life that just occurred. So if you're 16, you don't want to be treated like a 12-year-old. If you are 40 and want to take a leading role in the business, you don't want to be treated like a junior partner. In both instances, you want a new relationship with the people around you," says Edward Monte, Ph.D., director of the Couple and Family Therapy Program at the Crozer Chester Medical Center in Upland, Pennsylvania.

Midlife crisis isn't believed to be linked to hormonal changes. In fact, at least 40 common stressful midlife events, including death of a parent, divorce, and job change, can combine to unleash a crisis, Dr. Brim says. But however it occurs, it does change how you see yourself and the world, Dr. Felder says.

"Somewhere between ages 40 and 50, people begin to see life differently," Dr. Felder says. "Instead of seeing the years since birth, they being to consider how many years they have left. They develop a real sense of time urgency. That can be extremely depressing or highly motivating."

Damage Control

A midlife transition doesn't occur overnight and navigating through it can take years, Dr. Monte says. But if you prepare yourself, you can sail through just fine.

"You can come through midlife feeling better about yourself, more alive, and younger in some ways," Dr. Goldstein says. "Midlife is an opportunity to have a new beginning. It's a chance to pursue some of the dreams, passions, and hopes you didn't have time to explore at earlier points in your life."

Here are a few ways to avoid a crisis and help you make a smooth midlife transition.

Rediscover the wonder years. What did you like to do as a child? If you had a favorite book when you were young, reread it. If you liked to play field hockey or baseball, go to a high school game. "It may sound silly, but it has a real psychological purpose," says Susan Olson, Ph.D., director of psychological services at the Southwest Bariatric Nutrition Center in Tempe, Arizona. "Doing these childlike things will help you realize that you really don't have to mourn your youth because it's still within you to a certain extent. Once you realize that, your energy levels will literally surge."

Get a little help from your friends. Contact your best friend from high school or college, Dr. Olson suggests. "It will rekindle old feelings and bring perspective to your current life," she says. "It may help you realize that you're mourning a time that wasn't as ideal as you once believed."

Do lunch. Take at least one person who you know has been through a midlife crisis to lunch. Ask her which of the urges she resisted and which ones she followed through on and why, Dr. Felder recommends. It may give you some insight into your own situation.

Keep a half-full glass. Think positive, because being older can be neat, says Stanley Teitelbaum, Ph.D., a clinical psychologist in private practice in New York City. Instead of concentrating on lost energy or sex appeal, consider what you have now that you didn't have at 20, such as a satisfying career, a loving marriage, a supportive family, or independence. "Life really does begin at 40 for many people. Yes, you're older, but the things you have now may outweigh or counteract the things you had in the past," he says.

Switch gears. One good way to be a leader, help others, and build your self-esteem is to become a role model to others—whether it's a young colleague at work or your own children. A woman who is an editor at a daily newspaper could help a young female reporter polish her writing skills and groom herself for a future management position. "Instead of being the star of the show, why not get satisfaction from helping others shine in the spotlight?" Dr. Teitelbaum says.

Share your feelings. People who express their feelings will do better during midlife than those who clam up. In fact, if you can't articulate what you want from your relationship, you're likely to destroy it.

Arrange a time each week to discuss your feelings in a nonthreatening way.

The Telltale Signs

Are you heading for a midlife crisis? To find out, we asked Ross Goldstein, Ph.D., a San Francisco psychologist and author of *Fortysomething: Claiming the Power and Passion of Your Midlife Years*, to develop this test. Answer the following statements yes or no. Scoring follows.

1. My future looks as positive now as it always has.
2. My life is as rewarding to me as I expected it to be.
3. Security is becoming more important to me.
4. Sometimes I feel excitement is missing in my life.
5. I am more flexible in my values today than I was 10 years ago.
6. I get angry about the struggle to find "satisfaction" in life.
7. It feels like time is running out on me.
8. I wish there were an effective way of making all the tension and stress go away.
9. I am more sure of who I am today than ever before.
10. Balancing my work and family is becoming more difficult.
11. Sometimes I feel exhausted from the struggle of "making it."
12. I have a hard time accepting that I am as old as I am.
13. I miss the excitement and adventure of my earlier years.
14. My work is as satisfying as it has always been.
15. I am more aware of my health as I grow older.

Give yourself two points for each "yes" to questions 3, 4, 6, 7, 8, 10, 11, 12, 13, and 15 and two points for each "no" answer to questions 1, 2, 5, 9, and 14. Total your score.

0 to 8. Your life is running smoothly. Your philosophy: If it isn't broke, why fix it?

10 to 16. Occasionally, you yearn for a day at the beach, but in general, you feel secure and comfortable with your life. Your outlook: You're ready to make a few minor midlife course adjustments, but you don't yearn to sail off to Tahiti with a co-worker.

18 or more. Who is that worn-out person in the mirror, and why is she still working at a job that seems as grueling as watching an IRS agent audit a tax return? Your dilemma: How to make significant changes in your life without sacrificing the best of what you have. Career counseling may help.

If, for example, you fantasize about other people, you might say, "I love you, and I'm attracted to my co-worker. It doesn't mean I love you less, but maybe it means something is missing in our relationship. Can we talk about it?" Dr. Monte explains: "The key is to discuss the topic in a way that doesn't cause either of you to panic and think your relationship is doomed."

Say happy birthday to you. Say your 40th birthday is approaching. Stop dreading it, Dr. Goldstein says. Instead, embrace the moment. Rituals such as birthdays, anniversaries, and class reunions help us unleash feelings, reflect on who we are, and where we are going in life. Use these natural pauses to rest, observe the vista, chart or correct your course, and move on, he suggests. It's also an excellent time to share feelings and seek the support of family and friends.

Don't panic. "Making impulsive decisions during the midlife almost always ends up creating a bigger mess and, in some cases, disaster," Dr. Felder says. "If you think you need to resolve these midlife issues in the next 2 weeks, you're not going to get happy solutions. You need a plan that will allow you 6 months or a year to experiment with new options and that has room in it for you to stumble and fall at least a couple of times."

To get started, take a sheet of paper and divide it into three columns, Dr. Olson suggests. In the first column, list the goals you had as a child, such as "I want to be on the Supreme Court." In the second column, write down which of those goals you should abandon, such as "I'll never be a judge." In the last column, list new goals that you'd like to accomplish in the next 5 years, such as "I'd like to resign from my firm and start my own private practice."

OSTEOPOROSIS

When Bones Lose
Their Strength

Your bones seem like steel girders—strong, permanent, a structure you can depend on.

But for 1 in every 4 women and 1 in 10 men, this skeletal structure is eroding, the girders weakening and wearing away.

The cause is osteoporosis.

Osteoporosis is a disease of thinning bones, fractured hips, and hunched spines, a disease of aging. Everybody loses some bone over time, usually at the rate of 1 percent a year. But in people with osteoporosis, the loss is a lot faster than normal, and bones can become so brittle and fragile that they break when you step off a curb or bump your hip on the edge of a table. In fact, the bones in your spine—your vertebrae—can even break under their own weight.

These fractures might be painless or misinterpreted as muscle problems—at least at first. "A person may have back pain that hurts for a while and then goes away. She may attribute it to a muscle spasm when she really has a compression fracture," says Clifford Rosen, M.D., director of the Maine Center for Osteoporosis Research and Education in Bangor.

Osteoporosis is particularly a problem if you're a woman because you have less bone to start with, and during menopause, there's a dropoff in the production of the female hormone estrogen, which holds calcium in your bones like a dam.

Fortunately, this is also a disease that you can prevent—if you understand the causes and take the right steps today.

Are You a Candidate?

If you're a woman whose mother has osteoporosis, you may also be prone to these frightening fractures, says Dr. Rosen. "Up to 70 percent of your peak bone mass, which you reach in your twenties, is determined by heredity," he says. Very small or thin women are also more susceptible to osteoporosis, he adds, since they have less bone mass than other women.

One of the other big causes of osteoporosis—for women and men—is too little calcium in the diet. Although estimates of how many people are short on this basic bone-building nutrient vary from 10 to 25 percent, experts agree that calcium deficiency is extremely common. Another nutrient vital to bone health is vitamin D, because it aids in the absorption of calcium. If you're not getting enough vitamin D, your body won't be able to take advantage of even generous amounts of calcium.

Even if your diet is in good shape, if you don't get the right kind of exercise, your bones may become more porous—and more easily broken.

Heavy smoking or a drinking habit also can contribute to osteoporosis, as can certain prescription medicines, which may also erode bone strength, particularly if taken for many years or in extremely high doses.

What's Your Risk?

It's not difficult to evaluate your risk of developing osteoporosis, says Susan Allen, M.D., Ph.D., assistant professor of internal medicine at the University of Missouri-Columbia School of Medicine. Start with the following questions.

1. Do you have a small, thin frame, or are you Caucasian or Asian?
2. Do you have relatives with osteoporosis?
3. If you're a woman, have you reached menopause or had an early or surgically induced menopause?
4. Do you take high doses of thyroid medication or cortisonelike drugs for asthma, arthritis, or cancer?
5. Do you avoid eating many dairy products and other sources of calcium?
6. Are you not getting regular weight-bearing exercise such as brisk walking?
7. Do you smoke cigarettes or drink alcohol heavily?

If you answered yes to two or more of these questions, your risk for developing osteoporosis is high, Dr. Allen says. It's time to talk to your doctor about developing a lifelong prevention plan.

Healthy Habits for Life and Limb

The good news is that the right exercise and diet choices can put a check on osteoporosis. And even if you're getting a late start, you can take steps to halt further bone loss at any age.

Here's how to beef up your bones.

Pump up your calcium. Calcium is to your bones what air is to your lungs—the element they need to be healthy. Ninety-nine percent of the calcium in your diet goes straight to your bones. If you don't get enough calcium, you can't make enough bone—it's as simple as that.

Women should get at least 1,000 milligrams before menopause and 1,500 milligrams after menopause. Men need about 1,000 milligrams of calcium a day throughout their lives. Although eating the right foods is the best way to get calcium, what matters most is that you take in the recommended amount, says Dr. Rosen. If that's through food, fine; if it's through a combination of food and calcium supplements, fine. Just make sure the numbers add up.

Ounce for ounce, milk and milk products are the best sources of dietary calcium. One 8-ounce serving of nonfat yogurt provides about 450 milligrams of calcium. One cup of skim milk offers more than 300 milligrams. Many other foods contain calcium, but the nutrient isn't as easily absorbed from these foods as it is from dairy products.

If you decide to take a calcium supplement, choose one that's in the form of citrate or aspartate. These are easiest for your body to absorb, says Samantha Brody, N.D., a naturopathic doctor specializing in women's health in Portland, Oregon.

Don't forget the D. Vitamin D helps your body process calcium. Without enough vitamin D, your body absorbs about 10 percent of the calcium it takes in; with vitamin D, it can absorb 80 to 90 percent, says Michael F. Holick, M.D., Ph.D., director of the Vitamin D, Skin and Bone Research Laboratory at Boston University Medical Center. "Vitamin D tells the small intestine 'Here comes the calcium. Open up and let it in,'" explains Dr. Holick. The recommended amount of vitamin D is 5 micrograms or 200 international units per day—easily found in fortified foods such as milk, breads, and cereals.

Besides getting some of your daily vitamin D through food, your body can make it from sunshine, which triggers a vitamin D manufacturing process in your skin. Five to 15 minutes of bright sunshine every day, before you apply sunscreen, will fill most people's needs, says Dr. Rosen. But if you live north of New York City, you can't depend on the sun. In that case, you'll need to be sure you're getting enough vitamin D from dietary sources.

Maximize magnesium. Magnesium transports calcium to bones and also helps convert vitamin D to its active form in the body. To figure out how much magnesium you need, just take your calcium dose and divide it in half, suggests Lorilee Schoenbeck, N.D., a naturopathic doctor with the Champlain Centers for Natural Medicine in Shelburne and Middlebury, Vermont. If you're taking 1,000 milligrams of calcium, for instance, you should take about 500 milligrams of magnesium.

The form of magnesium that your body is best able to absorb is magnesium aspartate, says Dr. Brody.

Review your medication. Certain medications—thyroid medications; anti-inflammatory steroids such as hydrocortisone (Locoid), cortisone (Cortone Acetate), and prednisone (Key-Pred 50); anticonvulsants such as phenytoin (Dilantin), depressants such as phenobarbital (Barbita); and the diuretic furosemide (Lasix)—can cause osteoporosis, particularly when they're taken regularly in high doses over a number of years. Thyroid medications in normal doses should pose no problem, however, says Dr. Rosen, and the risk from diuretics can be offset by taking additional calcium. The most serious osteoporosis risk is from steroids, Dr. Rosen says. If you require long-term steroid medication, your doctor may recommend additional anti-osteoporosis medication such as calcitonin (Cibacalcin) or hormone replacement therapy in addition to calcium and vitamin D supplements, he says.

Add something special. Vitamin K is a bit of a forgotten vitamin. It certainly doesn't get much mention in the media, but it's very important for maintaining bone health. It helps reduce the amount of calcium you lose through urine, says Dr. Schoenbeck.

Vitamin K is also crucial to the formation of osteocalcin, a protein that is the matrix upon which calcium is put into the bone. "Vitamin K is kind of like the foundation that calcium builds on," Dr. Schoenbeck says.

The Daily Value for vitamin K is 80 micrograms. Since this vitamin is abundant in green leafy vegetables and whole grains, a diet rich in these foods may supply you with your daily quota.

Boost your boron. Boron, a trace mineral that is found in many vegetables and fruits, helps reduce the amount of calcium and possibly magnesium that you excrete in your urine. It may also help to slightly raise estrogen levels, which could prevent bone loss as well, says Dr. Schoenbeck. Because of that same estrogen-increasing property, however, women with breast cancer should avoid it, she says. A safe daily amount for women with no breast cancer history is 3 milligrams, says Dr. Schoenbeck.

Go easy on alcohol. "Alcohol actually poisons the cells that build bone," says Susan Allen, M.D., Ph.D., assistant professor of internal medicine at the University of Missouri-Columbia School of Medicine. A beer or glass of wine now and then probably won't cause you much harm. But avoid drinking to excess, she says—more than two to three drinks a day.

Don't smoke. Yes, here's yet another way that smoking can harm your health. It lowers your levels of estrogen for women and testosterone for men, says Barbara S. Levine, Ph.D., associate clinical professor of nutrition in medicine and director of the Calcium Information Center at Cornell University Medical College in New York City. And lower levels of these essential hormones mean less protection against bone loss.

Spine-Strengthening Exercises

Doing exercises that stretch your spine as straight as possible will strengthen the vertebrae most vulnerable to osteoporosis. Try these back extension exercises suggested by Susan Allen, M.D., Ph.D., assistant professor of internal medicine at the University of Missouri-Columbia School of Medicine.

"Do as many of these exercises as you can, once in the morning and once at night," says Dr. Allen.

• Lie on your back with your knees bent. Bring both knees as close as possible to your chest and hold (with your hands supporting your knees) for 5 seconds, then lower your feet slowly to the floor. Then bring one knee up to your chest as far as you can, hold for 5 seconds, and lower it slowly to the floor. Alternate right and left legs for 10 repetitions each.

• Lie on your back with your knees bent. Press the small of your back against the floor and hold for 5 seconds. Repeat 10 times.

• Lie on your back with your knees bent. Place your arms across your middle, cupping the opposite elbow with each hand. Raise your head and shoulders as far as you can without sitting up. Hold for 3 seconds. Repeat 10 times.

• Lie on your back with your legs straight and your arms at your sides. Raise your head and shoulders as far as you can without sitting up. Hold for 3 seconds. Repeat 10 times.

Interior Bodybuilding

An exercise program not only builds muscle, it strengthens your bones, too. And it improves your agility and reflexes so you're less likely to fall and break a bone, says Dr. Allen. Here are the best ways to exercise your bones.

Take up a weight-bearing exercise. To strengthen bones, you need activities in which you're bearing weight on your bones, Dr. Allen says. Weight-bearing exercises include brisk walking, jogging, and dancing. These actually stimulate bone cells to build more bone, particularly in your back and hips, where you most need it, Dr. Allen says.

You're doing a weight-bearing exercise if your feet are hitting the ground with at least the impact that brisk walking produces, says Dr. Rosen. "Basically, you can count on any exercise that makes heavy use of gravity," he says. "Swimming doesn't, for example, but most aerobics classes and tennis do."

Pump some iron. Lifting weights is also an ideal way to build bone strength, because it increases the weight of gravity on your bones. Any lifting done in a standing position is particularly helpful for the spine and hips.

Work out regularly. Once you've found the weight-bearing exercises you like, keep at them for 30 minutes to 1 hour three to four times a week, Dr. Allen says.

Concentrate on the back and hips. If you're exercising for weight loss and muscle tone, you're probably doing something for your upper body, and that's good. But remember, says Dr. Allen, the bones that are most vulnerable to osteoporosis are the hips and the spinal vertebrae in the mid- to lower back. Walking, jogging, and aerobic dancing are particularly helpful for your back and hips, she says.

OVERWEIGHT

Getting Yourself Down to Size

See that slender woman leading the aerobics class? There used to be 200 pounds on her five-foot-five frame. Can you believe it?

Those were heavy days for Karen Faye, a nurse who got in shape and is now the owner of Body Basics Aerobics Workout in Tyngsboro, Massachusetts.

"I was mentally and physically exhausted all the time, which just added to the burden of being overweight," she recalls. Like many women, she struggled with her weight from adolescence on. "I remember that when I was 16 and went to the beach with my mother, the boys whistled at my mother, not at me. I didn't feel like the young person I was supposed to be."

That feeling of being older than her years stayed with her well into adulthood, for as long as she was overweight, Faye says. "Mentally, I was a young person—I had three little children and a thin husband who could still fit into his Marine uniform. But physically, I felt like my own grandmother, and I couldn't believe what was happening to me. I felt the real me was trapped in an older person's body."

For years, Faye thought that her thyroid problem was the cause of her weight. But when she hit 200 pounds, she says, "I saw the handwriting on the artery wall. And it was my artery." She went on a low-fat eating and exercise regimen. Within 8 months, she lost 80 pounds, became fit for the first time in her life, and has maintained her weight for more than a decade.

After she got her weight under control, she became a fitness consultant and opened Body Basics Aerobics Workout. In August 1993, she won the physical fitness award at the Mrs. United States pageant, competing with some women who were nearly 20 years younger.

As Faye knows, being overweight is a burden on body and soul. You feel you've lost your youth and vitality. And you've opened yourself up to ailments of aging such as heart disease, high blood pressure, diabetes, arthritis, and high cholesterol—not to mention the backaches and other pains caused by carrying around more than you should.

There is a cancer connection as well. "When you're overweight, you also have increased risk for several cancers, including cancer of the endometrium, uterus, cervix, ovaries, and gallbladder," says John Foreyt, Ph.D., director of the Nutrition Research Clinic at Baylor College of Medicine in Houston.

Bigger Isn't Better

Of the age-related diseases, high blood pressure has a strong link to being overweight. When a heart has to work overtime to carry extra pounds, blood pressure shoots skyward. The Framingham Heart Study, which followed over 5,200 healthy men and women in Framingham, Massachusetts, from 1948 to the present, found that overweight people who pared their pounds lowered their blood pressure readings dramatically. A 15 percent decrease in weight resulted in a 10 percent decrease in blood pressure.

Type 2 diabetes is also tied to being overweight. Carrying those extra pounds directly affects the body's ability to utilize blood sugar. Many overweight people with diabetes who need regular medication find that once they drop 20 or more pounds, they may also drop their prescriptions.

The connection between overweight and arthritis is fairly obvious: The more pounds you carry, the more pressure you put on your joints. The Framingham Knee Osteoarthritis Study, using data gathered from the same group of 5,200 residents of Framingham, Massachusetts, showed that overweight people who lost just 11 pounds reduced their risk of developing arthritic knees by almost 50 percent.

And when it comes to cancer, particularly breast cancer, losing those extra pounds may give you extra protection. Research from the federal Centers for Disease Control and Prevention in Atlanta shows a particular danger for women who are 25 percent or more over their optimal weights at the time their breast cancer is diagnosed. These women face a 42 percent greater risk that the cancer will return.

Being overweight may also increase a woman's risk of developing breast cancer, says Dr. Foreyt. "A high-fat diet leads to obesity, and fat in the diet is associated with an increased risk of breast cancer," he says.

Aging Ups the Ante

Most of us have already realized that it's gets harder to lose weight the older we get. That's because our metabolism, the process by which our bodies burn calories, slows down over time. Reubin Andres, M.D., clinical director of the National Institute on Aging in Bethesda, Maryland, believes it is harmless to gain about 5 pounds each decade after age 20—but only if you are in good health to start with and remain free of ailments such as diabetes and heart disease. But many experts say any weight gain should be avoided throughout the years.

Research also shows that it's best to keep the weight off. After following a group of Harvard University alumni for 27 years, researchers found the lowest mortality rate among men who were 20 percent below the average weight for men of similar age and height. This finding held firm even after the researchers accounted for underweight from smoking or illness, which they believe may have distorted the results of previous studies.

What's a Healthy Weight, Anyway?

You don't need to be a slave to the scale. "Your healthy weight is what's produced by healthy eating and healthy exercise," says John Foreyt, Ph.D., director of the Nutrition Research Clinic at Baylor College of Medicine in Houston. "That's your goal, period."

But maybe you'd feel better with a weight range to aim for. If so, the chart below, from the federal government, will give you a general idea of where you should stand. These guidelines were prepared for both men and women; women will generally fall toward the lower end of each range.

Height	Weight (lb.) Age 19–34	Age 35 and up
5' 0"	97–128	108–138
5' 1"	101–132	111–143
5' 2"	104–137	115–148
5' 3"	107–141	119–152
5' 4"	111–146	122–157
5' 5"	114–150	126–162
5' 6"	118–155	130–167
5' 7"	121–160	134–172
5' 8"	125–164	138–178
5' 9"	129–169	142–183
5' 10"	132–174	146–188
5' 11"	136–179	151–194
6' 0"	140–184	155–199
6' 1"	144–189	159–205
6' 2"	148–195	164–210
6' 3"	152–200	168–216
6' 4"	156–205	173–222
6' 5"	160–211	177–228
6' 6"	164–216	182–234

The study also showed that men who were only slightly overweight—2 to 6 percent over their desirable weights—still had a significantly greater chance of dying from heart disease and that men who weighed 20 percent more than their desirable weights actually doubled their risk.

But regardless of where you fit on the charts, if you feel you're struggling with more than a few extra pounds and you don't have thyroid or other health problems, you may be eating too much—particularly fatty foods—and exercising too little.

What to do about it? Well, you could put yourself on a crash diet. But that probably won't get you anything but frustration. "Diets just don't work," says Janet Polivy, Ph.D., professor of psychology at the University of Toronto Faculty of Medicine. "Diets become popular because they work for a week or two and everyone says, 'You gotta try it.' Well, speak to those people in a year or two, and you'll find they've failed." When you fall for one of those speedy 5-pounds-a-week programs, you lose it all right—but you lose pounds of fluid, not fat. And as soon as you abandon the diet, the weight comes right back on.

In the long run, what works best to achieve a healthy weight is to modify your eating habits and to get more exercise.

It worked for Karen Faye. "Now I'm a grandmother," Faye says. "But since I've lost the weight, when people see me with my 25-year-old son, they think he's my boyfriend! If I can do it, you can do it."

Setting the Stage

The first step toward successful weight loss is accepting yourself as you are right now, says Thomas A. Wadden, Ph.D., associate professor of psychology and director of the Weight and Eating Disorders Program at the University of Pennsylvania in Philadelphia. Then you have to draw up a strategy for taking control of your weight. Here's how.

Make a long-term commitment. The key to healthy and successful weight loss at any age, experts say, is to make the changes gradually. Losing no more than ½ pound a week is ideal, says George Blackburn, M.D., Ph.D., associate professor of surgery at Harvard Medical School and chief of the Nutrition/Metabolism Laboratory at New England Deaconess Hospital, both in Boston. So aim to attain a healthy weight a year from now, not next week, he says.

Don't try to be a model. Never mind that professional models are often as skinny as straws. Many of them are teenagers in heavy makeup. "You have to recognize that you can't look like those skinny little models in the magazines, and middle age is a good time to do this," says Dr. Wadden. Once you let go of unrealistic fantasies and accept the notion that it's unfair to model yourself after an adolescent, then you can get on with a healthy and attainable weight loss plan, he says.

Surround yourself with support. A good support system is a key to successful weight loss, says Dr. Foreyt. Ask your family and friends to cheer you on. Maybe they could join you in eating low-fat, healthful meals.

Trimming the Tummy That Won't Quit

Even when you've been watching your weight diligently, you still may have a stubbornly protruding stomach. It's often a natural consequence of aging for both women and men, research shows. For women, it's often from repeated dieting—regained weight tends to be deposited on the belly, researchers say. Or it may be a lingering reminder of pregnancy. You can flatten your stomach without complicated exercise gizmos and gadgets, however. Here's how.

Don't belly up to the bar. There really is such a thing as a beer belly and cutting your alcohol intake may be the key to flattening it. In a large study, women and men who drank more than two alcoholic drinks a day had the largest waist-to-hip ratios, which is how doctors quantify potbellies.

Stamp out the cigarettes. In a study, researchers at Stanford University School of Medicine in Stanford, California, and the University of California, San Diego, detected a similar effect for smoking. There were twice as many fat abdomens among those who lit up as among nonsmokers. See your doctor for help in quitting.

Start huffing. Maybe belly dancing is just what that belly needs. To burn off a belly, exercise must do two things, says Bryant Stamford, Ph.D., director of the Health Promotion Center at the University of Louisville in Kentucky. First, it must start out vigorously to trigger a substantial adrenaline release, which frees fat to be used for fuel. You can get this effect from brisk walking, he says. Then the vigorous activity must be followed by prolonged aerobic exercise that will burn up the liberated fat. Walking at a comfortable pace fits the bill. So could a spate of hard housework followed by some steady raking. "Just step up the pace now and then to boost adrenaline output," he says.

Firm it up. Once the fat is whittled away by low-fat eating and aerobic exercise, daily abdominal exercises can really help to improve your shape, Dr. Stamford says. Start with isometric squeezes: Tense your abdominal muscles to the maximum and hold for 6 to 10 seconds. Relax, then repeat several times. Later, he says, you can move to crunches: Lie on your back with your legs apart, knees bent, and feet flat on the floor. Cross your arms on your chest. Lift your head up toward the ceiling. Keep going until you can lift your shoulder blades slightly off the ground. Hold for 2 seconds, then lie back down. Build up gradually to 10 repetitions a set.

"Form a neighborhood group that walks together, or look to the YMCA, the Jewish Community Center, or your local church or college for weight loss support groups," Dr. Foreyt says. "And groups such as Weight Watchers, which teach self-maintenance, can be very, very useful." If you tend to lose control and overeat compulsively or go on big food binges followed by a sense of shame, an Overeaters Anonymous group or professional counseling can be a tremendous help, he says.

Pay attention to your emotional needs. Sometimes you can confuse hunger with other feelings, especially if you're feeling depressed or stressed or just responding to a luscious photo spread in a gourmet food magazine. If it's not your stomach talking, you need to figure out what kinds of emotions or discomforts are triggering your urge for food, Dr. Foreyt says. Then develop a problem-solving approach. "How can you answer that need without eating? Walk around the block, call a friend, meditate, take a bath, brush your teeth, or gargle with mouthwash," he says. "This breaks the chain and develops an alternate behavior pattern."

Boycott the fat box. If you watch more than 3 hours of television a day, you double your risk of being saddled with extra pounds, says Larry A. Tucker, Ph.D., professor and director of health promotion at Brigham Young University in Provo, Utah. Slouched on the couch, you're not burning many calories, and you're likely to be taking in more by eating fattening snacks. So turn off the tube (plus the junk food habit that usually comes with it) to boost your weight loss campaign.

Nourish Yourself Thin

The latest nutrition research shows that there really is a whole new way to lose weight—without dieting and without hunger. It's based on understanding which kinds of food revitalize you and give you real energy and which foods go right to your thighs. You may be surprised to find that the most crucial changes don't require that you eat less—just differently. Here's how.

Forgo excess fat. Dietary fat makes us gain weight because it's stored in the body far more easily than either carbohydrates or protein, says Peter D. Vash, M.D., assistant clinical professor of medicine at the University of California, Los Angeles. The body burns carbohydrates and protein for fuel almost immediately, while the more calorie-dense fat burns slower and is more likely to be left over—on you.

Start by cutting fat in the obvious places: Eat fewer fatty meats, fried foods, high-fat dairy products, and desserts. Also, beware of salads slathered in oil or other fatty dressings. It's recommended that you keep your total calories from fat to 25 percent or less of your daily diet.

"A high-fat diet has been linked to obesity, which in turn is associated with an increased risk of various cancers. Prudence says that a high-fat diet is a factor in so many illnesses that it only makes sense to eat low-fat foods instead," says Dr. Foreyt.

Drown it. "Drinking generous amounts of water is overwhelmingly the number-one way to reduce appetite," says Dr. Blackburn. Not only does water keep your stomach feeling fuller, but also many people think they're having food cravings when in fact they're thirsty, he says. So aim for 8 cups of fluids daily, sipping ½ cup at a time.

When you're sipping away through the day, keep in mind that caffeine—in cola, coffee, or tea—has its drawbacks. Caffeine is a diuretic, which removes water from the body. For that reason, most doctors recommend that people on weight loss programs drink no more than three caffeinated beverages a day.

Count on carbs. Don't go hungry. When you replace the excess fat calories you've been eating with foods such as carbohydrates, you can actually eat more and still lose pounds. In one study at the University of Illinois at Chicago, people on moderately high-fat diets were told to maintain their weights for 20 weeks while switching to low-fat, high-carbohydrate diets. They ate all they wanted and still lost more than 11 percent of their body fat and 2 percent of their weight. So enjoy plenty of carbohydrate-rich pasta (without fatty sauces), low-fat cereals, breads, beans, fresh vegetables, and fruits to fill you up while you're losing weight.

Allow a few splurges. If you feel that all you're saying to yourself about food is no-no, you may eventually let slips turn into a downhill slide, says Susan Kayman, R.D., Dr.P.H., a dietitian and consultant with the Kaiser Permanente Medical Group in Oakland, California. That's why she advocates following the 80/20 rule. If you eat low-fat 80 percent of the time, then when you're dining with friends, out on the town, or over at the in-laws, enjoy an occasional higher-fat treat without beating yourself up about it, she says.

Break up the deadly duo. That's fats and sweets. When the body gets a jolt of sugar, it releases lots of insulin in response. Because insulin is a storage-prone hormone, it opens up fat cells, preparing them for fat storage. So when you eat sugar, keep your fat intake low. Also, fats and sugar taken together can turn up your appetite to unmanageable levels. Eating sweets leads to an increase in the amount of sugar in the blood, which, because of a chain of reactions in the body, pumps up your appetite, says Dr. Wadden. So soothe your sweet tooth with juicy fresh fruit or a bowl of low-fat sugared cereal instead of doughnuts and candy bars.

Stay with it. Here's a fat-fighting tip to hang on to: If you stick with it, you'll actually lose your taste for high-fat foods after a while. A 4-year study of more than 2,000 people at the Fred Hutchinson Cancer Research Center at the University of Washington in Seattle showed that people who limit their fat intakes lose their taste for fat in 6 months or less, eventually finding fatty foods unpleasant to eat.

Eat often. Some researchers support the idea of grazing—eating numerous small meals throughout the day instead of three larger meals—to control appetite and prevent bingeing. "But you cannot graze on M&M's, potato chips, and Häagen-Dazs," says James Kenney, R.D., Ph.D., a nutrition research specialist at the Pritikin Longevity Center in Santa Monica, California. "If you graze on low-fat, high-fiber foods that aren't packed with calories, such as carrots, apples, peaches, oranges, and red peppers, you'll keep your appetite down."

Satisfaction Guaranteed

Controlling appetite is perhaps the key to successfully losing weight, according to a study at the University of Sydney in Australia. Researchers there have identified a number of "high-satisfaction" foods that help keep you feeling fuller longer. In the accompanying table, anything with a rating of 100 or better is considered satisfying. Foods that scored less than 100 tend not to stick around, so you'll probably wind up eating more of them—and gaining weight.

Food	Rating	Food	Rating
Potatoes	323	Crackers	127
Fish	225	Cookies	120
Oatmeal	209	White pasta	119
Oranges	202	Bananas	118
Apples	197	Cornflakes	118
Whole-wheat pasta	188	Jelly beans	118
Steak	176	French fries	116
Baked beans	168	White bread	100
Grapes	162	Ice cream	96
Grain bread	154	Potato chips	91
Popcorn	154	Yogurt	88
Bran cereal	151	Peanuts	84
Eggs	150	Candy bar	70
Cheese	146	Doughnut	68
White rice	138	Cake	65
Lentils	133	Croissant	47
Brown rice	132		

Turn up the heat. Be lavish with hot spices such as cayenne pepper and horseradish to boost your metabolic rate, which may help your body burn more calories, says Dr. Kenney. "When people eat hot foods, they often sweat, a sure sign of increased metabolic rate. And the faster the metabolic rate, the more heat produced by the body. Remember, whatever warms you up in turn slims you down," he says. But be sure to avoid high-fat dishes, even if they're loaded with spices.

Start with soup. A soup appetizer tends to reduce the amount you eat at a meal, several studies suggest. In one study from Johns Hopkins University in Baltimore, people who had soup before a meal ate 25 percent fewer calories of the entrée than those who started the meal with cheese and crackers. It may be the volume of space that soup takes up in the stomach or the fact that most of soup's calories come from carbohydrates rather than fat, researchers say. Or there may be a psychological factor at work, Dr. Kenney says. "Hot soup is very relaxing if you have a nervous, gnawing appetite."

Ride out a craving. When the urge strikes for a chocolate eclair, don't confuse the craving with a command, says Linda Crawford, an eating behavior specialist at Green Mountain at Fox Run, a residential weight and health management center in Ludlow, Vermont. Though many people think cravings keep getting stronger until they're irresistible, research shows that food cravings actually start and escalate, then peak and subside. Distract yourself with a walk or something else incompatible with eating, Crawford says, and ride out the craving. "Just like with surfing," she says, "the more you practice riding a craving wave, the easier it becomes." But if you still have the craving after 20 minutes, go ahead and satisfy it with a small portion—and enjoy it, she advises.

A Weight Loss Workout Strategy

Adopting a healthier diet will help you lose weight, but you'll acquire a firmer figure faster—and keep it—if you combine your healthy new eating habits with exercise.

Exercise also strengthens your heart and arteries, and it boosts your self-confidence—in short, it will counteract many of the harmful effects of being overweight. Exercise can even help to curb your appetite.

If you're unaccustomed to exercising, see your doctor before you get started. After you have the okay, you'll be ready. Here are some tips to get you going.

Keep it up. "The best predictor of long-term weight management is regular aerobic activity, which boosts your heart rate," says Dr. Foreyt. "Brisk walking is a great choice because it's very easy for most people to do on a regular basis. But the effectiveness of any aerobic activity for weight control has been proven repeatedly." Any kind of daily exercise helps. Thirty minutes of aerobic exercise burns flab and tones muscles—as long as you do it regularly.

Burn by building. Aerobic exercise should always be part of your weight loss plan, but when you add resistance training such as weight lifting, you'll keep your weight down with the help of "hungry muscles. Muscle tissue needs more calories," says Janet Walberg-Rankin, Ph.D., associate professor in the Exercise Science Program in the Division of Health and Physical Education at Virginia Polytechnic Institute and State University in Blacksburg. "So if you increase muscle mass while you lose fat, you boost your ability to burn fuel." That means your new, ravenous muscle will be grinding away calories even when you're in a meeting or waiting in line at the bank, she says.

"Resistance training isn't just about lifting barbells," adds Dr. Foreyt, though

The Batwing Problem

A beautiful sundress catches your eye. Uh-oh . . . wait a minute. It's sleeveless. You give your flabby upper arms a squeeze, just to make sure they're still with you.

Charmingly dubbed batwings by doctors, these slabs of skin and fat have three main causes, says Alan Matarasso, M.D., a plastic surgeon at Manhattan Eye, Ear, and Throat Hospital in New York City. First, you may have inherited a tendency to deposit fat on the underside of your upper arms. Second, if you've gained and lost weight repeatedly over the years, your skin has stretched and contracted so many times that it has lost some of its elasticity. Third, that's loose, thin skin under there. It's as sensitive as the delicate skin on your inner thigh, Dr. Matarasso says. "It's thinner and looser than skin on the outer arm or abdomen," he says.

How to trim your wings? Any exercise that strengthens your triceps muscle—the one running along the back of your arm from underarm to elbow—will help, Dr. Matarasso says. Any trainer will be able to show you several, he says, but here's one to try.

In a standing position, hold a dumbbell weighing between 3 and 5 pounds in front of you with both hands, with your elbows slightly bent. Slowly raise the dumbbell straight up over your head. This is your starting position. Bending your elbows, lower the dumbbell to the back of your neck, then raise it back up to the starting position above your head. Continue to raise and lower the weight slowly, working up to sets of 10 repetitions.

---

that's great for firming the arms. To really work the different groups of muscles, your best bet is to go to a gym and ask a trainer to show you how to circuit train, he says. You use a series of different weight machines to work muscles in the neck, arms, chest, and legs. You can accomplish the same thing by working with free weights at home, he says. "Putting your muscles against something that doesn't yield—that's resistance."

Shake Weight Woes with Supplements

Once you've adopted good exercise and eating habits, you may find that supplements also can work in your favor. Some nutritional and herbal supplements can help suppress your appetite, alternative medicine experts say. There also are supplements that will help increase the rate at which you burn calories. Here are some of the best.

Fill up with fiber. Taking a daily fiber supplement will expand your stomach and make you feel full, says Jennifer Brett, N.D., a naturopathic doctor at the Wilton Naturopathic Center in Stratford, Connecticut. "When your stomach feels full, it sends a signal to your brain, telling it that you don't need to eat as much," she says. "Supplements diminish hunger pangs."

The best fiber supplements for weight loss are psyllium and glucomannan because they are rich in soluble fiber, says Dr. Brett. Take one glucomannan pill 20 minutes before each meal, she says, or two or three capsules of psyllium before meals. Drink at least 8 ounces of water with each dose to prevent constipation.

Get lean with chromium. Research shows that chromium picolinate, a supplemental form of chromium, can build muscle mass and reduce fat in people who exercise. Chromium also helps your body turn carbohydrates and fats into energy. Moreover, it improves the effectiveness of insulin, the hormone that allows cells to pick up blood sugar that your body needs for fuel from the bloodstream. As a result, blood sugar levels are kept under control. Your energy soars, you crave fewer sweets, and your body's sensitivity to insulin increases, which is key for successful weight loss, says Dr. Brett.

Dr. Brett suggests taking 200 to 400 micrograms of chromium picolinate daily, but before you take doses that high, you should consult your physician.

Burn fat with kelp. Kelp may help whittle away extra pounds when combined with a low-fat diet and daily aerobic exercise, says Ellen Evert Hopman, a professional member of the American Herbalists Guild, a lay homeopath in Amherst, Massachusetts, and author of *Tree Medicine, Tree Magic*. Kelp is believed to stimulate a hormone produced in the thyroid gland that's responsible for boosting metabolism, so you'll burn more calories by the hour, says Hopman.

While kelp is safe for most people, you should check with your doctor before taking it if you have a thyroid disorder, high blood pressure, or heart problems, says Hopman.

PROSTATE PROBLEMS

Corralling the Male Menace

Lately, your urinary tract is acting like a workaholic. It wakes you up in the middle of the night, interrupts your lunch, even yanks you out of important meetings, and sends you scurrying to the nearest bathroom. Yet though you're in the men's room a lot these days, you never feel you've finished what you went there to do.

You could blame your bladder, but in all probability, your prostate is the problem.

The prostate, a small gland about the size of a walnut, is wrapped around the urethra, the tube that drains the bladder. The prostate produces semen and secretes it into the urethra, providing the liquid medium that sperm cells need for nourishment and mobility. Usually the prostate works so well that you don't even notice it. But as you approach your midforties, your prostate may change.

Because of a variety of hormonal changes associated with aging, the gland may start growing and putting pressure on your urethra. This condition is called benign prostatic hyperplasia (BPH), and like it or not, you have a 50 percent chance of developing BPH at some time during your lifetime.

As the prostate balloons because of BPH, you may feel the urge to urinate more frequently, or your bladder may feel full after you've finished urinating. Or your stream may be weak or you may find it difficult to get things going and keep things flowing. In worst cases, the prostate can swell to the size of a grapefruit and pinch off urine flow, says Thomas Stanisic, M.D., a urologist in private practice in Ashland, Kentucky. Then you may need an operation called transurethral resection of the prostate. In this procedure, the doctor inserts a tiny tube into the urethra and shaves away the portion of the prostate that's pressing on the urethra. It's a painful procedure that can take a few months to fully recover from.

Fortunately, BPH is treatable. Not only that, there are things you can do to help minimize the problems it causes if you're willing to make a few adjustments in your diet and lifestyle.

Small Gland, Big Problems

Doctors aren't sure why the prostate grows as you age. Some researchers believe the gland's tendency to swell may have something to do with the male hormone testosterone. Eunuchs don't get BPH. For the rest of the male population, however, the condition is common. It affects up to 15 percent of men over age 40 and 60 percent over age 50.

"Testosterone fuels the prostate," says Kenneth Goldberg, M.D., founder and director of the Male Health Institute in Irving, Texas. "We've found that if you can reduce testosterone levels, you slow down the growth of the prostate."

One key way some doctors believe you can lower testosterone is to reduce your cholesterol. Cholesterol is converted to testosterone in the body. It has been observed that enlarged prostate tissue is very high in cholesterol. Some doctors claim an improvement in symptoms, if not in prostate size, by getting patients to lower their total blood cholesterol levels to 200 mg/dl or less.

You can improve your cholesterol by eating less food that is high in saturated fats, such as red meat and dairy products, and by consuming more food that is high in monounsaturated fat, such as olive oil, salmon, and tuna. Limit yourself to one 3-ounce serving of meat, fish, or poultry a day, suggests Dr. Goldberg. That's about the size of a cassette tape.

Another key way to control your testosterone: Eat more vegetables. Male hormone levels drop with a vegetarian diet and that may explain why BPH is rare in cultures whose diets are largely vegetarian, Dr. Goldberg says.

Taming the Wild Prostate

Beyond the testosterone connection, some doctors believe you can reduce the possibility and impact of prostate problems by taking these steps.

Ejaculate regularly. Doing so may keep prostatic ducts from getting clogged and backed up. "It can only help," Dr. Goldberg says.

Lose that waist. Men with 43-inch waists or greater are 50 percent more likely than normal-weight men to report symptoms of prostate enlargement or to have surgery for this condition, Harvard University researchers report. Losing about 7 inches of waistline, about 35 pounds in most cases, could be a method of treating and preventing prostate enlargement, they say.

Get enough zinc. Men with prostate problems tend to have low concentrations of zinc in their bodies, says Paul M. Block, M.D., a urologist in private practice in Phoenix. The Daily Value of zinc is 15 milligrams. Taking zinc supplements or eating foods rich in zinc, including oysters and herring can help. Oatmeal, wheat bran, milk, peas, and nuts also contain the mineral.

Shrink it with saw palmetto. One of the most widespread herbal medicines used to reduce the size and irritating symptoms of an enlarged prostate is an extract of the berries of the saw palmetto. Studies show that up to 60 percent of men with mild to moderate BPH experience some relief from all major symptoms within the first 4 to 6 weeks of treatment with this herb. Take 160 milligrams

When the Cause Isn't BPH

While benign prostatic hyperplasia (BPH) is the most common cause of prostate problems, it's not the only cause. Infection and cancer can also strike the prostate gland.

The infection is known as bacterial prostatitis and it usually is caused by an infection that spreads from the bladder or urethra. Bacterial prostatitis can affect men of all ages.

Although doctors aren't sure how the infection enters the urinary tract, some suspect that an obstruction in the urethra or unprotected anal sex increase the risk. With bacterial prostatitis, you may have the urination problems common to BPH, but you also may have symptoms such as lower abdominal or back pain, discomfort in the testicles, and fever.

Bacterial prostatitis is relatively easy to treat, says Christopher M. Dixon, M.D., assistant professor of urology at the Medical College of Wisconsin in Milwaukee. Usually your doctor will prescribe antibiotics. In most cases, symptoms improve in about a week, but it may take up to 6 weeks to evict prostatitis from your body.

Prostate cancer is the most common cancer among men over age 50 and the second leading killer among cancers in men in the United States. More than half of all men over age 70 have it, says Thomas Stanisic, M.D., a urologist in private practice in Ashland, Kentucky.

Prostate cancer is rare in men younger than age 45 unless they have family histories of the disease. It is usually curable if detected early, Dr. Stanisic says.

But often this cancer grows silently within the gland without any symptoms until it has spread to the surrounding bone and tissue. That's why it's especially important for men over age 50 to get a digital rectal exam, which lets a doctor feel for lumps on the prostate, and a prostate-specific antigen blood test that detects a protein that seeps out of the prostate when there is a tumor present.

If cancer is discovered, your treatment will depend on several factors, including the size of the tumor, how fast it is growing, and whether the disease has spread beyond the prostate. Treatments include radiation, surgical removal of the prostate, and hormonal therapy to reduce testosterone levels.

If concerned about developing prostate cancer, fill up on fiber. A high-fiber diet helps reduce your risk of prostate cancer by slightly lowering your body's levels of reproductive hormones. In population studies, men who eat the most fiber, from beans, whole grains, fruits, and vegetables, are least likely to develop prostate cancer.

twice a day with meals until your symptoms improve, suggests Thomas Kruzel, N.D., a naturopathic doctor in Portland, Oregon. Then, he suggests, continue taking at least 160 milligrams daily as a maintenance dose.

Limit spicy foods and alcohol. Both of these may increase bladder irritation, particularly if you have BPH, Dr. Block says. Alcohol especially can be tough, since it's a central nervous system depressant that reduces muscle tone throughout the body, including in the bladder, causing it to retain urine.

Get your exercise. There's no prostate-specific workout, though drinking water, voiding on demand, and regular sexual relations help. But you should know that many physicians have observed that men in good shape are less likely to have prostate trouble than their sedentary brothers.

Don't sit for too long. That's your prostate you're sitting on all day, and sitting puts pressure on it, Dr. Goldberg says. Get up and walk around.

Let it go. If you need to urinate frequently, logic may tell you to train your bladder by waiting as long as you can. Logic has been wrong before, and it's wrong here. "You may actually harm yourself by waiting too long," says Patrick C. Walsh, M.D., professor and chairman of urology at Johns Hopkins University in Baltimore. "When urine backs up too far, it can damage the kidneys." Urinate as soon as you feel the need.

Avoid drinking after dark. Forgo liquids after 6:00 or 7:00 P.M. if your sleep has been interrupted frequently (say two or three times a night) by the urge to urinate, Dr. Block suggests. Day and night, limit drinks containing caffeine. These make you urinate more and increase bladder irritation, causing it to feel full even when it isn't.

Soak it. Sit in a warm bath for 20 minutes at least once a week, Dr. Block suggests. The heat will penetrate the pelvis and increase blood flow, reducing muscle spasms and possibly swelling.

Take fatty acids to maintain your prostate. Some naturopaths believe that men who supplement their diets with two essential fatty acids—linolenic acid and alpha-linolenic acid—can reverse BPH and kiss irritating symptoms goodbye. "Essential fatty acids can inhibit cell growth in the prostate, therefore stopping its growth. They can rebalance the appropriate fatty acid rations in the gland," says Ian Bier, N.D., a naturopathic doctor and licensed acupuncturist at the Institute for Advancement of Natural Medicine in Portsmouth, New Hampshire.

To get these essential oils, take 1,000 to 2,000 milligrams of fish oil daily for 1 to 2 weeks if you are being treated for BPH. To maintain prostate health, take 500 to 1,000 milligrams of fish oil a day.

Take the right meds. Two medications can help relieve the symptoms of BPH, Dr. Stanisic says. Finasteride (Proscar) reduces the size of the prostate by an average of 20 percent, which is enough to boost urine flow. Another drug, terazosin hydrochloride (Hytrin) relaxes muscles of the bladder neck and prostate to open up the urethra. Ask your doctor if these drugs can relieve your problem.

REACTION TIME

Reversing the Big Slowdown

There was a time not too long ago when in almost every situation, your response was as quick as a cat's. If you were playing tennis and your opponent hit a smash down the line—*whoosh*! You'd return it, no problem. If you knocked a piece of china off the counter—*zoom*! You'd catch it before it hit the ground. If someone asked you a question—*bang*! You had the answer in an instant.

But lately, there has been a lot less whoosh, zoom, and bang in your life. Tennis balls are flying past. Family heirlooms are hitting the floor. And TV quiz show contestants are hitting their buzzers while you're still trying to figure out what the heck the question was.

What's happening here?

Well, you're getting older—and probably a little slower. While you're not ready for the nursing home yet, it's an undeniable fact that your reflexes aren't what they used to be.

But don't worry. It happens to all of us. And there's a lot you can do about it.

The Secret to Speedy Reflexes

Even the fittest of the fit will eventually join the ain't-what-I-used-to-be group. "Everyone, including great athletes, reaches their peak fitness levels in the mid- to late twenties and then gradually declines," says Ralph Tarter, Ph.D., professor of psychiatry and neurology at the University of Pittsburgh School of Medicine. "As fitness goes, our metabolism slows, and with it, our ability to perform tasks requiring sustained strength and speed."

Lucky for us that we have a surefire defense against this downward decline: lifelong physical activity. When you exercise, the body increases its output of growth hormone, a substance that helps maintain muscle mass, bone density, and lean body composition.

Keep Your Reflexes in Gear

Ever notice how Jet Li and Jean-Claude van Damme duck and move in those action movies? Their quick reaction times showcase the coordination of mind, body, and vision. One of the best techniques you can use to hone and develop all three is practicing martial arts.

What's so special about the martial arts? For one thing, they call for physical fitness. Martial artists spend hours building strength, developing flexibility, and performing routines that condition the body for speed. For another, they demand maximum concentration of mind and vision: If you don't pay attention, you or someone else may get hurt. And they're motivational: The belt system of awards encourages you to improve your skills and speed.

According to Charles L. Richman, Ph.D., professor of psychology and director of the Martial Arts Program at Wake Forest University in Winston-Salem, North Carolina, there are more than 100 martial arts styles. All share certain basic postures and rudiments, with some subtle differences. Some, such as tae kwon do and kempo, are more aggressive and emphasize hard contact. Softer styles, such as aikido and judo, emphasize throwing and evading your opponent. And tai chi and kung fu focus on developing fluid, dancelike movements.

Since the late 1970s Dr. Richman has studied and taught tae kwon do, a Lorena martial art that emphasizes a dazzling array of spins, kicks, and punches. Now in his sixties, he knows firsthand just how intertwined aging, fitness, and reaction time really are. "Naturally, I have found my reflexes to be slowing when competing against younger, quicker individuals," he says. "However, I have been able to hold my own quite well, speedwise, against men in my own age group. Overall, I feel my reaction time is still quite good—much better than if I had not made tae kwon do a part of my life."

Martial arts programs can help almost anyone develop quicker reaction time, better coordination, and greater concentration, regardless of a person's age. It can even help performance in other activities. "Tae kwon do or any martial art demands physical fitness and mental discipline," says Dr. Richman. "Many principles used in self-defense apply in other sports as well, such as keeping your head still and eyes forward and moving your hips through contact. Since I have been practicing tae kwon do, my golf game has improved considerably."

Consult your phone directory for a martial arts school near you.

Robert Mazzeo, Ph.D., a kinesiologist (he studies human motion) at the University of Colorado in Boulder, studied this issue. He found that regularly active individuals had higher concentrations of growth hormone in their blood than people the same age who didn't exercise and than sedentary people who were much younger.

"Even the elderly will see an increase in growth hormone levels from exercise, and with it will come increased strength, balance, and speed," Dr. Mazzeo says.

Playing Those Mind Games

Your ability to react to stimuli is controlled by the brain. In a split second, it processes information and then sends impulse signals to our muscles. "As we age, we see little change in the speed of these impulses," says Lawrence Z. Stern, M.D., director of the Muscular Dystrophy Association's Mucio F. Delgado Clinic for Neuromuscular Disorders at the University of Arizona Health Sciences Center in Tucson. "The greatest delays are in the processing of information that is necessary to formulate the messages that tell the muscles what to do."

Why? First, as we age, we lose brain cells that help us process new information. Also, we have much more information and experiences in our heads than we did when we were younger. This slows down our ability to make snap judgments. And, truth be told, we get lazy; it becomes easier to rely on old familiar ways than to deal with new ones.

So how do you keep your mind sharp and your reactions quick?

Use it. "Stay mentally engaged by exposing yourself to demanding tasks and new challenges every single day," says Dr. Tarter. "When we constantly use the brain and push it to its full capacity, it stays faster, more alert, and more efficient." Another recommendation: Cut back on passive activities such as watching television, says Dr. Tarter.

Check your vision. Before you can mentally or physically react, you must have an accurate picture of the world outside. For that, we must rely on our senses, vision in particular. "Seventy-five to 80 percent of reaction time is directly related to good visual skills," says Arthur Seiderman, O.D., an Elkins Park, Pennsylvania, visual consultant to many professional athletes and author of *20/20 Is Not Enough*.

"That means more than just seeing objects clearly; it also means having the ability to detect, track, and recognize fast-moving objects."

Steer clear of alcohol and drugs. Everybody knows that drunk drivers are slow to react behind the wheel, but even one or two drinks can be enough to send your reaction time plummeting, says Dr. Stern. And if you regularly drink alcoholic beverages or take any medication that affects the central nervous system, it could put your mind and body in a constant state of slow-mo.

Don't smoke. Tobacco saps speed in more ways than one, says Dr. Tarter.

Setting Your Sights

An optometrist or ophthalmologist can put you on a program to improve the clarity and quality of your vision. In the meantime, Arthur Seiderman, O.D., an Elkins Park, Pennsylvania, visual consultant to many professional athletes and author of *20/20 Is Not Enough*, recommends these exercises.

Have a ball. Cut out a variety of letters, small shapes, and colored pieces of paper, and tape them to a ball or beanbag. Then play a round of catch or bounce the ball off a wall, spotting and calling out one or more of the colors, shapes, or objects before you catch it.

Go for a spin. If you still have a record player, try this one: Cut a piece of cardboard into the shape of a disc, paste different-size letters, numbers, words, or figures on it, and put it on a turntable. Set the speed at 33⅓ rpm and call out the information on the disc for 1 to 3 minutes. When it gets easier, increase the speed to 45 rpm, then 78 rpm.

Box to the beat. Draw a large box with 16 squares on a chalkboard or piece of paper. Place the numbers 1 through 16 in the squares in random order. Turn on a musical metronome or other rhythm-making device, and point to each of the numbers in numerical order, keeping time with the beat. Try it again in backward order, then repeat.

Flip some flash cards. For this you'll need 50 3- by 5-inch cards. Draw a black dot in the center of each card, below the top edge. Write a different two-digit number on each side of the dot, about ½ inch from the dot.

Mark another card with a different pair of two-digit numbers, each placed ¾ inch away from the dot. Continue marking each card, spacing the numbers at ¼-inch intervals until you reach the far corners; then work back toward the center dot.

Hold the stack of cards 14 to 16 inches in front of you, then flip through the stack while focusing on the center dot and call out the numbers on the card.

It should get increasingly difficult to identify the numbers as they are spaced farther from the center. Start slowly, then build up your flipping speed.

We all know the effect it has on our cardiovascular systems. If our lungs and hearts don't work efficiently, neither will our bones and muscles. Smoking also dramatically reduces the amount of oxygen in our bloodstreams, and the brain needs a steady supply of fresh oxygen to stay in good working order.

Catch some Zzzs. A good night's sleep is nature's way of recharging our mental batteries. "Regular quality sleep every night is essential for the brain to stay alert and perform cognitive tasks at maximal levels," says Dr. Stern.

Zap some aliens. Video and computer games have been shown to dramatically improve mental and motor skills, says Dr. Tarter. "They are often used to help rehab patients develop speed, and even pilots these days practice on video simulators before they climb in the cockpit."

If beeps, buzzes, and explosions aren't your cup of tea, try some other fast-paced activity, such as Ping-Pong.

RESPIRATORY DISEASES

Keeping Them at Bay

You hike along a path that leads to a snow-covered peak. Far below is a picture-perfect village, seemingly cut off from time. Above is silent, glacier-cold rock and sky.

Drawing the crisp mountain air deep into your lungs, you hold it, exhale as long as you can, then repeat the process over and over again until every cell in your body is flooded with fresh, clean air.

Most of us would like lungs that can withstand a workout like this. We don't want to suck air on every hill as though we're 100 years old. We don't want to cough every time we take deep breaths. And we don't want to wheeze.

And we don't have to, says Robert Bethel, M.D., a staff physician at the National Jewish Center for Immunology and Respiratory Medicine in Denver.

Our lungs are made to last through any workout well into our seventies. Smoking, of course, can change that scenario, clogging up the lungs and making us gasp for air. Colds, flu, pneumonia, and other infectious diseases can do the same, but only temporarily. Other diseases can also affect the lungs, but these are less common.

Strengthening Your Natural Defenses

Every day, your respiratory system draws in approximately 9,500 quarts of air and mixes it with up to 10,600 quarts of blood pumped by the heart into the lungs. Your lungs send oxygen through arterial highways to support the rest of the body and to provide an exhaust system for gaseous metabolic garbage such as carbon dioxide.

Since your lungs are internal organs that draw in the microorganisms of the outside world with every breath, the strength of their natural defense system is particularly important in maintaining oxygen flow to and from the rest of your body. Fortunately for most of us, the lungs' defensive players, including mucus and hairlike filaments called cilia, can sweep pollens, dust, viruses, and bacteria out of the airway.

Most of the time they do a great job. But sometimes they're undermined by irritants such as cigarette smoke or overwhelmed by invading microbes.

More than 14 million men and women suffer from chronic obstructive pulmonary disease, which includes both chronic bronchitis and emphysema. And in any given year, 7 to 8 million men and women will have asthma, 129 million will have the flu, 4 million will have pneumonia, and practically every one of us will have some kind of cold virus.

How can you protect your lungs from the diseases and irritants that can slow you down? Here's what experts say.

Keep your cilia sober. Drinking interferes with the cleansing mechanisms that keep your lungs free of disease-causing germs, says Steven R. Mostow, M.D., chairman of the American Thoracic Society's Committee on the Prevention of Pneumonia and Influenza and professor of medicine at the University of Colorado at Denver. "The respiratory system's cilia get drunk right along with the rest of you," he explains. If you're used to having one or two drinks on a daily basis, your cilia will be okay. But if you suddenly decide to drink more than you usually do, your cilia won't be able to do their job.

Make it moist. To keep your respiratory system in fighting trim, humidify your environment in winter with a humidifier, says Dr. Mostow. The increased moisture will help the cilia sweep out dust, viruses, bacteria, and pollens.

Work your lungs. Don't just work your biceps. Get into an aerobic exercise program that works your heart and lungs, says Dr. Mostow. It will help keep your lungs functioning at peak efficiency. Walking, running, and swimming for 20 minutes at least three times a week will certainly do the job, but check with your doctor before you start, so she can tailor your exercise prescription specifically to your needs.

Stay away from smokes. Smoking a cigarette or even being in a room where others are smoking can damage your lungs, says Dr. Bethel. The smoke may cause your body's natural defense system to release an enzyme that, in trying to attack the smoke's chemicals, literally digests the lung. Not only does this set the stage for future diseases, but breathing can be immediately impaired.

Fighting Sniffles and Sneezes

Colds, upper respiratory infections, and bronchitis can be caused by any one of numerous microorganisms that can make you feel as though you lost the ability to breathe.

You get these diseases by inhaling somebody else's germs or touching someone that has a virus, then touching your eyes or nose, allowing the germs to enter your body.

Once the virus has invaded, it sets up shop in your throat and begins churning out baby viruses by the hundreds. These viruses spread throughout your body and trigger those beloved cold symptoms: a stuffy, drippy nose, sore throat, aches and pains, and cough.

There's no way to cure a cold as of yet, but here's how you can deal with its symptoms.

Eat five-alarm chili and curry. Hot peppers and spices such as curry and chili powder cause mucous membrane secretions. The extra fluid can thin out thick phlegm in your nasal passages and lubricate a sore, itchy throat.

Steam and sip. Sip chicken soup or linger in a steamy shower, suggests Thomas A. Gossel, Ph.D., dean of the College of Pharmacy and professor of pharmacology and toxicology at Ohio Northern University in Ada. The fluids you drink or inhale dilute the mucus in your nose and upper throat to help make breathing easier. Use decongestant sprays at bedtime for no more than 5 days to avoid inflaming tissues.

Try the big D. The D in many over-the-counter cough suppressants (such as Robitussin DM) is dextromethorphan. Doctors swear by it. Just make sure you follow package directions.

Suck on zinc. Zinc's ability to zap a cold has been suspected for years. And at least one study, at Dartmouth College in Hanover, New Hampshire, indicates that zinc tablets can cut the duration of a cold by 42 percent. But not any zinc tablet will do. You need those marked "zinc gluconate with glycine."

Eat some herbs. Echinacea and goldenseal, taken in combination, are top cold and flu fighters, says Kristy Fassler, N.D., a naturopathic doctor in Portsmouth, New Hampshire. Echinacea stimulates the production of natural killer cells that fight viral infections. Goldenseal helps break up nasal and chest congestion and also reduces the swelling of mucous membranes, Dr. Fassler says.

Numb your throat. Suck on over-the-counter throat lozenges to numb and soothe your throat, suggests Dr. Gossel. Or aim a medicated spray at the back of your throat, hold your breath, and squirt. Follow package directions for both lozenges and sprays.

Purge pain. Try aspirin, acetaminophen, or ibuprofen to relieve the aches and pains of a cold, says Dr. Gossel.

Fight malaise. The too-tired-to-move feeling that usually accompanies a cold is often caused by dehydration, according to Dr. Gossel. Try drinking at least eight glasses of water a day to prevent it.

Chill out. A study at Carnegie Mellon University in Pittsburgh indicates that the more stress you're under, the more likely you are to get a visit from any cold bug in the vicinity.

The researchers asked 394 men and women between the ages of 18 and 54 about any stress in their lives—recent bereavement, going on a diet, changing jobs, losing money, little sleep, and arguing with family members—and then divided them into five groups. Each group received custom-made nose drops containing one of five viruses known to cause colds.

The result? Those who had the most stress in their lives were five times more likely to get colds than those who had the least.

Coping with Emphysema and Bronchitis

One disease likely to send your respiratory system into an early retirement is chronic obstructive pulmonary disease. It includes chronic bronchitis, a condition in which the air sacs of the lungs are destroyed, and emphysema, a condition in which lung elasticity is lost and air is unable to flow freely in and out through the airway. It does not include the common bronchitis you might get with a cold—that's simply an irritation of the bronchial tubes that causes a few days of coughing and then goes away.

Both chronic bronchitis—roughly defined as a daily wet cough that lasts for 3 months or more—and emphysema are usually caused by smoking. With both conditions, you're likely to be short of breath, have limited ability to exert yourself, hack up mucus, and cough. Both conditions are on the rise. The number of people who have these diseases has increased 41 percent in the last 10 years, and chronic bronchitis and emphysema make up the largest number of respiratory illnesses (other than colds) in people between the ages of 30 and 45. Because more men than women smoke, men are nearly twice as likely as women to get emphysema, but women are rapidly catching up. When it comes to chronic bronchitis, women are more likely to get it. Emphysema and chronic bronchitis together kill approximately 75,000 people a year.

There's no cure for chronic bronchitis or emphysema, but the following strategies can lessen the shortness of breath that eventually comes from an obstructed airway and make life with the diseases a little easier.

Avoid people who sneeze. Any type of respiratory infection can make emphysema and chronic bronchitis worse, says Dr. Bethel. As much as possible, avoid crowded areas or people who have infections. See your doctor if an illness such as a cold or flu is aggravating your breathing problems.

Get your shots. Prevent the complications of influenza and bacterial pneumonia by getting immunized against both flu and pneumonia, says Dr. Bethel.

Learn to save your breath. If you have emphysema, ask your doctor to recommend both an occupational therapist and a physical therapist in your local area.

"An occupational therapist can work with people who are short of breath and who are limited in their day-to-day activities," says Dr. Bethel. "The therapist can teach people more energy-efficient ways of doing those activities."

A physical therapist can develop an exercise program that will train your body to use its available oxygen more efficiently. The result will be that the little oxygen you have will go farther.

Dilate your airway. Your doctor may prescribe medications to dilate your airway to its fullest, says Dr. Bethel. Use them according to directions.

Asthma: An Increasingly Deadly Disease

Asthma is different from chronic bronchitis and emphysema in that its obstruction of the airway is both intermittent and reversible.

TB: It's Back

Tuberculosis (TB), a bacterial lung infection that scientists thought they had virtually eliminated in the United States, is not only alive and well but also thriving.

While the disease had been declining since the late 1940s, the number of cases of TB has since risen.

The cause? Rampant spread of the bacteria that causes TB among those who have AIDS, those who are homeless, and those who have newly emigrated to the United States—plus the development of drug-resistant strains of the bacteria.

TB is spread by airborne droplets in sneezes, coughs, and just plain breathing. The bacteria are inhaled into the lungs. In those with strong immune systems, the bacteria are surrounded by a legion of bacterial fighters that render them harmless. In others, the bacteria settle into the lungs and multiply. With time, they may destroy extensive parts of the lungs and leave cavities. Eventually, the lungs look like Swiss cheese.

Today, 10 million Americans carry the disease, many without the typical symptoms of cough, fatigue, and weight loss.

"I think the general population is at risk," says Robert Bethel, M.D., a staff physician at the National Jewish Center for Immunology and Respiratory Medicine in Denver. "To a large extent, you can't control whether or not you're exposed to TB.

"Not that I want to be an alarmist," Dr. Bethel hastens to add. "But if you're on a bus, subway, or airline with someone who has active TB and who is coughing, then the people around that person are exposed and vulnerable."

Fortunately, a complicated long-term drug regimen can usually fight TB into a dormant stage. But early treatment is important. If you think you've been exposed to TB, check with your doctor. A simple skin test or chest x-ray can usually determine whether or not you have the disease.

During an asthma attack, the airway constricts, the airway walls thicken with inflammation, and mucus accumulates within the airway. The result is an obstructed airway that makes you feel as though you were choking to death. But after an attack, the airway usually returns to normal. Unfortunately, years of these attacks can lead to permanent airway damage.

If you've never had asthma before, breathe easy. Once you're past age 30, you're unlikely to develop it, says Harold S. Nelson, M.D., senior staff physician at the National Jewish Center for Immunology and Respiratory Medicine and a member of the National Asthma Education Expert Panel of the National Heart, Lung and Blood Institute.

"Asthma tends to run in families," says Dr. Bethel. "There may be a predisposition in some people, but we think that asthma is caused by an inflammation of the airway.

"All the mechanisms aren't clear," he adds. "Sometimes the inflammation is caused by allergens that people inhale. Sometimes it's workplace exposures. Exposure to a large number of agents—solder used in the electronics industry or fumes from the making of plastics—may sensitize the airway and make someone asthmatic. Many times people develop asthma, and it's not clear what caused it."

What is clear, doctors agree, is that asthma, which affects about 12 million Americans, is becoming more prevalent and more deadly every year. About 5,000 people die from it each year—and the death rate climbs with age.

What's behind the increase in asthma numbers and deaths is still a mystery, reports the American Lung Association. Any number of things can trigger an asthma attack, including allergies, cigarette smoke and other irritants, a viral infection in your respiratory system, and heartburn, which can result in coughing and spasms in your lungs. Even strong emotions and hard exercise—especially in cold weather—can cause troubles, Dr. Nelson says.

New or recurring cases of asthma can start off feeling like regular respiratory tract infections, Dr. Nelson says. If you begin to develop wheezing, tightness in your chest, or shortness of breath, see a doctor immediately.

If you're diagnosed with asthma, doctors can prescribe medication to ease the symptoms. Inhalers containing corticosteroids are the most effective way of reducing swelling and helping you breathe easier. Over-the-counter drugs rarely have much effect, Dr. Nelson says.

"This is not something you should treat by yourself," he says. "Asthma is much too serious for that." Here's what experts suggest to handle the disease.

Avoid pollution. "There's evidence that living in polluted environments increases the incidence of lung diseases such as asthma," says Dr. Bethel. That's why you should try to avoid heavily polluted areas such as industrial districts and urban highways.

Air quality is frequently monitored by various agencies to see if it complies with federal and state standards. To find out how badly the area in which you live or work is polluted, call your state's environmental agency. The people there have the information at hand or can refer you to someone who does.

Breathe through a scarf. Breathing in cold, dry air can constrict the airway and induce wheezing, coughing, and shortness of breath. The solution? Wear a scarf that you can draw up over your mouth and nose to breathe through during cold spells. And try to breathe mostly through your nose. Breathing through your nose warms and humidifies the air before it reaches the lungs.

Head for the kitchen. A review of what 9,000 adults eat every day revealed that higher vitamin C and niacin intakes were associated with fewer cases of wheezing. Good sources of vitamin C include black currants, guava, orange juice, and red bell peppers. Good sources of niacin include chicken breast, water-packed tuna, and swordfish.

Try magnesium for relief. Quite of bit of research has linked magnesium with the improvement of asthma symptoms. "Magnesium definitely has an anti-spasmodic effect on the smooth muscle of the upper respiratory tracts," says Claudia Cooke, M.D., a holistic doctor in New York City. Since asthma is aggravated by spasms in the smooth muscles, which are involuntary muscles, magnesium's antispasmodic effects can be beneficial.

Use an early warning system. The home peak-flow meter, a device that measures your breathing capacity, can help identify what's a normal flow and what's not, says Dr. Nelson. Since airflow sometimes drops a couple of hours or days before an attack, the peak-flow meter can give you an early warning that lets you ward off the attack with medication prescribed by your doctor.

Ask your doctor about where to get a peak-flow meter and how to use it.

Take the right medication. Prescription medications that treat asthma include anti-inflammatory drugs that suppress airway inflammation, such as steroids, as well as bronchodilators that dilate the airway itself.

But noting that some people use only bronchodilators, Dr. Nelson adds, "Anyone with more than the mildest occasional asthma needs to be on anti-inflammatory treatment rather than just bronchodilators. Together, they will decrease symptoms, probably decrease the number of acute episodes that would otherwise need hospital treatment, decrease the need for bronchodilators, and, doctors hope, prevent the long-term development of irreversible obstruction."

Surviving Flu and Pneumonia

Neither flu nor the most common forms of pneumonia are likely to damage your lungs, but they can make you so short of breath that you feel you can't even make it up a flight of stairs.

Flu, which generally causes fever, headache, sore throat, nasal congestion, muscle aches, and a feeling of exhaustion, typically strikes between December and March. It's caused by one of two virus strains, A or B, that usually manage to infect anywhere from 33 to 52 percent of Americans each year. Because flu affects older folks so severely, it is the sixth leading cause of death in the United States.

Fortunately, both flu and the most deadly and common types of pneumonia can frequently be prevented or successfully be treated without permanently damaging your lungs. Here's how.

Be alert for signs of danger. Some types of pneumonia, such as staph or klebsiella, can seriously damage the lung, says Dr. Mostow, and "your lung is never the same afterward." So see your doctor quickly if you have a fever, breathlessness, or a nagging cough that won't go away.

Defend yourself against pneumonia. The pneumonia vaccine doesn't prevent pneumonia, says Dr. Mostow, but it can prevent you from dying when pneumonia strikes. The vaccine is effective against 23 different types of bacterial germs—the kinds that are responsible for 90 percent of pneumonia deaths. You need to get it only once in your life.

Protect against flu. The flu vaccine is highly effective, says Dr. Mostow. Anyone with chronic lung or heart disease, diabetes, impaired immunity, kidney disease, anemia, or another blood problem should get the vaccine every year in the fall, as should anyone over age 65 and anyone who's involved in the care of patients.

Who should not get the shot? Since the vaccine is incubated in eggs, those who are allergic to eggs should avoid it. In general, if you can eat eggs, you can safely receive a flu shot.

Visit your family physician. If you forget to get your flu shot, there are two prescription antiviral drugs that can stop flu in its tracks, says Dr. Mostow. One is amantadine (Symmetrel) and the other is rimantadine (Flumadine). These two compounds are active against influenza A, the only flu virus that kills. Just one caveat: You must get them from your doctor within 48 hours of when you come down with the flu.

If you forget to get the pneumonia vaccine—or if you're unlucky enough to run into one of the pneumonias that's not in the vaccine—your doctor will prescribe an antibiotic that is specifically designed to kill the virus or bacteria that have attacked, says Dr. Mostow.

Skin Cancer

The Dark Side of the Sun

Remember summers on the patio with an aluminum foil reflector and nothing but an itsy-bitsy bathing suit between you and the sun? Or slathering baby oil all over yourself in hopes of getting a deep, dark tan?

Ouch. The truth is, just one bad burn in childhood doubles your risk of skin cancer as an adult. Add a few more decades of sun exposure—even if you've always tanned without burning—and your risk goes up even more, along with the cosmetic age of your skin, which will look older because of sun damage. Fair-skinned, light-eyed ancestors also boost your chances. And if a parent or grandparent has had a skin cancer removed, you may be next in line.

Like many people, you probably give a lot of attention to the appearance of your skin. If it looks good, you assume it's healthy. That's why skin cancer can be such a shock—it seems like an ambush from nowhere. (It can be 20 years between the initial sun damage and the cancer.) And these days many of us are being ambushed in our late forties or early fifties instead of in our seventies and later, the ages that used to supply the majority of victims. Researchers speculate that damage to the planet's ozone layer, which protects us from the worst of the sun's radiation, is one likely reason.

Fortunately, while skin cancer is scary, it's also nearly 100 percent curable, as long as it's caught in time. And best of all, it's preventable.

The Various Breeds

The two most common forms of skin cancer are known as basal cell and squamous cell. They very rarely spread, though if they're stubborn, they can recur, says Thomas Griffin, M.D., a dermatologist at Graduate Hospital of Philadelphia and clinical assistant professor of dermatology at the University of Pennsylvania School of Medicine in Philadelphia. They appear as small bumps on the skin, usually on sun-exposed areas including your back, which receives radiation right through light fabrics. They can be flesh-toned or brown to gray, and some have

Tanning Parlors: Fountains of Aging

Don't buy the hype that tanning under a sunlamp or on a tanning bed is somehow safer than the radiation you get from the sun. Or that a "base tan" you acquire in a tanning parlor will somehow protect you from deeper sun damage.

Both claims are dangerously false, says Vincent DeLeo, M.D., associate professor of dermatology at Columbia-Presbyterian Medical Center in New York City.

"Tanning parlors and sunlamps are the most worthless things you can pay money for—and very damaging to the skin," he says. A report from the National Institutes of Health says that some tanning lamps generate over five times more ultraviolet radiation (UVA) than you'd get sitting for the same amount of time on a beach at the equator.

If you feel desperate for the golden look, use a self-tanning lotion, suggests Dr. DeLeo. But don't forget to use a sunscreen, too.

tiny ulcers at the center of the growth that bleed easily. Squamous cell cancers may also have a hard spot within the growth.

The shark of skin cancers is melanoma. It occurs much less frequently than other skin cancers, but it can be fatal. Once melanoma grows deeper than 1 millimeter into the skin, it has a higher risk of spreading to other organs. It may start from a mole, though it can also begin in a large, flat brown freckle or bleeding spot.

Although men have a higher rate of melanoma than women, it is increasing more rapidly in young women than in any other age group, says David J. Leffell, M.D., chief of dermatologic surgery at Yale University School of Medicine in New Haven, Connecticut. "We're not sure why, but it may be that women now in their thirties had enormous sun exposure in the 1960s when they were children," he says.

Yet doctors say skin cancer is cause for caution, not alarm. Although it appears more often as you get older, you have high odds of outrunning skin cancer for two reasons. One—it's easy to diagnose, and two—in most cases it's curable.

Reducing Your Odds

Even if you've spent quite a few summers in the sun, you can dramatically reduce your chances of developing skin cancer by controlling your exposure from now on. You also need to know how to detect cancer on sun-exposed skin or in an abnormal mole before it grows to the danger point. Here are the top tactics for saving your skin.

Screen it. Wear a full-spectrum sunscreen that blocks both kinds of ultraviolet radiation (UVA and UVB)—and wear it every day, summer and winter, says Perry Robins, M.D., associate professor of dermatology at New York University in New York City, president of the Skin Cancer Foundation, and author of *Sun Sense*. Check to be sure that your sunscreen has a sun protection factor (SPF) of at least 15.

Spend noon indoors. Try to limit your outdoor activities during the hours when the sun's rays are the strongest—from 10:00 A.M. to 2:00 P.M., says Dr. Griffin.

Check for changes. Examine your skin thoroughly twice a year, with a hand mirror or with help from a friend or spouse. Look for any kind of spot that changes, says Dr. Robins. The change can be in color, texture, or size (the spot gets bigger), or the spot can begin to bleed, he says. If you have a family history of skin cancer or you've had severe sunburns, ask your dermatologist to "map" your body for potential trouble spots and to keep track of any changes with followup visits.

Memorize the ABCDs. This will help you monitor moles for signs of melanoma, says Vincent DeLeo, M.D., associate professor of dermatology at Columbia-Presbyterian Medical Center in New York City:

- A is for asymmetry (no symmetrical shape).
- B is for border (an irregular border).
- C is for color change (a dark area arises within a mole, or a mole shows areas of lightening).
- D is for diameter (the mole gets larger or is larger than a pencil eraser).

If you have any of the ABCDs, get to a doctor immediately, says Dr. DeLeo.

Take vitamin E. There is some scientific evidence that taking the natural form of vitamin E can decrease the damage done by the sun to the skin, says Karen Burke, M.D., Ph.D., a dermatologic surgeon and dermatologist in private practice in New York City. So it may help to prevent the conditions that could lead to skin cancer. She recommends a vitamin E supplement of 400 international units a day as a dose that may help with protection. Be sure to get the natural form of the vitamin—it should say so on the label and will contain d- (not dl-) alpha tocopherol or d-alpha tocopheryl acetate or succinate, says Dr. Burke. But if you are considering taking vitamin E in amounts above 200 international units, discuss this with your doctor first.

Apply vitamin C to your skin. "Vitamin C can't block the sun, but it can help reduce the damage from the rays that do get through your sunscreen," says Sheldon Pinnell, M.D., the J. Lamar Callaway professor of dermatology at Duke University Medical Center in Durham, North Carolina. Vitamin C also helps to reduce the weakening of the skin's immune system from overexposure to the sun, a problem that has been found in more than 90 percent of people who get skin cancer.

A Safe Tan in a Tube

Today's self-tanning lotions won't turn you the awful streaky orange that skin dyes did years ago, thank goodness. The new breeds of tan-in-a-bottle are easy to apply, look natural, and won't harm your skin.

A self-tanner actually interacts with your skin to turn it a natural, golden-looking color, says Yveline Duchesne, international training director for New York City–based Clarins Cosmetics. The tan fades gradually as you shed your dead skin cells, usually within a few days.

The main active ingredient in self-tanning lotions is a chemical called dihydroxyacetone (DHA). DHA combines with certain amino acids and keratin on the very superficial cell layers of skin to produce the color.

With the new products, you can be attractively tanned without damage to your skin—if you continue to wear sunscreen. Most self-tanners have sunscreen with only a low sun protection factor (SPF), so it's best to also use your own sunscreen of SPF 15 or higher. The best timing? Since self-tanners take a few hours to develop, apply them the night before, Duchesne suggests. Then apply your sunscreen the next morning, at least an hour before going out.

Other tips for making the most of your self-tanner:

Always allergy-test. Before you try a self-tanner all over, apply the lotion to a small patch of skin and leave it on overnight to see if your skin is sensitive to DHA. (If it reacts, a bronzing gel or tinted sunscreen is your best bet for color.)

Exfoliate before you apply. DHA can take unevenly in areas where there's a buildup of dead cells. Be sure to include hands, elbows, and knees.

Start at the top. Work down from your forehead, covering all exposed areas, but skip the eyebrows, where color can concentrate. Apply evenly, including your ears and under your jaw.

Moisturize the rough spots. Elbows and knees will look more natural if you moisturize first and apply self-tanner lightly.

Wait for results. How often you reapply, not how much, determines the depth of your tan. It takes from 3 to 5 hours for color to develop, so don't reapply until you've seen the full results.

Let it dry. Wait a half-hour before dressing or going to bed, since some tanners can stain fabric.

Wash up. Wash your hands after you apply your self-tanner, or you'll end up with tan palms.

Ascorbic acid is the only form of vitamin C the body can use, and to be effective, it must be formulated properly, he says. It is found in several products, including SkinCeuticals Topical Vitamin C High Potency Serum 15. These products are available without prescription from dermatologists, plastic surgeons, and licensed skin-care professionals, according to Dr. Pinnell.

Early Detection, Early Cure

What happens when your early detection efforts pay off? You've called your dermatologist's attention to a growth, and she confirms that it must be removed.

For most cancers, a local anesthetic is all that you'll need, and the removal won't leave a noticeable scar. Depending on the depth and nature of the growth, your doctor will use one or a combination of procedures. They include burning, scraping, freezing, and cutting out the growth. Some shallow cancers can be treated with a topical chemotherapy cream.

For difficult or recurring cancers, a surgeon can remove malignant cells in very thin layers, leaving healthy skin untouched. Even melanoma has a potent new enemy—a melanoma cell vaccine that significantly increases survival rates.

SLEEP APNEA

The Snooze That Can Leave You Breathless

There's nothing restorative about a night's sleep if it involves relentless interrupted breaths and choked gasps. But that's exactly what happens night after night to millions of people who have a disorder known as sleep apnea.

The scary thing about sleep apnea is that you may have it and not even know it. Unless, of course, you haven't been feeling quite your youthful, robust, happy-go-lucky self lately. It makes sense: Even if you're getting 8 hours of sleep a night, if you have sleep apnea, you gasp and wheeze during the night, waking yourself up ever so slightly each time. So 8 hours of sleep becomes a series of little, fitful pieces.

"These recurrent mini-arousals rob you of the full restorativeness of unfragmented deep sleep," says Stuart F. Quan, M.D., director of the Sleep Disorders Center at the University of Arizona in Tucson. "This chronic sleep deprivation leaves you extremely sleepy and lethargic during your waking hours."

Sleep apnea not only saps your energy but also can leave you feeling irritable, depressed, and even a little dopey. It can also take a toll on your physical appearance, producing baggy eyes, poor posture, and changes in the way you walk and talk. "Many people who are in their forties come into our offices with obstructive sleep breathing problems but they look, feel, and act 10 years older," says Richard Millman, M.D., director of the Sleep Disorders Center of Rhode Island Hospital in Providence.

Even if you're lucky enough to stay cheerful and keep your looks, you're not out of the woods yet. People with sleep apnea may experience sharp drops in their blood oxygen levels. This can foster serious health problems that we usually associate with aging, including high blood pressure, heart rhythm disturbances, heart attack, and stroke. On top of that, as many as one-third of all people with sleep apnea probably have experienced car accidents or dangerous mishaps on the job, says Willard Moran, M.D., clinical professor of otolaryngology at the University of Oklahoma College of Medicine in Oklahoma City.

Sleep apnea can put a severe strain on your relationships as well. The loud gasps and other noises have driven many spouses to separate bedrooms. And impotence is a problem for men. "Sleep deprivation inhibits a man's sexual interest and his ability to obtain an erection," says Dr. Quan. "The man is just too tired to keep his mind on the act, and he falls asleep."

When Your Airway Says No Way

Sleep apnea is caused by a closure of the tissues in the upper airway of the nose and throat. As we age, these muscles and tissues—including the tongue, the tonsils, the soft palate, and the uvula (the fleshy structure that dangles from the roof of the mouth)—get flabby and lose tone. When we sleep, they relax and close in upon themselves. If this closure is partial, the obstruction will only be partial, so when you breathe, the tissues vibrate against each other, producing the familiar sounds of a snore.

Now suppose that these same tissues over-relax, creating a total airway obstruction. This is sleep apnea. "Sleep apnea can be thought of as the most advanced form of snoring. The process in both is the same, only in sleep apnea, no air passes at all," says David N. F. Fairbanks, M.D., clinical professor of otolaryngology at the George Washington University School of Medicine and Health Sciences in Washington, D.C.

These pauses can last from 10 seconds to a minute. During that time, you struggle for air, but nothing happens until your brain jumpstarts your breathing by signaling a loud gasping or snorting response. The gasp wakes you up slightly, restores tone to the tissues, and opens the airway. When normal breathing resumes, you drift back to unconsciousness, only to have the process repeat.

Sleep apnea is usually years in the making. "It's extremely rare for severe apnea to develop out of the blue," says Christian Guilleminault, M.D., professor at the Stanford University School of Medicine Sleep Disorder Center in Palo Alto, California. "People will usually progress gradually over the years from heavy snoring to mild sleep apnea to more severe."

Sleep apnea can snag you at any age, but it's more likely to get you after you hit your thirties or forties. The age connection is obvious: As we age, we lose muscle tone, and our tissues get flabbier. We become less active and put on weight.

Certain conditions can bring on sleep apnea, too. Among them: bulky throat tissue; large tonsils, adenoids, or uvulas; tumors or cysts in the airway; a recessed jaw; or a nasal deformity. All these things can create blockages or cause the airway to collapse when you breathe.

Although obstructive sleep apnea affects people of all shapes and sizes, it is much more likely in heavyset people. Neck size seems to be a factor, too. A thick, fat neck promotes the collapse of the throat during sleep. A large number of men with sleep apnea have size 17 necks or larger, says Dr. Millman.

Don't Ignore a Snore

You may not think that snoring is a big deal, and it may not be. But persistent snorers need to be checked for sleep apnea, says James Rowley, M.D., assistant professor of medicine at Wayne State University School of Medicine and medical director of the Harper Hospital Sleep Disorders Center, both in Detroit.

If you don't have a bedmate to tell you details about your snoring, you will have to investigate on your own, says Barbara Phillips, M.D., medical director of the Samaritan Hospital Sleep Apnea Center and director of the University of Kentucky Sleep Clinic, both in Lexington. You can do this by putting a tape recorder with a timer next to your bed. Set the timer on the recorder so that it will turn on during the wee hours of the morning, preferably about 2 hours before you normally wake up. That is when your sleep is the deepest—and when your snores are most likely to be sounding like a rhino's mating call.

Here are some signs to look for, according to Dr. Rowley.

- Snoring is loud, frequent, and irregular sounding.
- Snoring keeps others awake, even people in other rooms.
- There are pauses in snoring that sound as if you have stopped breathing.
- You wake from sleep with a gasping or choking sensation.
- You wake up nonrefreshed or with a headache.
- You are exceedingly sleepy during the day—and doze off in highly inappropriate and even dangerous situations, such as at the desk right after lunch or behind the wheel of your car while waiting at a red light.

If you suspect that you have sleep apnea, see a doctor for advice on treatment options.

An Arsenal of Airway Openers

There is no cure for sleep apnea, but it is treatable. If these tips don't help nip it in the bud, your physician can refer you to a sleep or breathing specialist, who can prescribe a more specific treatment.

Slim down. Fat can press down on the neck, making the airway more prone to obstruction and decreasing the amount of air you obtain with each breath, says

Dr. Guilleminault. A weight loss of 10 to 25 percent can eliminate sleep apnea or significantly reduce the episodes.

Kick the habit. Cigarette smoke irritates the airway, causing it to swell and narrow, says A. Jay Block, M.D., professor of medicine and anesthesiology and chief of the pulmonary division at the University of Florida College of Medicine in Gainesville. It also increases mucus production in your nose.

Clear your nasal passages. People with nasal obstructions must inhale with greater effort, causing the throat and airway to constrict, says Dr. Millman. Open your nasal passages with an over-the-counter saline solution or ask your doctor about allergy treatment. Nonprescription nasal sprays (such as Afrin) are also good, but be careful—overusing them can make matters worse.

Lock up the liquor cabinet. Alcohol causes muscles and tissues to over-relax, says Dr. Millman. If you must drink, do so in moderation, and avoid it within 4 hours of bedtime.

Dump the downers. Many snorers perceive their excessive sleepiness as a sign of insomnia and turn to sleeping pills. This is the worst thing you can do, says Dr. Quan. Like alcohol, tranquilizers, sedatives, and other sleep-inducing medications will exacerbate your apnea by encouraging muscles and tissues to relax.

Don't burn the midnight oil. Sleep deprivation only makes you extra drowsy, which plunges you into a deeper sleep, over-relaxes your muscles, and brings on apnea, says Dr. Quan. Try to keep normal bedtimes.

Eat light. Large evening meals and midnight snacks can bring on heavier sleep, which results in increased muscle relaxation and a night full of gasping, says Dr. Fairbanks.

Back off. Apnea is more common when you're on your back, so get in the habit of sleeping on your stomach or your side, suggests Dr. Guilleminault. One thing you can try is a snore ball: Sew a pocket on the back of your pajama top and insert a tennis ball. This will condition you to keep off your back.

Put some slope in your sleep. It's wise to raise your head and shoulders while you sleep. But propping with pillows will only kink your neck and cut off your airway. Get around this by placing bricks or wood blocks under the bedposts to raise the head of your bed several inches, says Dr. Millman.

Try a tongue retainer. A sleep disorder center or an orthodontist can fit you with a variety of dental appliances to comfortably hold your tongue or pull your jaw forward so that your tongue doesn't fall into the back of your throat while you're sleeping, says Dr. Millman.

Mask your apnea. Perhaps the most effective apnea treatment is a home device called a continuous positive airway pressure machine. This is a mask that fits over your nose and provides air pressure to keep your throat from collapsing. The only drawback to the device, says Dr. Moran, is that many people don't enjoy the idea of going to bed looking like Darth Vader. A doctor must fit you for the device.

Be wary of medications. According to Dr. Moran, some doctors may prescribe stimulants to maintain tone in the airway while you sleep. But these drugs tend to prevent you from entering deep sleep, which is needed for good health.

Watch your blood pressure. Researchers aren't sure which comes first, high blood pressure or sleep apnea. They only know that when you have one condition, you stand a greater chance of having the other. If you believe you have sleep apnea, check your blood pressure regularly, suggests Barbara Phillips, M.D., medical director of the Samaritan Hospital Sleep Apnea Center and director of the University of Kentucky Sleep Clinic, both in Lexington. High blood pressure is a risk factor for stroke and heart disease.

Consider corrective surgery. As a last resort, physicians have a variety of surgical procedures at their disposal. They can remove tonsils, adenoids, and nasal blockages. One popular procedure called a uvulopalatopharyngoplasty (UPPP for short) removes, shortens, and tightens excess tissue in the airway. Surgery to correct setback jaws also has proven successful in keeping the tongue from falling back into the throat.

SMOKING

Clear the Air and Rejuvenate Your Life

If you're among the millions of people who started smoking as teenagers because they wanted to look and feel older, you got your wish—and maybe more than you bargained for. Nothing ages your appearance, spirit, and health more than America's most practiced and most dangerous vice.

Just ask Elizabeth Sherertz, M.D., a dermatologist and researcher at Bowman Gray School of Medicine of Wake Forest University in Winston-Salem, North Carolina.

"We found that on average, smokers tend to look between 5 and 10 years older than their actual ages because of the wrinkles caused by smoking," she says. "People who smoke are more likely to develop wrinkles, because smoking damages the elastic tissue that keeps skin tight and probably enhances the sun's damaging effects to the skin."

Or ask Richard Jenks, Ph.D., a sociologist at Indiana University Southeast in New Albany, who studies the effects of smoking on our emotional state. He found that once again, puffers suffer.

"Smokers know that their habit is a sure road to health problems, and they're actually even more likely than nonsmokers or ex-smokers to describe it as dirty," he says. "But what my study found was that smokers tend to feel they have less control over their lives, and feel less satisfied with their lives, than nonsmokers."

Or ask any other researcher or doctor who has ever studied the effects that smoking has on our physical and emotional well-being. Study after study—and there have been hundreds of them—backs up what experts already know: If it doesn't kill you—and one in five people worldwide dies from smoking-related diseases each year—it will most certainly take years off your life.

Says Margaret A. Chesney, Ph.D., a women's health and smoking researcher and professor at the University of California, San Francisco, School of Medicine, "If you want to radically slow down the aging process and live longer, stop smoking."

Quitting: A Key Problem for Women

The good news is Americans are aware of the dangers of smoking and many have quit. These days, fewer Americans are smoking than when the surgeon general released his report on the dangers of tobacco in 1964. In real numbers, about 24 percent of American women over age 18 smoke, down from the 34 percent who smoked in 1964. About 28 percent of American men smoke today—a drastic decrease from the 52 percent who smoked in 1964.

But quitting isn't easy, as you no doubt know if you smoke. It's especially difficult for women—both physically and psychologically. "There is evidence that equal numbers of men and women attempt to quit, but men succeed at about twice the rate," says Douglas E. Jorenby, Ph.D., coordinator of clinical activities for the Center for Tobacco Research and Intervention at the University of Wisconsin Medical School in Madison. "One reason is that women report more depression when they quit smoking, and we know from various studies that depression makes it more likely that you'll go back to smoking."

But, he adds, it seems as though women are less likely to want to quit. "Many women feel so overwhelmed by their families and jobs that a lot of them say cig-

No Weighty Move Here

For many people who want to quit smoking, the biggest fear is gaining weight.

Well, fret no more, because it's official: According to the Centers for Disease Control and Prevention in Atlanta, when you quit, the average weight gain is about 5 pounds. And the weight gain can be prevented through a careful diet and stress management. In fact, some people actually lose weight after they quit.

For many people, quitting smoking is part of an overall get-healthy program that includes regular exercise and improvements in diet, says Douglas E. Jorenby, Ph.D., coordinator of clinical activities for the Center for Tobacco Research and Intervention at the University of Wisconsin Medical School in Madison.

arettes are their only refuge. And they're hesitant to give that up, even though they know quitting has a big benefit to their health."

Women, particularly those under age 25, have become a major target market for cigarette companies. "One of the big messages behind the advertising to women is that smoking helps you control your weight," says Dr. Jorenby. "In one cigarette advertisement I saw, there was a photo of a model who was already pretty skinny. But the photo was distorted to make her look even thinner—thinner than any human being can really be. The message, which is targeted to women in their teens and early twenties, is obvious: Smoking helps you to be thin and glamorous."

Smokers Aren't Thinner

Despite what Madison Avenue would have you believe, smokers aren't thinner. True, nicotine slightly curbs the appetite, meaning that smokers consume fewer meals. But when they eat, smokers are more likely than nonsmokers to gravitate toward foods that are higher in calories and fat, says Doris Abood, Ed.D., associate professor of health education at Florida State University in Tallahassee. In her study, which examined the smoking, eating, drinking, and exercise habits of 1,820 people, she also found that smokers exercise less and consume more alcohol, which is notoriously high in calories. Dr. Abood and other researchers found that the more people smoke, the more bad habits they practice, and to a greater extent.

Still, regardless of these other habits, it's smoking itself that does the most damage, causing nearly 419,000 deaths a year. It also plays a leading role in scores of diseases, from cancer to colds, from heart disease to hip fractures. "The effects of smoking are distributed so much throughout the entire body that it has an impact on virtually any disease you can think of," says Dr. Jorenby.

How to Quit—For Good

If you quit, the benefits start accruing right away. Just 1 year after you stop smoking, your risk for heart disease is cut in half, and after 3 years, your risk becomes comparable to that of someone who never touched a cigarette. Your risks for other diseases, such as emphysema, bronchitis, and cancer, also diminish. Plus, you'll look and feel younger, with more energy and stamina and fewer wrinkles.

Sure, quitting is tough. Fewer than 10 percent of the 20 million smokers who try to quit each year actually succeed, says Rami Bachiman, director of community education for the American Lung Association of New York in New York City. There are various strategies to help you along—keeping your hands busy, chewing on carrot sticks, taking deep breaths of fresh air, drinking lots of water, or even rewarding yourself with a present. But here's how you can increase your chances of quitting successfully and not relapsing during those crucial first few weeks.

Do Shortcuts Work?

Nicotine patches and gum and hypnosis may take some of the sting out of the withdrawal symptoms that come with quitting but don't expect these aids to replace grit and determination.

Smokers who quit with the assistance of these tools are two to three times more likely to succeed than those doing it cold turkey. Although quitting cold turkey is the most popular method, it is also the least successful, having a success rate of only 5 percent. The smoker using nicotine gum or patches plus enrolling in a comprehensive behavioral smoking cessation program increases her chances of stopping and can anticipate a 1-year success rate of 23 to 40 percent. Meanwhile, there's a 15 percent success rate using hypnosis.

There are some side effects to nicotine patches and gum, which are prescribed by a doctor usually to heavy smokers who simply can't quit or who have had severe withdrawal symptoms when they've tried.

The patch, an adhesive square that secretes nicotine through the skin and into the bloodstream to help ease the pain of withdrawal, can cause itchiness and minor burning. And smoking even one cigarette while wearing the patch can cause a heart attack.

The effectiveness of the gum, meanwhile, is washed away if you eat or drink anything—especially diuretics such as coffee and cola—within 15 minutes of chewing it. And although the gum isn't supposed to be used after 4 months from your last cigarette, 1 in 12 smokers continue using it for over a year after quitting.

The bottom line: If you've tried to quit and failed in the past, ask your doctor about these products. But, says psychologist Mitchell Nides, Ph.D., of the University of California, Los Angeles, you have to "learn" how to be a nonsmoker, and that's something that no pharmaceutical can do by itself.

Log your progress. The first thing you should do is set a deadline up to 3 weeks away from when you'll have your last smoke. But in the meantime, log each cigarette you smoke—where you smoke and under what circumstances, advises Don R. Powell, Ph.D., president of the American Institute for Preventive Medicine in Farmington Hills, Michigan, and a former smoker. This will help you identify situations that cause you to smoke and then find alternative behaviors other than smoking cigarettes.

Delay the desire. If you are quitting gradually, each time you get the urge to smoke, hold off lighting up for 5 minutes, suggests Dr. Powell. After a few days, extend the delay to 10 minutes. After another few days, extend it to 15 minutes, and so on. "You'll find that the actual urge to smoke at any given moment fades relatively quickly," he says.

Seek support. Whether you're quitting cold turkey or doing it gradually by slowly decreasing the number of cigarettes you smoke, you'll probably fare better if you have a lot of encouragement. "Since they have a harder time quitting, women need as much support as they can get," says Dr. Jorenby. "Having some kind of group support can make a big difference in how you do, whether it's from friends and family or some sort of group therapy." There are probably groups in your area offering free counseling and group therapy for women trying to quit. Contact the local chapter of the American Heart Association for more information.

Drink orange juice. The hardest part of quitting cold turkey, which is the most popular method, is getting through the symptoms of nicotine withdrawal, which last 1 to 2 weeks. But you'll get over the irritability, anxiety, confusion, and trouble concentrating and sleeping that come with nicotine withdrawal a lot faster if you drink a lot of orange juice during that time.

That's because OJ makes your urine more acidic, which clears nicotine from your body faster, says Thomas Cooper, D.D.S., a nicotine dependency researcher and professor of oral health sciences at the University of Kentucky in Lexington. "Besides," adds Dr. Jorenby, "the citrus taste in your mouth makes the thought of having a cigarette pretty disgusting."

If you're quitting with the aid of doctor-prescribed nicotine gum or patches, however, avoid orange juice and other acidic drinks, because you want to keep nicotine in your system with these products.

Imagine it's the flu. "Before we had nicotine gum and patches, I used to tell people who were quitting smoking to imagine they were having the flu," says Dr. Jorenby. "A lot of withdrawal symptoms are similar to the flu: You fly off the handle easily, you have trouble concentrating, your stamina is down. And as with the flu, there's little you can do other than let it run its course. But you will get over it. As long as you don't relapse and have a cigarette, the withdrawal will be over and done within a week or two."

Stay out of bars. The greatest chance of relapsing occurs in bars, says Dr. Jorenby. "For many people, having a drink in one hand means having a cigarette in the other. I advise that anyone trying to quit stay out of bars for at least the first 2 weeks after they stop smoking." Instead, he advises, go to libraries, museums, and other public places where smoking is prohibited. "People who quit smoking don't have to swear off going to bars, but we know from many studies that they are at much higher risk of going back to smoking unless they stay away for the first few weeks."

Write a letter to a loved one. When a nicotine fit hits, pick up a pen instead of a butt and write a letter to a loved one explaining why smoking is more important than your life, suggests Robert Van de Castle, Ph.D., professor emeritus of behavioral medicine at the University of Virginia Medical Center in Charlottesville. In the letter, try to explain why you continue a habit that you know will kill you rather than quit and live to see a child graduate from college or get married or to witness other important events. When Dr. Van de Castle's patients try this letter, he says, they feel so selfish that it often gives them the courage to put up with withdrawal symptoms and stay smoke-free.

Reducing the Damage

Though kicking the habit is your number-one priority, there are measures you can take nutritionally to block smoking's path of destruction if you're finding it difficult to "butt out" once and for all.

Protect yourself with E. When it comes to protecting your body from smoking's nasty side effects, vitamin E, an antioxidant found in sunflower seeds, sweet potatoes, and kale, is a top performer. Vitamin E slows the progression of arteriosclerosis, a condition in which the coronary arteries harden from deposits of cholesterol, calcium, and scar tissue, gradually restricting blood flow and leading to heart disease. Additionally, investigators believe that vitamin E can protect tissues from smoke irritation and discourage the cell mutation that marks cancer and other tobacco-associated chronic diseases.

Experts recommend 100 to 200 international units of vitamin E a day.

Stock up on C. Found in strawberries, papaya, citrus fruits, and many other foods, vitamin C has been found to protect against a variety of cancers, as well as heart disease and stroke, says pharmacist Earl Mindell, R.Ph., Ph.D., professor of nutrition at Pacific Western University in Los Angeles and author of *Earl Mindell's Food as Medicine.*

Experts suggest smokers take 2,000 milligrams of vitamin C a day. This amount is considered safe but may cause diarrhea in some people.

Boost your beta-carotene. Abundant in orange and yellow fruits and vegetables, such as apricots, cantaloupes, carrots, pumpkins, and squash, beta-carotene seems to protect against "smokers' cancers"—those of the colon, kidneys, skin, and lungs, says James Scala, Ph.D., a nutritionist and author of *If You Can't/Won't Stop Smoking.* Study after study also shows that low levels of beta-carotene are associated with a greater cancer risk, including the risk of lung cancer.

Experts say smokers should get 16,500 to 50,000 international units of beta-carotene each day.

Prevent bone loss with calcium. Research shows that people, especially women, who smoke accelerate the bone loss that occurs naturally with age, putting them at greater risk for osteoporosis, a condition of brittle, easily fractured bones.

Though the only surefire way to stem this bone deterioration is to snuff your cigarette habit, some doctors recommend stepping up your calcium intake in the meantime to nourish your bones. And while it will help to increase your intake of calcium-filled foods, including low-fat dairy products and certain vegetables such as broccoli, the best way to get the 1,500 milligrams that experts recommend is through supplements.

Finish off with a multivitamin. "Because smoking depletes the body of all vitamins, smokers absolutely need to take a multivitamin/mineral supplement on top of their specific nutritional supplements," says Dr. Scala. He also stresses the importance of smokers adding more fruits and vegetables to their diets. "Smokers generally eat poor diets, which contributes to their nutritional deficiencies," he says.

SNORING

Not as Harmless as You Think

Here are three great unanswerable questions of our time: What was the purpose of Stonehenge? Did Oswald act alone? Why does a snorer only wake his spouse up and never himself?

Though science isn't sure how a person can rattle the rafters and keep right on snoozing, the cause of snoring is clearly understood.

When your air passageway constricts, the air flowing through it picks up speed, just the way a lazy river turns into whitewater when the riverbed narrows. The faster the air, the greater the turbulence. Greater turbulence vibrates the soft tissues in your throat—especially the back of your palate and your uvula, the thing that hangs down in the back of your mouth. Snoring is the sound of those tissues flapping in the accelerated breeze, says Hector P. Rodriguez, M.D., assistant professor of clinical otolaryngology/head and neck surgery at the Columbia University College of Physicians and Surgeons and director of the division of rhinology at Columbia-Presbyterian Medical Center, both in New York City.

Loud Nights, Foggy Days

For people who are mild or moderate snorers, snoring is more an irritation than a threat. But the industrial-strength window rattler does face the possibility of some very serious medical problems—problems that we usually expect to see in older adults.

One such problem is hearing loss. "We've recorded snoring as high as 85 decibels, almost the equivalent of a diesel engine," says Willard Moran, M.D., clinical professor of otolaryngology at the University of Oklahoma College of Medicine in Oklahoma City. "That much loudness at close distances night after night can damage your hearing and your spouse's as well."

The greatest health risk comes from the most advanced form of snoring

249

Spare Your Spouse

The man who snores will never be voted Mr. Popularity by those who must share sleeping quarters with him.

"Snoring has not only driven couples to the point of sleeping in separate bedrooms, it has also caused its fair share of bitter arguments and ugly divorces," says A. Jay Block, M.D., professor of medicine and anesthesiology and chief of the Pulmonary Division at the University of Florida College of Medicine in Gainesville. "Anything that you can do to make your spouse's night more bearable not only will reduce the number of kicks in the shin you receive, it may save your marriage." He recommends the following possible marriage-savers.

Buy her earplugs. Heavy-machine operators use them all the time. They are cheap, easy to use, and comfortable, and they work well even with really harsh snoring.

Install a white noise machine. Many department stores now sell electronic noise-filtering devices that produce barely audible sounds that help muffle other more offensive sounds in the room.

Make sure you're the last to go to bed. Let your spouse and anybody else in the house get into bed and drift off to sleep for awhile before you head to bed. Your snores are less likely to wake them once they're sound asleep.

---

known as obstructive sleep apnea. (For more information on sleep apnea, see page 237.) Sleep apnea makes your heart pump harder and deprives you of the benefits of deep-stage sleep.

Fortunately, not all snorers have sleep apnea. Still, even the heavy snorer may exhibit the aftereffects usually associated with full-blown apnea. He—and the snorer most often is a man—will wake with a throbbing headache and feel drowsy all day, possibly dozing off on the job or while driving.

In other ways, his behavior may start to resemble that of a much older man. He will be moody and sullen, will have difficulty with memory and mental tasks, and may lose his sex drive.

"The heavy snorer or apnea sufferer may even appear a bit senile," says Richard Millman, M.D., director of the Sleep Disorders Center of Rhode Island Hospital in Providence. "The real problem is that inadequate sleep and oxygen are robbing him of his alertness, concentration, and vigor."

The lack of oxygen in the blood and added strain on the heart can produce cardiovascular problems normally associated with old age, such as high blood pressure, heart failure, stroke, irregular heartbeat, and heart attack. "We can't say for certain that snoring necessarily ages you and that you will suffer from one of these problems if you snore," says Dr. Millman. "But a large number of men with long-term sleep breathing problems do look, act, and feel older than their true ages. And in general, snorers don't live as long as nonsnorers."

Snore No More

Snoring does not have to be a life sentence. Today, physicians specializing in sleep and breathing disorders can do wonders for almost all cases of snoring and sleep apnea. But even the heaviest of snorers may not need a doctor. The following tips may be all you need to quiet the storm once and for all.

Snuff that butt. As if you didn't already have enough reasons to quit smoking. Cigarette smoke greatly irritates the tissues of the nasal passages and upper airway, causing them to swell and obstruct airflow, says David N. F. Fairbanks, M.D., clinical professor of otolaryngology at the George Washington University School of Medicine and Health Sciences in Washington, D.C.

Lighten up. Your typical snorer is overweight. Carrying around a lot of excess pounds can mean that the person has fatty throat tissues, thus a smaller airway, says Barbara Phillips, M.D., medical director of the Samaritan Hospital Sleep Apnea Center and director of the University of Kentucky Sleep Clinic, both in Lexington. "The vast majority of patients who are willing to lose excess weight find that it helps," she says. Sometimes losing as little as 10 or 15 pounds can make a difference.

Eat light. Heavy meals right before you go to sleep can contribute to snoring, says Dr. Rodriguez. That's because the process of digestion causes muscles everywhere—including those in your throat—to relax. Relaxed throat muscles help seal off your throat, obstructing the flow of air and encouraging snoring. So try not to eat anything in the hour before you hit the sack. If you have to eat a late dinner, at least make it a light one—like soup and a sandwich.

Unclog your snoot. If your nose feels like it's stuffed to the rim, consider opening things up with an over-the-counter nasal spray (such as Afrin), suggests A. Jay Block, M.D., professor of medicine and anesthesiology and chief of the pulmonary division at the University of Florida College of Medicine in Gainesville.

But be careful. Overuse can backfire on you, clogging up your nose even worse. Follow the instructions in the package. And if your nasal passages seem to be blocked constantly, consult your doctor.

Don't drink and doze. Avoid drinking for 4 hours prior to going to bed, says Dr. Millman. Alcohol causes the muscles in the airway to over-relax.

Steer clear of sedatives. Sleeping pills and diazepam (Valium) relax your

Are You a Snorer?

If it weren't for kicks from irate bed partners, many people wouldn't have a clue that they're buzzing like chainsaws. But even with black-and-blue shins, some people need convincing.

One thing you or your spouse can do to find out for sure if you're snoring is to tape record your sleep, says David N.F. Fairbanks, M.D., clinical professor of otolaryngology at the George Washington University School of Medicine and Health Sciences in Washington, D.C.

Even without tape-recorded proof, you can get a sense of whether you have a snoring problem by seeing if you have symptoms like these: morning headaches, frequent awakenings and gaspings at night, daytime sleepiness, and dry morning mouth.

muscles and slacken tissues in the back of your throat, says Dr. Phillips.

Get off your back. Sleeping on your side may prevent your tongue and uvula from falling back into your airway, says Dr. Moran. One good way to make sure you don't roll over onto your back is to sew a pocket in the back of your pajamas and place a tennis ball inside. The ball will cause just enough discomfort to either wake you or encourage you to roll off your back.

Raise your head and shoulders. Sleeping on a slight slant can help prevent snoring by keeping the tongue from falling back into the airway. Don't prop your head with pillows, however. This will only kink the airway in your throat, making matters worse. Instead, says Dr. Millman, place a brick under each bedpost at the head of the bed to raise it 4 or 5 inches.

Try a whiplash collar. A neck brace may not be your version of an ideal bed partner, but it may keep your chin extended so that your neck won't kink and your throat stays open, says Dr. Fairbanks. To guard against a stiff neck the next morning, Dr. Fairbanks suggests using a foam collar rather than a plastic one. Foam cushions the neck better and is less restraining. But if you do have some morning kinks, it will help to gently stretch your neck muscles, give yourself a gentle massage, or take a warming shower, he says.

Hold your tongue. Many sleep disorder centers provide tongue-retaining devices that hold the tongue forward and keep the mouth closed while you sleep, says Dr. Millman. An orthodontist can also create a device that achieves the same effect by pulling the jaw forward at night.

Don't go short on sleep. Sleep deprivation makes snoring worse, says James Rowley, M.D., assistant professor of medicine at Wayne State University School of Medicine and medical director of the Harper Hospital Sleep Disorders Center, both in Detroit. Going to bed overly tired—either from lack of quality sleep or from too much physical activity—can cause snoring. If your airway muscles are tired, they will loosen up and vibrate.

Join the NFL. Ever notice those adhesive strips that some football players wear across the tops of their noses? The theory is that they open nasal passages and let the athletes get more air, which helps them pulverize opponents more effectively. The strips may help prevent snoring, too, says Dr. Phillips. Marketed under brand names such as Nozovent and Breathe Right, these nasal strips have been proven effective for some people who have snoring problems.

STRESS

Control Is the Cure

You can't get enough rest, and you can't get enough done. And your stomach is always wrapped up in a knot.

"Stress will do that to you," says Leah J. Dickstein, M.D., professor in the department of psychiatry and behavioral sciences at the University of Louisville School of Medicine in Kentucky and former president of the American Medical Women's Association. "It can really wear you out. And the real problem is that you could be paving the way for other troubles later on."

The American Institute of Stress in Yonkers, New York, estimates that 90 percent of all visits to doctors are for stress-related disorders. Stress has been linked to fatigue, hair loss, bad complexion, insomnia, disruption of the menstrual cycle, low libido, impotence, and lack of orgasm. There's even evidence that it can increase your risk of more serious problems such as high blood pressure and heart disease.

"Stress increases heart rate and blood pressure, therefore changing the inner lining of our blood vessels, making your blood more likely to clot," says Robert DiBianco, M.D., director of cardiology research at the Washington Adventist Hospital in Takoma Park, Maryland. "Stress may change the way cholesterol is handled by your blood vessels and, in doing so, may increase plaque formation."

Allen J. Elkin, Ph.D., director of the Stress Management and Counseling Center in New York City, puts it another way: "Stress speeds up your entire system and produces conditions in younger people that are more commonly associated with growing old. Virtually no part of your body can escape the ravages of stress."

There are several steps you can take to reduce the stress in your life. But before you can beat it, experts say you have to understand what stress is—and how it works.

You Can't Always Run

Despite its bad reputation, stress is one of your body's best defense systems. When you sense danger—such as a car coming at you—your body releases adrenaline and other chemicals that make you more alert, raise your blood pressure, and increase your strength, speed, and reaction time.

That's great if you're responding to a threat that requires physical action. Unfortunately, Dr. Dickstein says, your body doesn't recognize the difference between physical threats and mental ones. When you get nervous about meeting a deadline, for instance, you may produce the same stress chemicals as when you see that oncoming car. And if you don't burn off these chemicals through physical exertion, they can linger in the bloodstream and start causing problems.

Studies show that stress can reduce the power of your immune system. A study in Britain exposed 266 people, most of them in their thirties, to a common cold virus and then tracked who became sick. The study showed that 28.6 percent of those with few signs of stress caught the cold. But the figure jumped to 42.4 percent for those who were under high stress.

The reason? Stress may inhibit the disease-fighting cells in your bloodstream. "Everybody gets sick from time to time," Dr. Dickstein says. "But if you're under a lot of stress, a virus may get to you that you would have been able to fight off otherwise."

Other studies show that people who have trouble coping with stress may be at risk of building up dangerous abdominal fat. A study at Yale University in New Haven, Connecticut, of 42 obese women found that those with abdominal fat—so-called apple-shaped women—secreted more stress hormones than those with pear-shaped bodies, who carry extra weight on their hips. And doctors know that apple-shaped people are more at risk of heart disease.

Stress can be triggered by a variety of problems, even too much noise. In one study, 100 college students were given a standardized test on a computer. Half had terminals that emitted high-pitched sounds, while the other half didn't. The students with noisy computers scored 8.5 percent lower on the test. They worked faster and were more prone to mistakes—an indication that they were operating under stress, says Caroline Dow, Ph.D., assistant professor of communication at the University of Evansville in Indiana, who helped run the study.

Even society itself can stress us out. In fact, our jobs cause the majority of our stress, Dr. Dickstein says. But it doesn't stop there. After they leave work, women with careers typically must cook, clean, look after children, and be loving spouses. And that kind of double-barreled stress can be hard on your system. A Swedish study of men and women automobile plant managers between the ages of 30 and 50 showed that the blood pressure and levels of stress hormones went up for everyone during the workday. But when men went home, their blood pressure and stress readings dropped dramatically, while the women, with more left to do in the day, stayed higher.

Go Where Your Mind Takes You

Daydreaming has always gotten a bum rap—you probably can hear the echoes of your first-grade teacher telling you to pay attention—but daydreaming can be useful. Through a technique known as guided imagery, you can direct your daydreams and deliberately create images that promote wellness and give you a sense of calm.

"Guided imagery takes the mind to a purposeful fantasy or memory," explains Belleruth Naparstek, a licensed psychotherapist in Cleveland Heights, Ohio, and author of *Your Sixth Sense*, and the *Health Journeys* guided imagery audiotape series.

The idea behind guided imagery is simple. Think back to a time when you felt warm, safe, and loved, and invoke the sense memories of that time. If you can conjure the sights, sounds, tastes, smells, and feelings, your mind and body will respond accordingly. "If you visualize a time when you felt safe and prized, the body begins to reproduce the same stress-reducing biochemical response you had at that time," says Naparstek.

To guide your own imagery toward relaxing thoughts, Naparstek recommends the following steps.

• Wait until everyone is asleep or out of the house, then find a quiet space that you can call your own. If possible, turn off the ringer on the phone and add some soothing background music.

"That study encapsulates everything," says women's health researcher Margaret A. Chesney, Ph.D., professor at the University of California, San Francisco, School of Medicine. "It's psychological proof that women are going home to second jobs. Men know that there's a distinction—that they're off duty at home. Women are not off duty. They're under more duress."

The Road to Calm

There are a number of basic ways you can keep yourself from getting wound too tight. At the head of the list: Creating a sense of control. You have to understand that some stress is inevitable. In fact, a little stress helps you accomplish tasks and meet goals, Dr. Dickstein says. But too much from the wrong sources—such as arguments with spouses or unrealistic expectations at work or at home—

• Sit comfortably and think of a time when you felt very safe, loved, and protected. Perhaps you have memories of sitting on your grandmother's lap and hearing your favorite story. Or recall walking along the beach at sunrise. Whatever it is, take that memory and relive it in all of its sensory detail. If it is the beach scenario, for example: Was there water lapping at your ankles? Was warm sand squishing through your toes? Did the air smell salty? What sounds did you hear?

• Allow yourself to fantasize. Guided imagery doesn't have to be based on actual events in your life.

• Don't think that you have blown it if your mind drifts away from the scene you are re-creating. Just gently guide your attention back to the original sensory details. Your level of concentration will improve over time.

• Practice guided imagery twice a day for 10 to 15 minutes each time, preferably when you are waking up and falling asleep, says Naparstek.

• Put your hands in the same position on your body (for example, your stomach) every time you try guided imagery. That way, when you feel yourself getting stressed, you can put your hands on that spot, take a couple of breaths, and immediately cue your body to de-stress, says Naparstek.

can make you feel helpless and unable to cope. And that's when stress does most of its dirty work.

Here are some tips to help you put stress in check.

Work it out. Nothing eases stress more than exercise, according to David S. Holmes, Ph.D., professor of psychology at the University of Kansas in Lawrence. "Regular aerobic workouts reduce stress more effectively than meditation, psychiatric intervention, biofeedback, and conventional stress management," he says.

Exercise helps burn off all the stress-related chemicals in your system. During a workout, your body will also release mind-relaxing endorphins, Dr. Holmes says. And exercise strengthens your heart, too, further protecting you against the ravages of stress.

Research by Robert Thayer, Ph.D., professor of psychology at California State University, Long Beach, showed that 30 minutes of intense aerobic exercise immediately reduces body tension—and it does so even more effectively than moderate exercise such as walking.

Don't be listless. So many projects, so little time. To beat stress, you have to learn to prioritize, according to Lee Reinert, Ph.D., director and lecturer for the Brandywine Biobehavioral Center, a counseling center in Downingtown, Pennsylvania. At the start of each day, pick the single most important task to complete, then finish it.

If you're a person who makes to-do lists, never write one with more than five items. That way, you're more likely to get all the things done, and you'll feel a greater sense of accomplishment and control, Dr. Reinert says. Then you can go ahead and make a second five-item list. While you're at it, make a list of things that you can delegate to co-workers and family members. "Remember, you don't have to do everything by yourself," Dr. Reinert says. "You can find help and support from people around you."

Just say no. Sometimes you have to learn to draw the line. "Stressed-out people often can't assert themselves," says Joan Lerner, Ph.D., a counseling psychologist at the University of Pennsylvania Counseling Service in Philadelphia. "And so they swallow things. Instead of saying 'I don't want to do this' or 'I need some help,' they do it all themselves. Then they have even more to do."

If you're overbooked at work and your boss wants you to handle another task, give the boss a choice. "Say, 'I'd really like to take this on, but I can't do that without giving up something else. Which of these things would you like me to do?'"

Most bosses can take the hint, says Merrill Douglass, D.B.A., president of the Time Management Center in Marietta, Georgia, a company that trains individuals and corporations in the efficient use of time and energy, and coauthor of *Manage Your Time, Manage Your Work, Manage Yourself.* The same strategy works at home, with your spouse, children, relatives, and friends. If you have trouble saying no, start small. Tell your hubby to make his own sandwich. Or tell your daughter to find another ride home from volleyball practice.

Pad your schedule. "Realize that nearly everything will take longer than you anticipate," says Richard Swenson, M.D., author of *Margin: How to Create the Emotional, Physical, Financial and Time Reserves You Need.* By allotting yourself enough time to accomplish a task, you cut back on anxiety. In general, if meeting deadlines is a problem, always give yourself 20 percent more time than you think you need to do the task.

Trade in the Jag for a Hyundai. Living beyond your means can actually make you sick. A researcher at the University of Alabama in Tuscaloosa studied British census data on 8,000 households and found that families who tried to maintain lifestyles they couldn't afford were likely to have health problems.

Curb stress-producing foods and drinks. Limit your intake of caffeine, alcohol, high-fat foods, and sugar. Caffeine and alcohol can raise the levels of stress hormones in the blood and alter brain chemistry. And when you eat high-fat foods and sugar instead of nutritious foods, you lower the amount of vitamins and minerals in your diet, depleting your body of the essential nutrients that protect you from the dangers of stress.

Sit up straight. A good upright posture improves breathing and increases blood flow to the brain. We often slouch when stressed, which restricts breathing and blood flow and can magnify feelings of helplessness.

Get a grip. Keep a hand exerciser or a tennis ball in your desk at work and give it a few squeezes during tense times. "When stress shoots adrenaline into the bloodstream, that calls for muscle action," says Roger Cady, M.D., medical director of the Shealy Institute for Comprehensive Health Care in Springfield, Missouri. "Squeezing something provides a release that satisfies our bodies' fight-or-flee response."

Soak it away. Want to really relax your muscles? Soak in a hot tub. To get the most relaxation from a hot bath, soak for 15 minutes in water that's just a few degrees warmer than your body temperature, or about 100° to 101°F. But be careful: Longer soaks in warmer water can actually lower your blood pressure too much.

Tune out with a potato. If you want to unwind at the end of the day, eat a meal high in carbohydrates, says Judith Wurtman, Ph.D., a research scientist at the Massachusetts Institute of Technology in Cambridge and author of *Managing Your Mind and Mood with Food*. Carbohydrates trigger release of the brain neurotransmitter serotonin, which soothes you. Good sources of carbohydrates include rice, pasta, potatoes, breads, air-popped popcorn, and low-cal cookies. Dr. Wurtman says just 1½ ounces of carbohydrates, the amount in a baked potato or a cup of spaghetti or white rice, is enough to relieve the anxiety of a stressful day.

Try some fiber. "Stress often goes right to the gut," says George Blackburn, M.D., Ph.D., associate professor of surgery at Harvard Medical School and chief of the Nutrition/Metabolism Laboratory at New England Deaconess Hospital, both in Boston. That means cramps and constipation. To avoid these problems, Dr. Blackburn suggests eating more fiber to keep your digestive system moving. You should build up gradually to at least 25 grams of fiber per day. That means eating more fruits, vegetables, and grains. Try eating whole fruits instead of just juice at breakfast time, and try whole-grain cereals and fiber-fortified muffins.

Have a laugh. Humor is a proven stress reducer. Experts say a good laugh relaxes tense muscles, speeds more oxygen into your system, and lowers your blood pressure. So tune into your favorite sitcom on television. Read a funny book. Call a friend and chuckle for a few minutes. It even helps to force a laugh once in a while. You'll find your stress melting away almost instantly.

Hold your breath. This technique should help you relax in 30 seconds. Holding palm to palm, press your fingers together. Then take a deep breath and keep it in. Wait 5 seconds, then slowly exhale through your lips while letting your hands relax. Do this five or six times until you unwind.

Take a 10-minute holiday. Meditation is a great stress reliever, but sometimes it's hard to find the time or place for it. Dr. Reinert suggests taking a mini-vacation right at your desk or kitchen table instead. Just close your eyes, breathe

The Herbal Cures

After you've taken the basic steps to de-stress your life, you can try a variety of nutritional supplements as added stress protection. Certain vitamins and herbs can calm your nerves, increase stamina, and keep you mentally and physically strong in the midst of turmoil. Here are the best.

B-complex: The treasure trove of relief. The B vitamins can give you more energy, strip away fatigue, and manufacture brain chemicals responsible for keeping you alert and lifting your mood. If you want to combat stress, check with your doctor about taking a daily high-potency B-complex vitamin formula that includes 100 to 500 milligrams of pantothenic acid, 50 to 75 milligrams of vitamin B_6, and 500 micrograms of B_{12}, says Joseph E. Pizzorno, Jr., N.D., a naturopathic doctor and president of Bastyr University in Bothell, Washington.

Ginseng: A stress-busting powerhouse. Ginseng is considered the most notable medicinal herb used to restore vitality, boost energy, reduce fatigue, improve mental and physical performance, and protect the body from the negative effects of stress. There are several types of ginseng available, each with different potency. You can take 100 milligrams one to three times a day if you choose an Asian ginseng extract standardized to 5 to 7 percent ginsenosides, says Dr. Pizzorno. If you're taking a Siberian ginseng extract that is standardized to 0.8 percent eleutherosides, take 100 to 200 milligrams three times a day.

Kava kava: Cool out with it. This time-honored herb can calm your nerves and help you unwind. It also can preempt stress if you take it prior to an expected stressful situation. Take one capsule that contains between 40 and 70 milligrams of kavalactones two or three times a day, suggests Ray Sahelian, M.D., a physician in Marina del Rey, California, and author of *Kava: The Miracle Antianxiety Herb.* Start with the lower dosage first to determine whether you feel any of the soothing effects, he says. If you don't feel stress relief in 2 to 3 hours, you can take another capsule. Don't take kava on a daily basis for more than 4 weeks. And don't use kava if you have liver problems.

deeply (from your stomach), and picture yourself lying on a beach in Mexico. Feel the warmth of the sun. Hear the waves. Smell the salt air. "Just put a little distance between yourself and your stress," Dr. Reinert says. "A few minutes a day can be a great help."

Keep the noise down. If you work, live, or play in a high-noise area, consider wearing earplugs. Make sure the ones you buy reduce sound by at least 20 decibels, says Ernest Peterson, Ph.D., associate professor of otolaryngology at the University of Miami School of Medicine.

You can also use sounds to your advantage. Try listening to gentle music, with flutes or other soft-sounding instruments, says Emmett Miller, M.D., a nationally known stress expert and medical director of the Cancer Support and Education Center in Menlo Park, California. He also suggests taking walks in quiet places and listening to leaves rustle or streams babble. Recordings of ocean waves or gentle rainstorms also help, he says.

STROKE

It's Not Too Early for Prevention

Of all the thieves of youth, stroke is the swiftest and most tragic. In an instant, a vital, vibrant person can lose the ability to speak, to move freely—even to think clearly.

And despite its reputation as an older person's problem—an older man's problem at that—stroke doesn't discriminate.

More than 8,000 American women and more than 15,000 American men between the ages of 30 and 44 suffer strokes each year. Nearly one in every three strokes is fatal. And the aging effects on those who survive can be brutal. Survivors could suffer brain damage affecting speech, memory, thought patterns, and behavior. Sometimes there is temporary—or permanent—paralysis.

The good news is that you can significantly cut your risk of stroke. "We're beginning to realize that stroke is not an inevitable process," says Michael Walker, M.D., director for the division of stroke and trauma at the National Institute of Neurological Disorders and Stroke in Bethesda, Maryland. "It's preventable, and it is treatable."

It may mean eating more fruits and vegetables, exercising a few times a week, and staying vigilant about your blood pressure. But when you weigh the options, it's not a bad tradeoff.

Cause and Effect

Stroke is a sudden severe illness that attacks the brain. There are two basic types. Ischemic strokes, which account for about 80 percent of all strokes, happen when blood flow to a part of the brain is cut off, causing brain cells to die from lack of oxygen. This frequently occurs because of hardening and clogging in your carotid arteries, which feed blood from your neck to your head. Ischemic strokes can also be caused by atrial fibrillation, an irregular heartbeat that leads to clots that may travel through your body and lodge in the brain's arteries.

Hemorrhagic strokes account for the remaining 20 percent. These strokes are caused by bleeding from ruptures in either a blood vessel on the surface of your brain or an artery in the brain itself. These strokes can be even more deadly than ischemic strokes, with a mortality rate of close to 50 percent.

Women ages 30 to 44 are about half as likely to have strokes as men in the same age group, according to figures from the American Heart Association. African-Americans in general are at greater risk than Caucasians of dying from stroke. Family history of stroke can play a role, too, though just how much remains unclear. And the risk of stroke goes up as you age. American Heart Association statistics show that the incidence of stroke more than doubles each decade after a person reaches age 55.

Younger women have some protection against stroke because their bodies produce large amounts of estrogen. That helps keep cholesterol levels lower and checks the onset of atherosclerosis, or hardening of the arteries. After menopause, though, the rate of stroke rises quickly. By age 65, women and men have about the same incidence of stroke.

Pregnancy can cause a slight increase in stroke risk, though the odds are still quite low. There are a few reasons for this increased risk, says Harold Adams, Jr., M.D., professor of neurology at the University of Iowa Hospital and Clinic in Iowa City. A woman's blood clots differently during pregnancy. And her blood pressure also tends to be a bit higher. Studies also show that certain forms of birth control pills may slightly increase stroke risk, too—especially for smokers older than 35 or for women with high blood pressure.

Of course, you have no say over age or gender. But Dr. Adams says there are many risks you can definitely control.

High blood pressure, for example. Also known as hypertension, it's the single most important risk factor for stroke. "About half of all strokes are caused by high blood pressure," says Edward S. Cooper, M.D., past president of the American Heart Association.

High blood pressure causes stroke by speeding up arteriosclerosis and damaging smaller blood vessels. And in Dr. Cooper's words, it can cause tiny blood vessels in your brain to "blow out like an overinflated tire."

Smoking also puts you at increased risk for stroke by accelerating clogging of the carotid arteries, says Jack P. Whisnant, M.D., chief investigator for a study of carotid artery disease at the Mayo Clinic in Rochester, Minnesota. Women who smoke are over 2.5 times more likely to suffer strokes than nonsmokers, according to a Harvard Nurses' Health Study that tracked 117,000 female registered nurses between the ages of 30 and 55 at entry to the study. The more that women in the study smoked, the greater their risk. Compared with nonsmokers, women who smoked 1 to 14 cigarettes per day had twice the risk of stroke, while women who smoked 35 to 44 cigarettes per day—about two packs—had a fourfold increase in risk. Those who smoked more than 45 cigarettes per day were 5.4 times more likely to suffer strokes.

People with diabetes are also at increased risk for stroke. And obese people and those with high blood cholesterol levels may be at higher risk of developing arteriosclerosis and thus having strokes.

Saving Yourself from Strokes

Strokes are still shrouded in mystery. They seem to strike without warning. Sometimes it's hard to tell when you're even in danger.

But early prevention can be the key to improving your chances of avoiding stroke. "The process leading to a stroke begins in your forties, even earlier, so now is the time to intervene," says David G. Sherman, M.D., head of neurology at the University of Texas Health Science Center at San Antonio.

To help lower your risk, try these tips.

Ease the pressure. Many people don't even know they have high blood pressure, because it has few outward signs. That's why the American Heart Association recommends having your blood pressure checked by a doctor or another health care professional at least once a year if your blood pressure is 130/85 or higher. If your blood pressure is lower, get it checked every 2 years. Many cases of high blood pressure begin developing between ages 35 and 45.

Research shows that controlling high blood pressure can cut your risk of stroke by as much as 40 percent. Any reading above 140/90 is considered high.

Your doctor will be able to prescribe treatments for high blood pressure, from dietary changes to getting more exercise to drug therapy. Follow the advice like your life depends on it. It might.

"Controlling hypertension is absolutely vital in stroke prevention," Dr. Adams says.

Kick the habit. The Nurses' Health Study showed that people who stopped smoking cut their stroke risk substantially. In fact, the risk of stroke dropped to normal levels for study subjects 2 to 4 years after they quit.

"Don't just cut back on cigarettes," Dr. Adams says. "There's no such thing as moderate smoking. You have to stop altogether, all the way, right now."

Go low with the Pill. For years, doctors warned women about birth control pills and increased stroke risk. But with the low-dose estrogen pills now in use, Dr. Adams says the risk of stroke is lower.

"We're seeing more and more evidence that low-dose estrogen oral contraceptives are safer," he says. "Low-dose estrogen is probably safe."

There are two caveats, however. Smoking and the Pill are a dangerous mix—especially for women over age 35. And high blood pressure, combined with the Pill, can also increase stroke risk. "If you have those risk factors, birth control pills are not advisable," Dr. Adams says.

Stroke Warning Signs

Quick action can mean the difference between tragedy and recovery when it comes to stroke. Heed these warning signs, says the American Heart Association:

- Sudden weakness or numbness in the face, arm, or leg on one side of the body
- Loss of speech, or trouble talking or understanding speech
- Sudden dimness or loss of vision, particularly in only one eye
- Sudden severe headache with no known cause
- Unexplained dizziness, unsteadiness, or sudden falls, especially along with any of the previous symptoms.

If you notice any of these symptoms, get help immediately by calling 911 or the emergency phone number for your area. A study of response times showed that people with stroke signs who called this emergency number got to the hospital two to three times faster than those who called their doctors or tried to transport themselves to the hospital. And with stroke, minutes matter.

What seems like a stroke may actually turn out to be a transient ischemic attack (TIA). These are sometimes called temporary strokes, since the symptoms quickly disappear. But you shouldn't ignore a TIA, since it is the single most important warning of impending stroke, according to Harold Adams, Jr., M.D., professor of neurology at the University of Iowa Hospital and Clinic in Iowa City.

Check your neck. Ask your doctor to listen for a bruit, a whooshing sound in the carotid arteries in your neck. This is caused by partial blockage and turbulence in the crucial blood vessels that feed oxygen to the brain.

"This is especially important if you have arteriosclerosis causing blocked blood vessels elsewhere in your body," says Patricia Grady, Ph.D., acting director of the National Institute of Neurological Disorders and Stroke.

Also, make sure the doctor checks your heart. Treating atrial fibrillation can reduce stroke risk by up to 80 percent.

Get some exercise. Physical inactivity may be a risk factor for stroke, but a total exercise time of at least 20 minutes a day, three times a week, could reduce your risk for stroke. Walking, tennis, bicycling, stairclimbing, aerobics, and even gardening and Ping Pong can be potential stroke busters.

A British study showed that the sooner you start exercising, the better. People who started exercising between ages 15 and 25 had a 63 percent reduction in their risk for stroke. Even if you're a little late getting started, you can still benefit from exercise: The study showed that people who began exercising between ages 25 and 40 reduced their risk by 57 percent and that people who started exercising between ages 40 and 55 cut their risk by 37 percent.

"Exercise has so many benefits," Dr. Adams says. "If you're not exercising, you could be robbing yourself of years later on."

Crunch some carrots. The same Nurses' Health Study that looked at smoking also discovered a link between the nutrient beta-carotene and stroke.

"We found a 22 percent reduction in the risk of heart attack and a 40 percent reduction in stroke for those women with high intakes of fruits and vegetables rich in beta-carotene compared with those with low intakes," says JoAnn E. Manson, M.D., co-principal investigator of the cardiovascular component of the Nurses' Health Study, who is co-director of women's health at Brigham and Women's Hospital and associate professor of medicine at Harvard Medical School, both in Boston.

Just one large carrot, which has 15 milligrams of beta-carotene, provides the amount of the nutrient that was associated with the lowest risk in the study. Other foods that worked were sweet potatoes, mangoes, apricots, and spinach. Beta-carotene can be found in most dark green and orange fruits and vegetables.

Pass the potassium. Researchers at the University of California, San Diego, have found that adding a single daily serving of potassium-rich food to your diet could cut your risk of fatal stroke by as much as 40 percent. The reason for the benefit isn't completely clear. Although potassium is known to help lower blood pressure, the amount of potassium the test subjects ate had little direct effect on their blood pressure readings. Studies at the University of Mississippi Medical Center in Jackson showed that potassium may help prevent the formation of blood clots, one of the primary factors in heart attack and stroke.

If you're looking for a high-powered potassium boost, eat a baked potato every day. Potatoes are one of the richest sources of potassium. Other foods rich in potassium include dried apricots, lima beans, Swiss chard, bananas, skim milk, roasted chestnuts, okra, and oranges.

Know about aspirin. Aspirin might help ward off ischemic stroke by thinning potential blood clots, Dr. Adams says. But unless you already have a risk factor, such as arteriosclerosis or a prior stroke, it may not do you much good. In fact, research shows that aspirin might be linked to a slightly higher incidence of hemorrhagic stroke.

Just how much aspirin you should take also remains debatable. Some studies have found benefits with an 81-milligram daily dose (a children's aspirin). Others tout a 325-milligram daily dose (a regular-strength adult aspirin). And some researchers say that as many as three regular aspirin tablets daily may be necessary. The bottom line: See your doctor before you start an aspirin regimen for stroke prevention.

Keep it in balance. What's good for your heart is good for your brain. Keeping your cholesterol in check can slow arteriosclerosis and ward off ischemic stroke. So eat a low-fat diet. The current recommendation from most doctors and researchers is to limit fat to no more than 25 percent of your total calories. Pay particular attention to eating less saturated fat by choosing lean meats and low-fat dairy products.

"Along with exercise and quitting smoking, what you eat is key to preventing stroke," Dr. Adams says. "What we're talking about is a good diet that will help lessen the risk of hardening of the arteries." This diet doesn't need to be extreme, he says. It does need to be well balanced and low in fat.

Get some of the "good oils." You may want to substitute monounsaturated or polyunsaturated fats for the saturated fats in your diet, says Joel Simon, M.D., assistant professor of medicine at the University of California, San Francisco, School of Medicine.

He found the men with high concentrations of alpha-linolenic acid (a polyunsaturated fatty acid in the same family as fatty acids in fish) in their blood had a lower risk of stroke. "Alpha-linolenic acid may decrease the risk of stroke by affecting blood viscosity and clotting," says Dr. Simon. Important sources of alpha-linolenic acid are flaxseed, canola, soybean, and walnut oils.

Toast your health—in moderation. Excess drinking means increased stroke risk. Numerous studies show that having more than four drinks a day greatly increases your chances of having a hemorrhagic stroke.

But some studies show a link between moderate alcohol intake and a slightly reduced risk of ischemic stroke, at least among whites.

"There may be something about alcohol that helps in small levels. It may prevent both heart attack and stroke. I'm not telling my patients to drink for their health," Dr. Adams says. "If you're not drinking now, I don't recommend starting. If you do have more than a couple of drinks a day, the potential complications of alcohol are probably going to hurt you in the long run. The key to alcohol use is moderation."

Drink black tea. A study from the Netherlands found that men who drank more than 4.7 cups of black tea a day were 69 percent less likely to have a stroke than men who drank less than 2.6 cups a day. Black and green teas contain bioflavonoids, compounds that increase capillary strength, says Barry Taylor, N.D., a naturopathic doctor with the New England Family Health Center in Weston, Massachusetts.

Look for pressure valves. There is a lot of evidence that stress contributes to high blood pressure. If you have a particularly stressful life *and* high blood pressure, find ways to relax, says Murray Goldstein, M.D., director of the United Cerebral Palsy Research and Education Foundation and a member of the board of directors of the National Stroke Association. Try meditation or imagery. An engrossing hobby can help: Woodworking or gardening may take your mind off the stressors in your life.

A beagle can lower blood pressure, too. A number of studies have shown that interacting with pets can help put people at ease. Pet ownership changes your perspective and directs your attention to affection interactions, says Dr. Goldstein.

Watch your neck. People sometimes have strokes after their necks have been hyperextended or twisted. That movement can tear the lining of one of the four arteries going to the brain, causing a clot to form inside the artery. "This kind of stroke has been reported in women whose neck has been extended over a sink at the hairdresser, in drivers who sharply turn their necks, and, rarely, as a result of chiropractic neck adjustment," says Dr. Goldstein.

At the hairdresser, make sure you have a pillow under your neck or you may prefer to lean forward over the sink, instead of backward. When driving, turn your head slowly. If you experience any lightheadedness during a chiropractic adjustment, ask the doctor to stop immediately.

TYPE A PERSONALITY

This "A" Is for Aging

You have never liked losing—not at the office, not on the tennis court, not even when one of the kids gets lucky and beats you at Chutes and Ladders. And you don't like wasting time, either—especially when it's because of something you can't control, such as a slow-moving driver on the freeway or a slow-talking co-worker. With all the hurdles life puts in your path, it's no wonder you can't hold your temper anymore.

Whoa! Time out! These are some of the classic signs of Type A behavior. If you're running your motor at 150 miles per hour, 24 hours a day, it may be time to re-examine some goals and habits and your outlook on life. Because if you don't, you could be setting yourself up for problems—from headache to heart disease—that will erode your body's youthful edge.

"Type A behavior is very hard on your system," says C. David Jenkins, Ph.D., professor of preventive medicine and community health at the University of Texas Medical Branch at Galveston. "You're putting yourself under a lot of needless pressure. And believe me, that will take its toll in the long run, in ways you may not expect."

Anxious, Angry—And at Risk

The American Heart Association lists six characteristics of Type A people. They love competition, attempt to achieve many poorly defined goals, have a strong need for recognition and advancement, are always in a hurry, show intense concentration and alertness, and are prone to anger.

Fewer than half of the people in America are Type A, but the figure is creeping higher, Dr. Jenkins says. If you're a salesperson, newspaper reporter, or air traffic controller or in another high-pressure job, the odds are that you were drawn to your field by Type A tendencies. In fact, even if you weren't Type A to start with, Dr. Jenkins says that the demands of these jobs can push you in that direction.

The key problem with Type A behavior is stress. Hard-driving men and women put themselves under constant strain, and their bodies react in pressure-packed ways. Studies show that Type A people are more likely to grind their teeth, which can lead to jaw pain, headaches, and dental troubles. Because of stress, they also may suffer from chronic muscle fatigue and soreness in their necks and shoulders.

A study of 72 female college students in Ohio showed that Type A women may also face more anxiety and depression than other women—while at the same time receiving less support from friends and family. Researchers speculate that this may happen because society tends to shun and isolate competitive, hard-driving women, even as it encourages men with the same traits.

Scientists are even exploring a possible link between cancer and Type A behavior. There's no concrete evidence on this one. But a continuing study of 3,154 American men shows that Type A behavior might predispose people to develop cancer. Scientists think that this may happen because stress suppresses the immune system, making the body less able to fight off disease.

Then there's heart disease. A study at Harvard Medical School in Boston of about 500 men and women showed that the Type A's had a 50 percent higher risk of suffering heart attacks than their mellower Type B counterparts.

Dr. Jenkins says the process probably works like this: Every time you lie on the horn at an intersection or argue with your boss, your body produces a stress hormone called noradrenaline. This sparks your body, making you more alert and raising your blood pressure temporarily. Dr. Jenkins says it can also cause minor damage to the lining of your blood vessels. As your body repairs the blood vessels, they pick up cholesterol flowing in your bloodstream. Over time, this patchwork can lead to a buildup of cholesterol in your arteries—setting you up for blockages and heart attacks.

A-mazing Solutions

You can't really "cure" Type A personality, Dr. Jenkins says. Not that you'd want to; there's really nothing wrong with a touch of assertiveness and a sturdy work ethic. But you may want to change some daily habits and attitudes to help lower your risk of Type A health trouble. Here are a few suggestions to get started.

Aim lower. Sure, you want to succeed at everything. But there are only 24 hours in a day—and sometimes something has to give. So be a little more choosy. "I think setting realistic goals is the most important thing a Type A person can do," says Lee Reinert, Ph.D., director and lecturer for the Brandywine Biobehavioral Center, a counseling center in Downingtown, Pennsylvania. "Goals make you focus on what's important, instead of whatever crisis is facing you at the moment."

At the start of each week, make a list of things you feel you absolutely must do. Each time you write something down, ask yourself what would happen if you didn't do it. If you can't come up with a legitimate concern, scratch that item off the list. Now comes the tough part: Cut the final list by five items. You may try delegating a few of the items to your spouse, children, or co-workers. "What's left is a more achievable set of tasks," Dr. Reinert says. "You'll get a greater sense of accomplishment this way, and you won't be chasing after brushfires that keep popping up."

Try aerobics. You'll sweat the stress a little less if you work out regularly. Aerobic exercise relieves stress and can ward off its long-term consequences, says David S. Holmes, Ph.D., professor of psychology at the University of Kansas in Lawrence.

One word of caution, however: Don't overdo it. Because they tend to over-train, Type A people get injured more during exercise, reports *Sports Medicine Digest*. In fact, Type A athletes lose twice as much training time as others to injury. "Get a good workout. Raise your heart rate, but don't try to win at all costs. Don't keep trying to beat your own record," Dr. Jenkins says.

Account for your anger. Keeping journals can help you discover the root of your aggressiveness and anger, Dr. Reinert says. "A lot of times, you're not really mad at what's going on right now. You're upset about more of a core issue—maybe an unhappy family relationship," she says.

Writing down your thoughts and feelings may help you discover what's really angering you. It can also help you detect patterns. Maybe you always get mad when you're waiting in line. Or when Marla in accounting won't let you get a word in at the staff meeting. If you anticipate these moments, you can either find ways to avoid them or ask yourself whether they're really important enough to blow your stack over.

Make amends. Is that little old lady in the slow-moving Buick really trying to make you mad? Was she awake deep into the night plotting ways to make you late? Or is she just a little old lady who needs to use a little extra caution to drive these days?

In his book *Anger Kills*, Redford B. Williams, M.D., director of the Behavioral Medicine Research Center and professor of psychiatry at Duke University Medical Center in Durham, North Carolina, suggests putting yourself in the other person's shoes. When you look at the world from the perspective of the people who anger you, you'll probably be a little less cynical about them—and a little less Type A in the process. Dr. Williams also suggests doing some volunteer work as a way to relieve hostility and gain empathy for other people.

Come up for air. Type A people typically schedule their days to the millisecond. That leaves no margin for error—and sets you up for extra stress when things go wrong. So try to give yourself a 10 percent pad. If you work a 10-hour day, leave at least 1 hour free to deal with the unexpected. If that sounds like an awfully big block of time, Dr. Reinert suggests setting aside 5 or 6 minutes per hour instead.

These cooldown periods can help you organize your thoughts and create new plans of attack. They can also spark creativity, making the rest of the workday more productive. "If you don't have a little downtime, you're not giving yourself a chance to absorb all the information that's flying at you," Dr. Reinert says. "You'll be more creative and efficient if you just take time to process."

Pay attention to your body. Find another 10 or 15 minutes a day to check in with your body. Sit on a comfortable chair in a quiet room, close your eyes, and breathe deeply. Tense, then release, the muscles in your feet. Then do your calves. Work up your body, paying special attention to the areas that feel tight or are throbbing (especially your shoulders and neck). "This is a great stress reducer," Dr. Reinert says. "It lets your body relax. And it shows you how needlessly tense you become during the day."

ULCERS

Taming the Fire Within

Not long ago the best advice for preventing ulcers was the Never-Do-Anything-Fun Wellness Program. Spicy food like tacos and pizza were forbidden. And worry itself was deemed worrisome because it implies stress, another suspected cause of ulcers.

Well, you can reschedule the chili fest without giving it another worry. Science now knows that although pepperoni and pressure are not necessarily good for your health, they are not entirely to blame for ulcers. The major cause is a bacteria—*Helicobacter pylori*, to be precise. A secondary cause of ulcers: overuse of common painkilling drugs.

In both cases, the real damage occurs because the lining of your stomach is exposed to the juices your stomach produces.

How We Set Ourselves Up

Ulcers form when digestive juices—acids, really—start burning through the delicate pink lining of your digestive organs. This is usually the result of a deterioration in a protective layer that covers the lining of the stomach and duodenum, the top part of the small intestine.

Gastric ulcers, which show up more frequently in women and usually after age 50, occur in the stomach, and symptoms include a burning or "hungry" feeling in the stomach or under the breastbone, a vague uneasiness of the stomach, and even chronic nausea. Duodenal ulcers, which are more common among men, hit lower, in the upper portion of the small intestine. With duodenal ulcers, pain is often relieved after eating; with gastric ulcers, it's not.

Either type of ulcer can lead to stools that are black or maroon and foul-smelling and to vomiting what appears to be coffee-ground material.

Many times the deterioration of the stomach lining is linked to an infection in the upper gastrointestinal tract caused by *H. pylori*. The bacteria is so common among ulcer sufferers that it is found in the stomachs of nearly all people with duodenal ulcers and in four out of five people with gastric ulcers.

"These bacteria are more common as you age," says William B. Ruderman, M.D., chairman of the department of gastroenterology at the Cleveland Clinic Florida in Fort Lauderdale. "For one thing, exposure to these bacteria increases over time. And your body's defenses may get impaired over time."

The other major reason people develop ulcers is taking too many painkillers for long-term conditions such as arthritis. "Probably the worst offenders, simply because they're the most frequently used, are aspirin and other nonsteroidal anti-inflammatory drugs (NSAIDs) available over the counter," says Jorge Herrera, M.D., associate professor of medicine at the University of South Alabama College of Medicine in Mobile. "If you take any of these drugs for more than 3 months at a time, you increase your risk of ulcers significantly."

NSAIDs do their dirty work by inhibiting the production of mucus and protective acid-neutralizing agents. Aspirin can also weaken the stomach lining and cause bleeding. "In fact, many patients don't even realize they have ulcers because of the painkillers in the drugs they take," adds Dr. Herrera. "Sometimes they come into the office for problems with bleeding or their stools, and only then do they realize they have ulcers."

How to Help Yourself

If you think you have an ulcer, see your doctor. A doctor can prescribe drugs that reduce acid secretions and ease pain, as well as antibiotics for *H. pylori*. In the meantime, here's what you can do to prevent ulcers or to lessen their severity.

Choose Tylenol. For headaches and other minor aches and pains, take acetaminophen, which is in products such as Tylenol, rather than ibuprofen, commonly sold as Advil and Nuprin. Ibuprofen is an anti-inflammatory, and products containing it can cause ulcers, says Dr. Herrera. "Sure, they have painkilling ingredients, but so do other medications that won't lead to ulcers. So if you have a headache or other minor problem that requires a painkiller, take Tylenol." And stay away from aspirin, since it can do even more damage than ibuprofen. Aspirin can weaken the stomach lining and cause bleeding.

Be smoke-free. "Smoking increases the potential for ulcers in people who are predisposed to them," says Lawrence S. Friedman, M.D., associate professor of medicine at Harvard Medical School and associate physician in the gastrointestinal unit at Massachusetts General Hospital, both in Boston.

Not only does smoking increase your risk of developing ulcers, but smokers are more likely to sustain serious ulcer complications like perforation. Furthermore, the antibiotic treatment that fights *H. pylori* is less effective for smokers compared to nonsmokers, and once healed, a smoker's ulcer is more likely to recur. Quitting is your best move.

Limit your alcohol. Alcohol alone generally won't cause ulcers, but avoid alcohol in excess because it can damage the stomach lining, says Dr. Friedman.

"If you think you have an ulcer, drinking alcohol is most unwise," agrees Malcolm Robinson, M.D., clinical professor of medicine at the University of Oklahoma and medical director of the Oklahoma Foundation for Digestive Research, both in Oklahoma City.

Fortify with fiber. There is some evidence that a high-fiber diet may be helpful in preventing ulcers, according to Dr. Friedman. A study by Harvard researchers found that people who averaged 30 grams of fiber a day cut their risk of duodenal ulcers in half. Though it isn't clear if fiber can inhibit the recurrence of ulcers, it is worth trying since a high-fiber diet has plenty of other health benefits, he says.

Some good sources of fiber? Dried pears, apples, and peaches, and many kinds of beans, including lima beans, kidney beans, navy beans, and black beans.

Become an onion lover. Not only is this pungent food not harmful to ulcer sufferers, it is actually beneficial as an ulcer preventive. Scientists believe the sulfur compounds in onions attack the *H. pylori* bacterium. Experts suggest that eating half an onion a day may be beneficial, so try to include it whenever possible in your salads, sandwiches, and cooking.

Mellow out. While stress alone won't cause an ulcer, people who view their lives as being too stressful are up to three times more likely to develop ulcers than those who learn to roll with life's punches, says Robert Anda, M.D., of the National Center for Chronic Disease Prevention and Health Promotion in Atlanta. But since we're all under stress, why do some of us get ulcers and others don't?

"It's how you interpret stress," says Dr. Anda. When you feel the weight of the world is on your shoulders and perceive stressful events as negative, you're a prime candidate for ulcers, because this perception results in the production of more stomach acids. On the other hand, people who acknowledge they have stress but view it as a fact of everyday life and don't let it overwhelm them are less likely to get ulcers.

Many people who react negatively to stress find it helps to talk about their problems with good friends, to do regular meditation or relaxation exercises, or even to start regular exercise programs, says Howard Mertz, M.D., assistant professor of medicine at the University of California, Los Angeles, UCLA School of Medicine.

Hold the milk. The old remedy of drinking milk for an ulcer may actually do more harm than good, says Richard W. McCallum, M.D., professor of medicine and chief of gastroenterology at the University of Virginia School of Medicine in Charlottesville. That's because while milk may initially have a neutralizing effect on these acids, after 30 minutes or so, you get a "rebound effect" in which the calcium and protein from the milk actually stimulate acid production.

Quaff some cabbage juice. Cabbage juice is high in glutamine, an amino acid that helps stomach cells regenerate. It also stimulates your body to produce a substance that actually protects the stomach lining. A good way to get glutamine is through drinking about a liter of fresh raw cabbage juice every day, says Priscilla Skerry, N.D., a naturopathic and homeopathic physician in Portland, Maine. To make your own juice, she suggests slicing then juicing or blending a green cabbage. You also can find glutamine supplements in most health food stores.

Feel great with ginger. Ginger is considered an herbal remedy to help protect against ulcers. Take it in capsules, in root form, or as tea, says Mindy Green, director of education services at the Herb Research Foundation in Boulder, Colorado. You will find ginger in these forms at many drugstores and natural food stores. Note: While fresh ginger is safe when used as a spice, some forms of ginger aren't recommended for everyone. Ginger may increase bile secretion, so if you have gallstones, do not use therapeutic amounts of dried ginger or ginger powder without guidance from a health care practitioner.

UNWANTED HAIR

Hair, Hair, Go Away

You may not have noticed it when you were young, when a little peach fuzz on smooth, childish skin didn't matter a bit. But now that you're older, you may find the hair is more profuse or suddenly darker. You may remember a loving aunt whose smile carried a pronounced shadow—but surely, you haven't reached her age already!

Perhaps you have. Or maybe the unwanted hair has simply come on sooner. In any case, it makes you feel aged and unattractive, as though your body is sabotaging your beauty. It's a common problem for a lot of women, though a lot of us would rather die than admit it.

Often it's genetically based, doctors say. If your family tree has Mediterranean roots, you may develop a dark, downy crop on your upper lip or below the "sideburn" hairline. Sometimes just a few stubborn whiskerlike hairs will appear, often on the chin.

But the most common cause of excess hair growth as women get older is the hormonal changes of menopause, says Victor Newcomer, M.D., professor of dermatology at the University of California, Los Angeles, UCLA School of Medicine. "Most women have a little down on the upper lip after puberty, and in brunettes, it can be very heavy. But after menopause, it really kicks in with coarse, fibrous hairs." That's because the effects of the male hormone androgen (which every woman has) become more pronounced when levels of the female hormone estrogen drop. The androgen then is free to stimulate more hair growth, he says.

If excess facial or body hair isn't common among the women in your family, your hair growth possibly could be from medications you are taking, says Seth L. Matarasso, M.D., assistant professor of dermatology at the University of California, San Francisco, School of Medicine. Sometimes blood pressure medicine, steroids for arthritis, diuretics (water pills), or birth control pills can stimulate hair growth, he says.

If hair growth of more than a few hairs appears suddenly, Dr. Matarasso says, see your doctor for endocrinological tests. Although it's very rare, unusual hair growth in women may indicate a thyroid or hormonal problem.

And though leg and arm hair is normal, it's very unusual to have any hair growth on the cheeks or forehead. Hair in these areas could result from several causes, including disease in the ovaries or in the pituitary or adrenal glands, says Dr. Newcomer. Some rare liver diseases may also stimulate hair growth on the cheeks or forehead, he says.

Whether the hair is age-related or not, there are several ways to deal with it.

Gentle and Not-So-Gentle Methods

So how do you get the excess fleece to flee? Here are some suggestions.

Bleach away. With hair that's dark but not too heavy, try a facial hair bleach that you can buy at your pharmacy, says Dr. Newcomer. Bleaching may make the hair less noticeable, so there's no need to remove it.

But if the hair growth bothers you or you feel you would look better and smoother-skinned without it, here are some other temporary solutions.

Shave away the hair. You may have heard that shaving causes hair to grow back thicker but that's just a myth, says Dr. Matarasso. It's easy to be confused, because the growing-in hairs may look darker, he says. Usually your hairs cycle in a few at a time, but when they reach the surface of the skin all at once, the stubs will appear thick and feel rough, he says. There's not really more or thicker hair growing back.

The choice between an electric razor and a blade is up to you; whatever feels best, Dr. Matarasso says. They shave the same, although you use an electric razor on dry skin. If you use a blade, soak it in water for a few minutes first, then let your favorite shaving cream or gel sit on the skin for a moment or two before you shave, he says. It will soften the hair and give you smoother results. And if you're thinking of shaving a part of your face, there's no harm in that. But if facial growth is profuse, check with your doctor first to rule out medical causes.

Use tweezers. For just a few recurring hairs, one of the simplest removal methods is tweezing, with the aid of a magnifying mirror if you need it, says Dr. Newcomer. Some benefits of tweezing are that it is effective and you can do it in privacy. But even though tweezed hair follicles will eventually give up the ghost, it can take many years for that kind of permanent result, he says.

Try a depilatory. Chemical lotions such as Neet and Nair are perfectly fine to use, says Dr. Matarasso, as long as you patch-test a small area first to make sure you're not allergic to the product. "The chemicals aren't bad, but they can be abrasive," he says. They work by dissolving hair at or just below the skin line, so results last for up to 2 weeks, says Dr. Matarasso.

Depilatories are simple and painless to use, but some have nasty odors. You apply the thick lotion to the skin, wait for up to 15 minutes, and then rinse off with warm water. You want to avoid using it near your eyes or pubic area.

If you use a depilatory on your face, apply only a little at first. Don't leave it

Electrolysis: The Permanent Solution—
Eventually

There's one way to remove hair permanently and that's professional electrolysis. This method is appropriate for hair on any area of the body, from the upper lip to the nipple area to the toes—anything but eyelashes, nose, and ears—although it's painful and time-consuming. Here's what you'll experience in a licensed electrolysist's office at fees that range from $15 to $100, depending on the length of the session.

The electrolysist cleans your skin with alcohol, guides a sterile electric needle into the hair follicle, and turns on the current. The current will destroy the hair follicle, but sometimes it takes multiple sessions. And some women find the treatments simply too painful to tolerate. What motivates many of them to endure the process is that if you persist with the treatments, the hair will eventually stop growing back.

For a small area of unwanted hair, it might be worth it, says Seth L. Matarasso, M.D., assistant professor of dermatology at the University of California, San Francisco, School of Medicine. But there are risks involved. There is some possibility of pigment change in your skin, slight scarring, or folliculitis, an inflammation of the hair follicles, he says. And though it's highly unlikely with the sterilization techniques used by most professional electrolysists, there is the potential to spread disease, including hepatitis, he says.

Your best protections against infection are to be sure your electrolysist uses a new needle each time and to ask her to wear latex gloves, says Victor Newcomer, M.D., professor of dermatology at the University of California, Los Angeles, UCLA School of Medicine.

If you've wondered whether the home electrolysis units you see in mail order catalogs work just as well as salon equipment, experts are skeptical.

"Some of these units are supposed to work painlessly with radio waves and destroy the hair follicle at the base," says Carole Walderman, a cosmetologist and esthetician and president of Von Lee International School of Aesthetics and Makeup in Baltimore. "But hair is not a conductor of electricity, so how could this method destroy the hair root?"

Even when the galvanic current from regular electrolysis machines cauterizes the follicles directly, Walderman says, you still get up to 90 percent regrowth, which is why repeated treatments are necessary to permanently remove the hair.

on too long, or you'll wind up with a rash, says Dr. Newcomer. "If you're an oily-skinned brunette, you can tolerate it longer. But thin-skinned blondes have less tolerance" to the chemicals, he says. The texture of the hair also makes a difference in how depilatories work. Big, coarse hair takes longer to dissolve, and fine hair comes off easier, he says.

Consider waxing, at least once. You've probably heard hair waxing compared to Band-Aid removal, but it's a little more challenging than that. The delightful side of waxing (and the reason so many women grin and bear it) is that you'll have hair-free skin for about 6 weeks afterward. And the new growth is soft and silky at first.

Waxing is appropriate for any area of the body—face, arms, legs, and even the bikini area. But be very careful near the groin, Dr. Newcomer says. "The wax can get tangled up in the pubic area, and you can't get it off," he says.

How does it work? At a salon, heated wax is applied to your skin with a wooden spatula. When the wax hardens, the technician yanks off the strips, lifting away the hair. You'll be treated to a soothing lotion afterward, but some women find the process quite painful. You can buy do-it-yourself waxing kits for face or body at a pharmacy, but, as Dr. Newcomer says, "it takes a brave soul to pull off that strip."

Is the pain of pulled hair a little too intense? "Go see your dermatologist about an hour before you wax and have him numb your skin with a local anesthetic," says Dr. Matarasso. "You'll hardly feel a thing."

If you'd like to try waxing and you happen to use the anti-wrinkling cream tretinoin (Retin-A) or any skin lotion containing glycolic acid, be sure to stop using it a few days before waxing, says Dr. Matarasso. These preparations are exfoliants and actually remove the outer two layers of skin, making the skin much more sensitive, he says. "If you wax on top of denuded skin, you'll give yourself a rip-roaring wound," he says. "You can take off a significant amount of the skin."

Also keep in mind that you have to wait until hair grows back to ¼ inch long before you can have it waxed again. This could be a problem in summer, when you might want to go bare-legged.

Avoid the mitts and electric coils. Don't use the pumicelike hair removal mitts sold in many salons and pharmacies, says Dr. Matarasso. "They really are quite abrasive and can injure your skin," he says. The mitts "just mechanically break off the hair, like another crude razor," says Dr. Newcomer.

The vibrating coils work by lifting up many hairs at once and pulling them out from their roots. Unlike waxing, which pulls out hair quickly against the direction of growth, the coils yank hair in every direction. "It's mechanized or group tweezing," says Dr. Matarasso. "Some women who use it are very stoic. The vast majority of people find this method too painful, and it doesn't leave you hair-free that much longer than shaving or a depilatory."

VARICOSE VEINS

You Don't Have to Live with Them

Who doesn't hate varicose veins, whether they're small and spidery or bulgy blue ropes? Varicose veins creep up the legs of over half of us after age 40, and they're a potent reminder of aging. All of a sudden, wearing shorts or a swimsuit isn't an automatic choice anymore.

What we call spider veins doctors call venous telangiectasia. They are actually dilated veins, often found on the upper calves and thighs. Both spider veins and varicose veins, which are usually found on the legs, are veins that are larger than they should be.

Although many people find spider veins just a cosmetic annoyance, larger varicose veins can be truly uncomfortable. Sometimes they cause a feeling of heaviness, tiredness, and chronic aching in the calves. They can trigger night cramps and restless legs that disturb sleep and leave you dragging and worn out. Swollen veins often become itchy and sore. And although it's rare, varicose veins may indicate a clot in a deeper leg vein.

Check Your Genes

Where do varicose veins come from? Your genes, for starters. You can inherit the tendency to form varicose veins from either side of the family.

But the fact is that varicose veins are up to six times more common in women than in men, which leads scientists to believe that female hormones play a strong role in their formation.

One theory suggests that when a woman is pregnant, her greater blood volume increases vein pressure. At the same time, her higher levels of the hormone progesterone may help dilate veins. Add to this the weight of the uterus pressing on pelvic veins, which, in turn, transmit more pressure to leg veins. It's the blueprint for varicose veins.

Menstruation can also cause pressure on the veins because of the increase in blood volume just before menstruation starts. It's why many women's legs may feel achy right before their periods.

Lifestyle factors can also aggravate vein problems. If you smoke, varicose veins are much more likely to creep up on you, because smoking affects blood flow by interfering with the regulation of fibrin, a blood-clotting protein. Although being heavy doesn't cause varicose veins directly, being 20 percent over your ideal weight can coax out varicose veins in those who have hereditary tendencies toward them. Lifting very heavy weights and running on hard surfaces may also hasten the appearance of varicose veins.

Sometimes the underlying problem is physiological. People with varicose veins have an inherited weakness in the valves inside the leg veins. These veins normally prevent blood from leaking back down as it flows up to the heart. If a valve leaks, gravity forces blood into lower veins when you stand up. Once this process is repeated enough times, vein walls can become permanently stretched.

"Whenever you're standing or sitting with your legs below the heart, gravity's working against you," explains Malcolm O. Perry, M.D., professor and chief of vascular surgery at Texas Tech University Health Sciences Center in Lubbock.

Fallout from a Low-Fiber Diet

There's one thing doctors know for sure about varicose veins: They are not a natural part of aging. In fact, Glenn Geelhoed, M.D., professor of surgery and international medical education at George Washington University Medical Center in Washington, D.C., has studied varicose veins in populations around the world and has found that in some Third World cultures, varicose veins are all but nonexistent, even in women who have borne children. He has also found that when these people move to countries such as the United States and adopt our habits—mainly, a low-fiber diet and a sedentary lifestyle—they start to develop varicose veins.

Too little fiber produces constipation and straining on the toilet and that may be where diet affects vein health most. Western populations on low-fiber diets pass smaller and harder stools than do Third World people, who have few varicose veins, Dr. Geelhoed notes. And when you strain in vain, that increases pressure in rectal veins, which in turn passes on more pressure to leg veins.

In fact, the famed Framingham Heart Study, which followed the lifestyles of residents of this Massachusetts town for over 40 years, found that the risk factors for varicose veins are the same as for heart disease—particularly being overweight and sedentary. The Framingham study also showed that compared with people without varicose veins, those with vein problems were more often obese, were less active, and had higher blood pressure.

They're Not Inevitable

If varicose veins run in the family but haven't yet turned up on you, there are many things you can do to help forestall them.

Shed some weight. If you are significantly overweight, a gradual, healthy weight loss plan can be your veins' biggest ally, says Alan Kanter, M.D., medical director of the Vein Center of Orange County in Irvine, California. Extra pounds put unnecessary pressure on your legs.

Fiber up your diet. Make sure your diet is high in fiber to keep bowels healthy and stools soft. This will prevent straining because of constipation, Dr. Kanter says. Fiber is found in abundance in fruits, vegetables, and whole grains.

Drink water. Another way to soften stools is to be sure you're well hydrated by drinking at least eight glasses of water a day, says Dr. Kanter.

Don't smoke. Or if you do, stop, says Dr. Geelhoed. Smoking increases your risk of developing underlying vein disease, which can contribute to varicose veins, he says.

Lift weights wisely. Weight-lifting exercise will help with weight control, but you need to do it right to avoid encouraging a vein problem, says Dr. Kanter. Use smaller weights and do more repetitions rather than straining with heavy weights, he says. Ask a trainer to set up a program for you.

Jog on gentle ground. Plan your running route along soft surfaces such as dirt, grass, or cinder track whenever possible, Dr. Kanter suggests. The impact of running on pavement can aggravate vein swelling.

Get a boost from bromelain. Bromelain, an enzyme that's extracted from green pineapple, can help prevent the development of the hard and lumpy skin found around varicose veins, says Joseph E. Pizzorno, Jr., N.D., a naturopathic physician and president of Bastyr College in Bothell, Washington.

Keep moving on the job. Don't sit for 2 or 3 hours straight while you work, says Dr. Perry. Be sure to get up and move around often to keep blood circulating. The Framingham study found that women who spent 8 or more hours a day in sedentary activities, sitting, or standing, had a much higher incidence of varicose veins.

Minds your Bs and Cs. Vitamin C helps your body manufacture two important connective tissues, collagen and elastin. "Both of these tissues help to keep vein walls strong and flexible," says Dr. Pizzorno. He recommends 500 to 3,000 milligrams of vitamin C daily.

Some doctors also recommend a combination of B vitamins, including folic acid, B_{12}, and B_6—available in supplements. These vitamins help prevent blood clots that can block varicose veins.

Get your gotu kola. The herb gotu kola is particularly good for varicose veins and also has a reputation as an anti-aging herb, says Roberta Bourgon, N.D., a naturopathic doctor at the Wellness Center in Billings, Montana. This herb seems to strengthen the sheath of tissue that wraps around veins, reduce the formation of scar tissue, and improve blood flow through affected limbs.

Removing the Webs

Some people call them spider veins—those visible red lines that usually crop up on the legs, especially the thighs, and seem to resemble the fragile patterns of a spider's web.

How do you get rid of them? If they're big enough, usually conventional sclerotherapy is the best bet, says Arthur Bertolino, M.D., associate clinical professor of dermatology at New York University Medical Center in New York City and a dermatologist in Ridgewood, New Jersey.

"The optimal size for treatment is at least as large as the line you'd write on a piece of paper with an ordinary ballpoint pen," he says. "If they're too small, you can't put a needle in."

If you have just a few tiny spiders, consider a cover-up makeup with a greenish base, which conceals red tones, Dr. Bertolino suggests.

But for more than a few on the face or legs, sclerotherapy is usually very successful, he says. A tiny needle is inserted into the vein, and a solution is injected. You can actually see the red network disappear as the clear solution enters the vein, he says.

Side effects? Occasionally, the solution will cause a temporary muscle cramp near the ankle or the back of the lower calf, which your doctor can massage away in a minute or two. Rarely, a skin ulcer may result from fluid that escapes a leaky vessel, or new spider veins called mats may form, he says. There may also be a brownish discoloration of the skin, which almost always fades completely on its own but can often be removed using a copper vapor laser.

The pulsed-dye laser is also used by some physicians to remove dilated facial capillaries, says David Green, M.D., a dermatologist at the Varicose Vein Center in Bethesda, Maryland. The light waves emitted by the laser are absorbed by hemoglobin molecules in the blood. "This vaporizes the hemoglobin, which turns the light energy into heat energy and 'fizzles' the vessel wall," he says.

Try taking 60 to 120 milligrams a day in capsules.

Lick the salt habit. Too much salt can make your legs swell and stress already damaged veins. Doctors suggest cutting back on salt by loading your diet with fresh fruits and vegetables, as well as whole grains. You'll also be upping your intake of potassium, magnesium, and calcium, three minerals that help reduce fluid retention.

Home Treatment for the Ones You Have

If you already have a few varicose veins developing, here's how to keep them under control.

Sleep on a slope. Put 6- by 6-inch blocks under the foot of your bed and leave them there, says Dr. Perry. This keeps blood from pooling in your legs at night. You can quickly adapt to the tilt.

Wear support hose. For a few small veins, choose high-quality support hose from a good clothing store and wear them regularly, says Dr. Perry. Support hose are available in knee-high, stocking, and panty-hose styles. The slight compression will help keep the veins down, he says. For more or larger veins, you may need to use gradient compression stockings, available over the counter in most drugstores.

Try gradient stockings. If the veins you have are fairly large, even good-quality support hose aren't enough, says Dr. Perry. Ask your doctor to prescribe custom-fitted gradient compression stockings instead. "They're hot and heavy, but they help," he says. Most women opt to wear them under pants for work and save the more sheer support hose for special occasions.

The Big Cover-Up

There are two basic medical treatments available for varicose veins: sclerotherapy (injection) and surgical removal (stripping).

The latest advance in both sclerotherapy and vein surgery is the use of sound wave technology, called duplex ultrasound imaging. The ultrasound equipment is used to locate deeper problem veins and to guide injections precisely, says Dr. Kanter. And ultrasound is both painless and safe.

Sclerotherapy involves injecting a solution into a vein, causing the vein's walls to be absorbed by the body. No anesthesia is needed, and "you can be up and about your business right afterward," says David Green, M.D., a dermatologist at the Varicose Vein Center in Bethesda, Maryland. A few weeks to months later, the vein shrivels to an invisible thread of scar tissue under the skin.

If you have had large varicose veins treated with sclerotherapy, you will need to wear gradient compression stockings for up to 6 weeks afterward, Dr. Green says.

Who's a candidate? Virtually anyone, as long as you are not pregnant and have no history of blood clotting disorders, Dr. Green says. But although the procedure is simple and effective, there are potential side effects. If the solution escapes the vein, it can cause an ulcer on the skin. And in up to 20 percent of patients, a brown line appears on the skin, following the course of the vein. In greater than 90 percent of these patients, the discoloration fades completely over months or a year or two, Dr. Green says.

Lasers can remove the discoloration when wielded by a physician skilled in using the copper vapor laser. One Australian study showed that 11 of 16 patients treated with copper vapor laser therapy for discoloration caused by sclerotherapy had significant improvement after 3 months.

Surgical stripping is sometimes recommended for severe varicose veins. Although some patients can undergo the surgery with local anesthesia, most surgeons prefer a light general anesthesia, Dr. Perry says. Many patients have the surgery as outpatients, going home late the same day. Compression stockings are worn for several weeks to months afterward.

Even though the affected veins are completely removed, there is no risk to your circulation, because other vessels can easily compensate for the loss of the superficial veins, Dr. Perry says.

While some scarring usually results from surgery, often long lengths of vein can be removed through several tiny incisions.

What are the advantages of surgery? Many vein specialists say that even large varicose veins can be effectively treated with sclerotherapy. But some vascular surgeons point out that there is a high rate of recurrence with the injection treatment, and multiple visits are often required if you have many affected veins. However, when ultrasound imaging is used to help guide the surgery, preliminary results show a higher success rate in fewer visits.

VISION CHANGES

Set Your Sights High

You've booked the corner table at Chez Chic, and it's time to wow the clients from out of town. The sommelier hands you the wine list. You sigh nonchalantly, make a joke about bad California Chablis, and open the list with a practiced touch of disdain.

Uh-oh. You can't read it. Your eyes won't focus on the fine print. So much for being nonchalant. You straighten your arms, hold the list a yard from your face, and start to squint.

Just like that, you've gone from deal maker to dear old grandma, sitting there reading a large-print version of *The Old Farmer's Almanac*. What's next—trifocals, knitting needles, a rocking chair?

Calm down. It's a fact of life that sooner or later, your vision is going to fade a bit. Nine in 10 people between ages 40 and 64 wear glasses or contact lenses to make reading and other close work a little easier.

But don't despair. You may be able to slow the process with regular eye exams, a healthful diet, and maybe even some do-it-yourself eye exercises. More importantly, you can take steps now to deal with serious vision problems such as glaucoma, cataracts, and macular degeneration that could lead to greatly reduced sight or even blindness.

Up Close and Blurry

Remember all the ladybugs in Mom's old flower garden? You'd pick them up gently and let them crawl on your fingers, holding them right up to your nose, and counting the little black dots on their backs.

Try that now. Odds are you couldn't tell a ladybug from a breath mint until it was 7 or 8 inches from your face. That's because the lenses in your eyes begin to stiffen with age. And the less they bend, the harder it is to focus on something close.

The condition is a form of farsightedness called presbyopia, and it's as inevitable as rain at a picnic. "There's really no way around it," says Richard

Bensinger, M.D., a Seattle-area ophthalmologist and spokesman for the American Academy of Ophthalmology. "It's easy to correct, but it means you're probably going to have to wear glasses or contact lenses."

If you do end up needing corrective lenses, the choice between glasses and contact lenses is usually up to you. "In most cases, it's just a matter of preference," Dr. Bensinger says. "Some people like glasses, which they can take off when they don't want them. And some like contact lenses, which allow them to see well without showing people that they need glasses."

Even if you eventually need bifocals, which help correct your vision both near and far, you don't have to advertise it to the world. Doctors have developed blended lenses that eliminate the telltale line across the center of each lens. You could also try bifocal contact lenses, which allow you to change focus as your eyes move up and down. Dr. Bensinger says they can be much more expensive than standard contacts, however, and warns that not everyone can adjust to them.

Your eye doctor might also prescribe so-called monovision contact lenses. You put a distance vision contact in your dominant eye (usually the right) and the reading contact in your other eye. "It's not as hard to adjust to as it sounds," Dr. Bensinger says. "You don't have to consciously adjust to it every time you change your focus." Monovision lenses are made like regular contacts and are less expensive than bifocal contacts, he says.

In addition to presbyopia, spots and floaters may appear more often as you get older. These are little specks or dots that pop up occasionally in your field of vi-

Common Eye Myths

Reading in dim light can damage your eyes. Myth. Low light can cause eye fatigue but will not harm your eyes.

Watching television hurts your eyes. Myth. There's no evidence that sitting too close to the television or watching for long periods causes any problems.

Too much reading wears out your eyes. Myth. Again, reading can make your eyes tired, but there's no evidence that it will hurt them in the long run.

Eating lots of carrots improves your vision. Semi-myth. You need vitamin A to see, but just a small amount—less than a carrot's worth a day. A healthful diet, with or without carrots, gives you all the vitamin A you need.

sion, then disappear after an hour or a day or more. Dr. Bensinger says they're caused when parts of the clear vitreous fluid that fills your eye get a little stringy or lumpy.

"Usually, it's nothing serious," Dr. Bensinger says. "The spots just drift down out of your vision, and that's it. But if you suddenly see lots of spots or flashes of lights in your eyes, that could be a sign that something more serious is wrong, and you should see a doctor immediately."

And if you live in especially dusty or windy areas, you may be at risk of developing pterygiums, which are fleshy, benign growths around the eyes. These can start growing in your midtwenties, usually on the sides of your eyes closest to your nose. Dr. Bensinger says they're just a cosmetic problem unless they grow large enough to block your sight. Pterygiums are easily removed with minor surgery.

Taking the Long View

Barring accidental injury, your eyes will probably serve you well right up to your midsixties. You may need a new set of reading glasses every few years, but you probably won't notice any serious deterioration of vision.

Still, experts warn that you should never take your eyes for granted. Most serious eye diseases are painless and show no symptoms for years. If you don't get your eyes examined on a regular basis, you may not know how bad things have gotten until it's too late to help. Here are some diseases to watch out for.

Glaucoma. This progressive disease causes 12 percent of all blindness in America. It is marked by increased fluid pressure in the eye, which, over the years, can cause irreversible damage to the nerves that send vision impulses to your brain.

Doctors don't know what causes most kinds of glaucoma, and they don't know how to cure it. Vision lost to glaucoma cannot be restored, but when detected early enough, glaucoma can be controlled. Eyedrops or oral tablets can sometimes help lower the pressure in the eye. If that fails, laser surgery may help unclog the eye's natural drains, allowing fluid to escape and lowering pressure. And if that doesn't work, eye surgeons can create an artificial drain to carry away the fluid.

In addition to any prescription medicines your doctor may prescribe, you can ask your doctor about ginkgo biloba, an herbal remedy that may help preserve vision, says Robert Ritch, M.D., medical director of the Glaucoma Foundation in New York City. "Gingko appears to increase blood flow to the eye and prevent the death of cells in the optic nerves," he says.

He recommends taking 120 milligrams of gingko twice a day for 2 months, then cutting back to 60 milligrams twice a day. Don't use ginkgo if you're taking monoamine oxidase inhibitor drugs like phenelzine sulfate (Nardil) or tranylcypromine (Partnate), or aspirin, nonsteroidal anti-inflammatory medications, or blood-thinning medications like warfarin (Coumadin).

Eye-robics: Exercises for Your Eyes

You work out every week to flatten your stomach, tighten your thighs, and firm up your arms. So why not take a few minutes to work out your eyes?

Not all experts think that exercises aid your eyes, but a growing number of vision therapists believe a few daily exercises can help keep your eyes younger.

"The logic behind vision therapy," says Steven Ritter, O.D., of the State University of New York College of Optometry in New York City, "is that if you can harm your visual system with close-up tasks, you should be able to rehabilitate it."

Vision therapists can prescribe as many as 280 different exercises. No single set can cure everybody's vision problems. But you can't go wrong with any of these.

Do the fine-print sprint. If you work at a computer terminal for hours at a time, try this: Tack a page of newsprint to a wall about 8 feet from where you ordinarily sit. Interrupt your work every 10 minutes or so and look up at the newspaper. Bring the print into focus. Then look back at the computer screen. Do this repeatedly for 30 seconds, about 6 times an hour. It could help eliminate the blurriness many people experience at the end of the workday.

Hit the wall. If you play handball, racquetball, squash, or tennis, this two-person exercise may come in handy. Stand 3 to 5 feet from a blank wall. Ask your partner to stand behind you and toss a tennis ball against the wall. When the ball caroms off the wall, try to catch it. This exercise can help improve your hand/eye coordination.

Read your thumb. Hold your thumb at arm's length. Move it in circles, X's, and crosses, closer and farther away. Follow it with your eyes. As you do so, keep as much of the room as possible in your field of vision.

An estimated 3 million Americans have glaucoma, and half of them don't even know it. Another 5 million to 10 million people have the eye pressure buildup that precedes the disease, and far fewer than half of them know it. The best advice for dealing with glaucoma? Find out if you have it—now. "The earlier this disease is picked up, the better able we'll be to control it," says Carl Kupfer, M.D., director of the National Eye Institute in Bethesda, Maryland. That means regular eye exams, especially if you're at high risk for glaucoma.

Continue the exercise with one eye closed. Repeat with the other eye. This can improve your peripheral vision.

Track the flashlight. This amusing exercise can improve your ability to track an object visually. It requires a partner and two flashlights. Stand in a darkened room facing a wall. Have your partner shine a flashlight on the wall and wave the disk of light in sweeping motions. Try to eclipse the circle of light with light from your flashlight while balancing a book on your head. This forces you to track the light with your eyes instead of moving your head.

Call the ball. Write letters or numbers on a softball or Styrofoam ball, then screw a hook into the top of it and hang it from the ceiling with string. The smaller the characters, the more difficult the exercise. Give the ball a push in any direction. Try to call out the numbers or letters you see. This exercise helps you keep a moving target in focus.

Bead a string. This exercise trains both eyes to converge on a target. It also trains your brain to not switch off one eye's vision. String three colored beads on a string 6 feet long. Fasten one end of the string to a wall at eye height, and hold the other end of the string to your nose. Slide one bead close to the wall, place the second bead 4 feet from your nose, and place the third bead 16 inches from your nose.

Look at the farthest bead. You will see two strings forming a V converging at the bead. Shift both eyes to the middle bead. Notice the X where the two strings seem to converge upon it. Shift both eyes to the nearest bead, and observe a similar X. Shift quickly from one bead to another, always observing the V or the X. If both eyes are working as a team, you should always see two strings crossing when you're focused on a bead. If your eyes aren't working together, you'll see different patterns or just one string.

Cataracts. Although they usually don't become a problem until you near retirement age, cataracts often start forming much earlier in life, especially if you have ever had an eye injury or have undergone such procedures as radiation treatment, chemotherapy, or an organ transplant.

Over the years, the once-clear lens in each eye may turn yellow because of protein buildup. In time, the lens may become milky white and translucent, clouding vision to the point where you need an artificial lens implant. This plastic replacement lens does not flex to focus light, as the original lens did. But with corrective glasses, your vision can be restored quite well. "While we can't yet cure cataracts, we can certainly provide patients with good sight," Dr. Bensinger says.

Cataracts, like glaucoma, may have a hereditary link. So if anyone in your family has had cataracts, you may be at higher risk and should have your eyes examined more often than the standard of every 3 years.

Macular degeneration. This insidious eye disease robs you of your fine visual skills. "In more advanced cases, you would be able to tell that someone was standing in front of you, but you couldn't tell who," Dr. Bensinger says. "You could see there was a bus coming down the street, but you couldn't tell which one, because you couldn't read the sign."

The cause remains unknown, but the condition somehow causes deterioration of the macula, the central part of the retina that's responsible for sharp focus. Unfortunately, there's little hope right now for restoring sight lost to macular degeneration, though laser surgery may help stabilize sight for a time. There is some hopeful news, though: Because macular degeneration strikes people who are over age 60 almost exclusively, you can start now—perhaps with the help of an improved diet—to ward it off before it starts.

Diabetic retinopathy. It primarily strikes people with diabetes and is the leading cause of blindness in people ages 20 to 50. Loss of vision begins to occur when blood vessels in the back of the eye leak, blurring vision and sometimes denying nutrients to the eye.

"If you have diabetes," Dr. Bensinger says, "I cannot urge you strongly enough to have your eyes checked regularly. It can literally save your sight."

Laser treatments can help slow the damage from leaking vessels. But again, help is available only if you get your eyes examined regularly. "Early detection of diabetic retinopathy is even more of a success story than testing for glaucoma," Dr. Kupfer says. If caught early, there's a 95 percent chance you can keep your sight for at least 5 years, Dr. Kupfer says.

Focusing on Prevention

You can't change your genes, so there's not much you can do about the biggest vision risk factor of all—heredity. Still, here's some advice to give you the best chance of staying 20/20 into the 21st century.

Get your eyes checked. Doctors just can't say this enough.

"Regular eye examinations are by far the most important thing you can do to help preserve your vision," Dr. Bensinger says.

If you are between ages 30 and 50 and have no previous eye problems, the American Academy of Ophthalmology suggests seeing an ophthalmologist every 3 years. If you have a family history of glaucoma or diabetes or are already wearing glasses or contact lenses, your doctor may suggest more frequent visits.

The academy suggests an immediate visit to the doctor for any of the following:

- Sudden vision changes in one or both eyes
- Unexplainable redness
- Seeing a number of spots or floaters or showers of sparks in the corners of your eyes
- Eye pain that won't go away
- Accidental contact with chemicals, especially lye.

Hide behind some shades. Sunglasses that block both UVA and UVB rays and visible blue light may help decrease the risk of cataracts, Dr. Bensinger says. Wraparound glasses that cover the sides of your eyes are a good idea, since they shield your eyes completely. And try to wear a hat with a visor to block direct sunlight from your eyes. "Exposure to sunlight drops the age at which you may develop cataracts," Dr. Bensinger says. "So if you're going to be outside, it makes sense to cut that sunlight as much as possible."

Stop smoking. Cancer. Wrinkles. Stinky clothes. Yellow teeth. Emphysema. If you really need another reason to quit, here it is: Cigarette smoking might cause cataracts. A Harvard Medical School study of 120,000 nurses showed that women who smoke 35 or more cigarettes a day have a 63 percent greater risk of developing cataracts.

The reason isn't known, but researchers speculate that smoking may reduce antioxidant levels in your blood, promoting cataract growth.

Walk it away. Regular aerobic exercise like walking can help lower pressure in the eye, increase blood flow to the optic nerve, and slow the progression of glaucoma, says Dr. Ritch.

In fact, research conducted at Oregon Health Sciences University in Portland on a group of sedentary people who began a program of brisk walking for 40 minutes three times a week found that those with glaucoma reduced their eye pressure by 20 percent. And those people who did not have glaucoma saw a 9 percent reduction in eye pressure.

Try some see-food. The links between diet and vision are still weak. But there's growing evidence that a substance called glutathione may help control the spread of macular degeneration. It's found in fresh green, red, and yellow vegetables. Canned or frozen vegetables lose all their glutathione in processing.

A report in the *American Journal of Clinical Nutrition* claimed that people who eat 3½ servings of fruits and vegetables every day have a lower risk of cataracts, too.

"Eating a healthy diet may delay the usual aging of the lens and so delay cataracts," says Paul F. Jacques, Sc.D., an epidemiologist with the U.S. Department of Agriculture Human Nutrition Research Center on Aging at Tufts University in Boston.

Make the most of milk. You wouldn't think to toast your eyes with a glass
continued on page 296

Test Your Vision at Home

More than 10 million Americans over age 25 suffer some loss of sight. Many don't even know it. These simple tests could help you discover whether your vision needs some attention.

Remember: The tests are not a substitute for a professional eye examination. They can only serve as a warning to see an eye doctor.

These tests were prepared by Prevent Blindness America. For more information, write or call: 500 East Remington Road, Schaumburg, IL 60173; (800) 331-2020.

Vision Test 1: Distance vision. If possible, have someone help you with this test. Don't take it if you're tired. And if you have glasses or contacts, be sure you're wearing them. (1) Position the chart on page 295 10 feet away from you, against a bare wall or door. Make sure the room is well lit and avoid glare from windows. (2) Lightly cover your left eye with a piece of paper. Keeping both eyes open, tell your assistant (or write down) where the opening is in each C on the chart. Start with the largest C and work down the page. Repeat with your right eye covered. (3) If you don't get all the C's correct on the next-to-bottom line, repeat the test another day.

Nearly half of all blindness can be prevented.
Everyone should have periodic eye examinations.

Ω Ɔ Ω U C   U Ɔ C U Ω

Vision Test 2: Near vision. Wear your contacts or glasses only if you use them to read. (1) Sit in a well-lit room away from window glare. (2) Keeping both eyes open, hold the near-vision test about 14 inches from your eyes. (3) Read the test sentence above, or write it down as it looks to you. (4) Write down where the openings are for each C. If you didn't get them all right, take the test another day.

continued on page 296

Test Your Vision at Home—Cont.

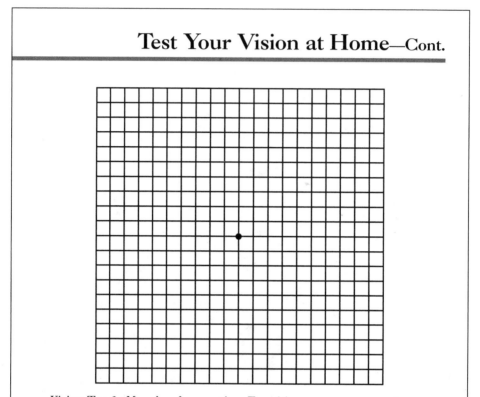

Vision Test 3: Macular degeneration. For this test, wear your glasses or contact lenses only if they're for reading. (1) Have someone hold the grid against a bare wall or door in a well-lit room without glare from windows. Make sure the center dot on the grid is at eye level. (2) Stand 14 inches from the grid. Look at the dot in the center of the grid and cover your left eye with a piece of paper. You should see all four corners of the grid. If the grid looks distorted or you see any blank spots or wavy lines, make a mental note of it. Repeat with your right eye covered.

of Bessie's best, but milk, along with chicken and yogurt, provides some of the best eye protection you can find.

All of these foods contain large amounts of riboflavin, a B vitamin that appears to help prevent cataracts from forming. The connection, once again, appears to be antioxidants. The body uses riboflavin to manufacture glutathione.

Play Popeye. Popeye used spinach to build strong muscles, but it works just as well for strengthening the eyes. In fact, studies show that spinach may be one of your best protections against cataracts.

Spinach, along with kale, broccoli, and other dark green, leafy vegetables, contains beta-carotene, lutein, and zeaxanthin. These three antioxidants can help stop damage to the eyes before cataracts form. They also concentrate in the fluids in the eyes, which means you're getting the protection right where you need it most.

Try the vision vitamins. Antioxidant vitamins A, C, and E showed promise as cataract fighters in the Harvard Nurses' Health Study. Studies also suggest that vitamins C and E can relieve low eye pressure and slow the development of glaucoma, Dr. Ritch says. He recommends taking 2,000 milligrams of vitamin C and 800 international units of vitamin E daily.

Seek out zinc, too. Though there's no hard evidence yet, Dr. Bensinger says taking multivitamin supplements containing zinc "is probably not a bad idea, as long as you're not spending too much money on fancy brands."

WORRY

Don't Agonize—Energize

You watch your little boy board the school bus every morning. Are the brakes okay? Will he be warm enough? Is he eating his lunch?

Off to work. Did that proposal make it to Dallas on time? The economy's so bad; are you going to be laid off? What will you do without a job?

Back home in time for the evening news. The ozone layer is disappearing. War, hunger, and violence are everywhere.

Life provides plenty to worry about. And sometimes it can become too much to handle. Maybe you're suffering from constant tension headaches or feeling tired all the time. Maybe worrying leaves your stomach in knots. Just a few years ago, you felt flush with youthful hope and optimism, ready to solve the planet's problems. But now you may be starting to feel powerless, worn out, unable to deal with even the smallest dilemmas.

"Worries are like a straitjacket," says Mary McClure Goulding, coauthor of *Not to Worry! How to Free Yourself from Unnecessary Anxiety and Channel Your Worries into Positive Action*. "You feel like you can't do anything, and so you don't. It's a totally unproductive way to spend the best years of your life. And it's something you need to change—and can change—starting immediately."

The Fearful Facts

We all worry. In fact, the average person spends about 5 percent of each waking day—about 48 minutes—worrying about one thing or another. Surveys show that the most common sources of worry for Americans are family and relationships, jobs and school, health and finances.

For as many as 6 percent of us, worrying becomes chronic. It can even evolve into a clinical condition called generalized anxiety disorder. People with this disorder worry about multiple problems at the same time, including things they have little or no control over, such as the weather or nuclear war. And they worry excessively. Chronic worriers report spending an average of 50 percent of each day worrying, and some report as much as 100 percent, says psychologist Jennifer L. Abel, Ph.D., associate director of the Stress and Anxiety Disorders Clinic at Pennsylvania State University in University Park. Chronic worry typically begins when you're in your twenties or thirties.

There's no evidence that worrying directly causes disease, says Timothy Brown, Psy.D., associate director of the Phobia and Anxiety Disorders Clinic at the State University of New York at Albany. Worry can lead to poor sleep in many cases, with resulting fatigue, restlessness, and irritability. But it's the psychological toll that's usually most devastating. "Worriers can't concentrate, get headaches, and may not be able to effectively confront and resolve their problems," he says.

Worriers almost always come from fretting families, Goulding says. You may have learned to worry by watching your mother, father, grandfather, or an aunt. Worriers may have low self-esteem, Goulding says, and have often been taught to repress feelings—especially happy ones.

All of which leads to a central problem: a feeling of helplessness. "You don't feel in control of your life," says Susan Jeffers, Ph.D., a psychologist and author of *Feel the Fear and Do It Anyway.* "You think everything is going to go wrong. That makes it hard to overcome even simple problems without great effort and anxiety."

A study of 24 American college students bears this out. When asked what would happen if they didn't get good grades, a group of nonworriers typically talked about ending up with bad jobs and earning less money. The chronic worriers talked about those same concerns. But then they took their worries much further. Some worried about becoming drug addicts. Others worried they would be in constant physical pain. And still others said they would die—or even end up in hell.

"At that point, you have to ask yourself whether worrying is worth the effort," Dr. Jeffers says. "You have to decide whether you're going to spend the rest of your life worrying about things or whether you're going to do something about it. It's a difficult decision, but hopefully, you'll choose the latter."

Winning over Worry

It takes years to build a world of worries. You may need a while to tear it all down. But time is on your side. A study of both young and elderly worriers showed that we tend to worry less as we grow older. The oldest of the 163 people studied by professors at the University of Massachusetts at Amherst were less anxious about social and financial problems and no more worried about health issues.

But why wait for things to get better? If you're ready to start banishing worry right now, here's some expert advice.

Think it through. Go ahead and fret a little. It's better than trying to suppress all the anxiety. "Give up trying to stop those unhappy thoughts," says Daniel Wegner, Ph.D., professor of psychology at the University of Virginia in

Charlottesville. "My research shows that the more you try to suppress unwanted thoughts, the more likely you are to become obsessed with them. That's particularly true when you're under a lot of pressure, stress, or mental overload. So just when you're trying to avoid unhappy thoughts, you'll actually get sadder than if you'd confront those unhappy thoughts head-on."

Dr. Jeffers likes to point out that 99 percent of what we worry about never happens. "Feel the fear. That's part of being human," she says. "But go out and do things anyway, knowing that most of your fears are unfounded."

Take your time. It's one thing to think about your problems. It's another to let them dominate your thoughts. Dr. Wegner says research on chronic worriers shows that if they spend time at night actively worrying about their problems, the degree of worrying in their lives goes down overall. "There's something boring, after all, about thoughts you spend an hour a night thinking about," he says.

Michael Vasey, Ph.D., assistant professor of psychology at Ohio State University in Columbus, suggests setting aside 30 minutes a day, always at the same place and time, to worry. "Focus on your worry for the entire period, and try to think of solutions to the problems," he says. If you're worried that you'll be fired, imagine the scenario—the firing and the consequences—and don't let the image drift away.

You'll probably be even more anxious at first. But things will improve. "If you practice focusing on worries and thinking of solutions for 30 minutes each day for several weeks, your anxiety will start to taper off," Dr. Vasey says. "You'll get better at generating solutions or realize it's not worth worrying about."

Write a new ending. People who worry can be amazingly creative, Goulding says. They turn any harmless scenario into a disaster by imagining the worst. Try putting that creativity to good use by turning your fears into fantasies. If you worry about a school bus crash, try picturing your little boy grabbing the wheel and steering everyone to safety. Then imagine the parade the town will hold for him. Maybe he'll even get the key to the city.

You're disarming your worries this way, Goulding says. By putting a happy or silly ending on a worry, you're allowing yourself a chance to be positive, she says. And that's a major step toward beating worry.

Tally your troubles. List all your worries. Are you afraid that it's going to rain on the family reunion this weekend? You can't control that, so Goulding suggests that you file it under the heading "Beyond My Skills." Do you worry that other people find you unattractive, even when you really know you're not? That goes on the "Creative Fiction" list.

What's the sense of worrying about things in these categories? "There isn't any," Goulding says. "Why worry about the weather? Why worry about things that aren't true?" Once you expose these thoughts as worthless worries, she says, it's easier to dismiss them.

Take action. Some worries are more legitimate. Are you concerned about your health? Well, list all the things you could do to improve things. Maybe you could start walking every day. Or eat better. Then decide which ones you're going

Calm the Worrier Within

Call her Fretful Fanny. She's the unhappy little doomsayer in your head who won't stop talking about things that can and will go wrong.

It's time to quiet her for good.

"You have to silence that voice of self-harassment," says Mary Mc-Clure Goulding, coauthor of *Not to Worry! How to Free Yourself from Unnecessary Anxiety and Channel Your Worries into Positive Action.* "If you listen to it, you'll always keep worrying."

Become aware of the voice. Sit in a quiet place and listen to your thoughts. When you start hearing negative thoughts, consciously replace them with positive ones. Affirmations—simple positive statements that you repeat frequently—might work. Try phrases such as, "There is nothing to fear," "I'm in control of my life," "I'll handle it," "Everything is working out perfectly."

"Repetition is the key. At first, you don't even need to believe what you're telling yourself," says Susan Jeffers, Ph.D., a psychologist and author of *Feel the Fear and Do It Anyway.* "Just talking positively changes our energy and helps us move forward."

Goulding suggests being more direct with your inner critic. Stand up, put your hands on your hips, and yell at Fanny: "Just shut up! I'm not listening to you anymore!" Curse, swear, do whatever feels good. "Drive that voice away," she says. "And then you can fill your mind with happier thoughts instead."

to do. The secret is doing, doing, doing. "When you're actively working on a solution, worry is less likely to be a problem," Dr. Jeffers says. "You'll begin to feel like you're the creator of your life, not a victim of it."

Find a friend. Tell someone special about your fears. "When you talk about your worries, it deflates those worries. They can't be suppressed. That cat's out of the bag. And thank goodness, it is just a cat and not some horrible monster," Dr. Wegner says.

Just be careful that your friend doesn't unintentionally make things worse. Out of kindness, she may tell you it's okay to worry or say, "Gee, I understand why you're so worried." Goulding says that might help reinforce your need to worry. If you decide to share your thoughts, make sure the other person agrees to be honest with you and helps you find positive, constructive ways to deal with your worries. If your confidante can't do that, find another ear.

WRINKLES

Draw the Line on Early Lines

Frowning with concentration, you're all business when you put on your makeup. You squint gently as you glide on a touch of eye shadow. You raise your eyebrows as you stroke on mascara and a sweep of blush. Then you pucker for lipstick. Nice. You reward yourself with a smile in the mirror.

Then it hits you. The frown is still there, along with the squint and the smile lines.

Wrinkles—already? Character is great, and you've always admired people who age with grace, but these lines feel premature—like a message from the future delivered too soon. You're just not ready for wrinkles.

Suddenly, you feel old. And maybe less attractive. You worry that a big smile will show your big wrinkles. You keep your eyes wide open, to erase those crow's-feet.

The Roots of the Ruts

Doctors say that the inevitable wrinkles from genetics and gravity really shouldn't arrive until you near your sixties. But they come a lot earlier—in the late twenties and thirties—for many of us. Here's why.

During the 1920s, French designer Coco Chanel came back from the tropics bronzed and glowing—and the centuries-old tradition of keeping skin in the shade was lost in the glare of the news. Fashion-conscious adults everywhere began to bask in the sun. In search of elegant tans, they started a new tradition: of sunburns and tanning booths—and skin cancer and early wrinkles. Even in naturally dark skin, sun damage causes 80 to 90 percent of the visible signs of aging, including wrinkles, doctors say.

The number-two cause of wrinkles is smoking, which speeds your skin's aging by up to 10 years. Smoking reduces blood flow to the skin, blunting its ability to repair damage. It also sets off enzymes that attack the tissues of your skin the way

302

meat tenderizer weakens the fibers of meat. And because skin gets a "memory" when it's folded in the same place over and over again, the mechanics of smoking cause wrinkles, too. Constant puckering to draw on a cigarette forms lip creases, and squinting against the smoke carves crow's-feet.

Some lines will form simply because we express emotion—with a ready smile or worried frown. The way you sleep can leave a wrinkle memory in your skin, too, especially if you snooze facedown.

But what can you do if you already have years of wrinkle-promoting habits behind you? Can the damage be undone? Yes, it can. You can prevent most new wrinkles from forming and remove the worst of the old ones with help from your doctor.

A New Wrinkle on Prevention

If you're determined to fight wrinkles, even if it means abandoning bronze for a paler, healthier beauty, here's where to begin.

Put up a chemical parasol. Sunscreen is your number-one weapon against further sun damage, says Albert M. Kligman, M.D., Ph.D., professor of dermatology at the University of Pennsylvania School of Medicine and an attending physician at the Hospital of the University of Pennsylvania, both in Philadelphia. Use a full-spectrum sunscreen that blocks both kinds of ultraviolet radiation (UVA and UVB), and use it every day, year-round, Dr. Kligman says. After you cleanse your skin in the morning, leave it slightly damp, and apply pea-size dabs of sunscreen on your cheeks and forehead, working it into the skin all over your face. Don't forget the backs of your hands, neck, and bustline.

Make sure your sunscreen is SPF 15 or higher. *SPF* stands for sun protection factor, and SPF 15, which most doctors recommend, means that you can stay out in the sun 15 times longer than you normally could before burning. Remember, too, that although daily use of SPF 15 sunscreen will protect you adequately while you dash in and out of buildings, for long hours in the outdoors you'll need to use higher-SPF products and reapply frequently.

Doctors disagree on how high to go with SPF numbers, however. Some say that numbers over 25 may give a false sense of security. While higher numbers do screen out the burning UVB rays, they may let in more UVA radiation. The UVA rays penetrate deeper into skin and cause most age-related changes such as wrinkles, says Melvin L. Elson, M.D., medical director of the Dermatology Center in Nashville.

Joseph Bark, M.D., a dermatologist in Lexington, Kentucky, and author of *Retin-A and Other Youth Miracles*, disagrees. He says research shows that skin will burn somewhat even with SPF 15 sunscreens, and he recommends using the highest SPF you can find, even for everyday use.

And read the sunscreen's contents. "The best of the broad-spectrum sunscreens (those that protect against UVA and UVB rays) contain titanium dioxide—

fine particles that stay in your skin and resist washing or rubbing off," says Dr. Kligman.

Don't rely on cosmetics. Your favorite cosmetic counter may offer foundations and moisturizers that contain low-SPF sunscreens, but these are too weak for real protection, Dr. Kligman says.

Protect your eye area. While you exercise, you don't want sunscreen to sting your eyes when you sweat. Try this workout tip from Melvin L. Elson, M.D., medical director of the Dermatology Center in Nashville. "Take a wax-based sunscreen made for lips and apply it around and over your eyes. It won't run," he says. You should also protect your eyes with a good pair of shades, preferably the wraparound kind. Make sure they shield UV radiation.

Dress for the sun. Innovative clothing manufacturers have come out with basic collections of shirts, swimsuits, and casual wear that are specially knit to prevent the sun's radiation from reaching your skin.

Dump that nasty habit. Yeah, yeah, you've been told before that smoking isn't cool anymore. Now you have one more reason to quit.

Feed your face. For general skin health, eat a balanced diet full of fruits, whole grains, and vegetables. You may also want to try supplements that have been proven to reduce sun damage to skin, says Karen E. Burke, M.D., Ph.D., a dermatologic surgeon and dermatologist in private practice in New York City. She recommends daily supplements of 100 micrograms of selenium (best taken as l-selenomethionine) plus 400 international units of vitamin E. Use the d-alpha tocopheryl acetate, d-alpha tocopheryl acid succinate, or d-alpha tocopherol form of vitamin E—not the "dl tocopherols" form, which is far less active. You should have no side effects from these safe doses, Dr. Burke says. Although research has not been designed specifically to link these nutrients with wrinkle repair, they may help, she adds.

Build collagen with C. Vitamin C, a nutrient known for its importance in the manufacture of collagen, is being touted by some experts as a key player in keeping the complexion smooth.

"Vitamin C is essential for connective tissue in the body, particularly for the layer where the collagen that maintains the integrity of your skin is made," explains Lorraine Meisner, Ph.D., professor of preventive medicine at the University of Wisconsin Medical School in Madison. "That's why people who eat adequate diets look younger than people who don't."

For a burst of vitamin C in your diet, you can go the traditional orange juice and citrus route, or you can create a vegetable medley of broccoli, brussels sprouts, and red bell peppers.

You also can apply topical vitamin C to your skin directly. This has been shown to prevent the free radical skin damage that occurs following exposure to ultraviolet rays from the sun. A 10 percent vitamin C lotion called Cellex-C is available without a prescription from dermatologists, plastic surgeons, and licensed aestheticians (full service beauty salon operators).

Take your measure in the mirror. Set a small hand mirror beside your telephone for a few days and watch yourself in conversation. You may have a few face-wrinkling habits you're not aware of, such as frowning or squinting while you mull something over. The mirror will help you learn to relax the facial muscles you're working overtime and to reduce expression lines.

Hit the bottle. If you must look like George Hamilton after a stint in the tropics, then try a bottled tan, suggests Seth L. Matarasso, M.D., assistant professor of dermatology at the University of California, San Francisco, School of Medicine. "Liquid tanners are getting much better, and their colors look more realistic," he says. But don't think the tanner protects you from the sun. You will still have to wear sunscreen.

No aerobics for your face. Although facial exercises have been touted in many beauty books, most of them actually increase wrinkling, says Dr. Burke. When you grimace or contort your face through exercises, you wind up working the same muscles that caused wrinkles in the first place, she says.

Sleep on your back. "It's the best position for a younger-looking, unlined face," says Gary Monheit, M.D., assistant professor of dermatology at the University of Alabama School of Medicine/University of Alabama in Birmingham. If you've been burrowing into your pillow face-first for years, lying on your back every night with a pillow under your knees may help you to change the habit.

Enhance your hormones. Although we all get wrinkles as we age, sometimes they seem to come on more suddenly after pregnancy, menopause, or emotional stress. These triggering events may upset the balance of hormones in the body. Proper regulation and production of these chemical messengers are essential to maintaining soft, elastic skin.

To prevent hormone imbalances, you can begin by eating more legumes and soy products such as tofu, says Michaal Gaszi, N.D., a naturopathic doctor in Ridgefield, Connecticut. These foods contain phytoestrogens, plant compounds that mimic the biological activities of female hormones.

Put on some fat. We mean essential fatty acids, of course. These acids, which are found in eggs, nuts, vegetables, butter, and whole milk, keep the skin healthy and help it fight off the effects of aging and sun exposure. For an extra boost, you can take a supplement of either 2 tablespoons of flaxseed oil per day or four capsules of evening primrose oil. These are both high in essential fatty acids.

"I'd probably start with the flaxseed oil and see how it works," says Dr. Gaszi. "It may take several months, however. Skin responds pretty slowly."

The ABCs of Wrinkle Repair

Now that you're committed to preventing new wrinkles, are you stuck with those you've already acquired? Not at all. There are many new developments in dermatology and plastic surgery that can remove your wrinkles. They range from prescription peeling lotions and creams to surface repairs and surgery.

Resetting the Clock with Retin-A

Retin-A is not just for acne.

"I don't know how to treat a patient for wrinkles without a prescription for Retin-A," says Melvin L. Elson, M.D., medical director of the Dermatology Center in Nashville. "Retin-A cream works by changing the skin to make it normal and smoother." It increases blood flow in the skin to give it a youthful, pink tone again and also attracts collagen-making cells closer to the surface of the skin, which tend to fill in wrinkles.

The effects of tretinoin (Retin-A) on wrinkles were discovered by Albert M. Kligman, M.D., Ph.D., professor of dermatology at the University of Pennsylvania School of Medicine and an attending physician at the Hospital of the University of Pennsylvania, both in Philadelphia. Many of his patients who were using Retin-A for severe acne pointed out their noticeably smoother, firmer skin. Since then, Retin-A's anti-aging effects have been proven in numerous studies, and Dr. Kligman recommends using it early in life to get a head start on wrinkle prevention.

"If you have a lot of wrinkles and you're young, even in your twenties, don't wait until you are 40 or 50 and have deep wrinkles and a lot of blotches," he says. "If you're a light-skinned person who had a normal childhood in America, you should start Retin-A early and get into a program that will last you the rest of your life."

Retin-A for wrinkles is sold in gel and cream forms in various strengths, and you and your dermatologist may need to experiment to find out which is right for you. At first, your skin may become irritated and flaky, but within a month or two, it should adapt. If you have very sensitive skin, try applying it once every third day and then every second day once your skin adjusts, or start with the lower strength (.025 percent cream) and increase gradually to higher concentrations, Dr. Kligman suggests. Or try a less irritating form of Retin-A, called Renova.

If you're committed to wrinkle fighting with Retin-A, you need to know that it's a lifelong relationship. If you stop using the drug, your fine wrinkles will return. And because Retin-A increases your skin's sensitivity to the sun, a daily regimen of sunscreen with a high SPF (sun protection factor) is vital.

But remember this: "You can't go out and get an unlimited amount of plastic surgery. Do as little as possible to get the maximum amount of improvement possible," says plastic surgeon Geoffrey Tobias, M.D., of Mount Sinai School of Medicine of the City University of New York. "You're never going to be 21 years old again or take 20 years off your face. But if two or three wrinkles bother you, take care of them. You'll look and feel better."

Consider this.

Smooth them with Retin-A. Tretinoin (Retin-A), derived from vitamin A, has earned its reputation as an excellent wrinkle smoother, particularly for the fine lines caused by years of indulging in the sun. But be warned: Retin-A cream is available only by prescription. The legions of similar-sounding ingredients in many cosmetics and lotions are only that: soundalikes. See your dermatologist. (For tips on using Retin-A, see page 306.)

Try AHA lotions. Your dermatologist has a gentle approach to wrinkle reduction, says Dr. Elson. Highly concentrated lotions made from alpha hydroxy acids (AHAs), derived from wine, milk, apples, lemons, or sugarcane, will gradually peel off the top layers of dead skin. "Over time, they will make crow's-feet and fine wrinkles less visible," says Dr. Elson. Some of the most popular lotions contain glycolic acid from sugarcane, which has small molecules that are easy for skin to absorb. Low-concentration AHAs are also available at your drugstore or cosmetics counter in some cleansers and moisturizers such as Avon's Anew Alpha Hydrox Skin Treatment System and Eucerin Plus Alphahydroxy Moisturing Lotion, but these are less effective than the higher-strength products your dermatologist can provide.

So far, AHAs offer the only real competition for Retin-A's wrinkle-fighting ability. AHA lotions give less dramatic results than Retin-A, but they are also less likely to irritate your skin.

Peel away the lines. Though the name may sound drastic, chemical peeling can be a fairly gentle procedure, says Sorrel S. Resnik, M.D., clinical professor of dermatology and cutaneous surgery at the University of Miami School of Medicine. The dermatologist wipes your face with acetone, a strong cleansing solvent, and then applies acid to your skin with a swab. The skin turns white and stings briefly as the acetone penetrates; then several layers of skin (and fine wrinkles) peel off a day or two later. Many doctors offer a series of three to six light acid peels at intervals of several weeks, for results that are only a little less effective than a medium or deep peel. With the series, you'll have less discomfort and a quicker healing time, usually only a few days. Trichloroacetic acid has a good record for safety and effectiveness, and glycolic acid, which is less penetrating, is also popular.

Very deep peels can be dangerous, says Dr. Resnik, and are usually offered only to people with extremely weathered, leathery skin. The chemical most often used for deep peels is phenol, which may cause cardiac or kidney problems. Phenol must be applied in the operating room because it requires close heart monitoring.

Amazing Face

In a business where the average model is washed up at 30, Gabrielle von Canal is a rarity. Blond-haired and blue-eyed, von Canal—now in her fifties—has been on the covers of *Harper's Bazaar*, *Town and Country*, *Woman's Day*, and *Prevention*. She is every bit as busy now as she was in her wrinkle-free twenties.

A model since 1963, von Canal is a firm believer in the cardinal rules of skin care. After gently cleansing and moisturizing, she applies a sunscreen with a sun protection factor (SPF) of 15 every day, regardless of the weather or the season.

Doing print ads for Oil of Olay, Revlon, Max Factor, and Lancome, among others, von Canal is living proof that true beauty has no age. "A woman becomes her most beautiful at 30. Something inside and out comes together at that age. If you have good genes and lead a healthy life, there's no reason you can't look terrific at 40 and 50."

Her career did hit one lull when she was in her thirties, she admits. "That's when you're considered too old to be young, yet too young to be older," she says. But in her forties, she got work again—in part because many older models left the profession for marriage and kids.

And von Canal has found her niche as a model whose good looks appeal to older women seeking youth-enhancing moisturizers and skin creams. But that doesn't mean the New York City resident has flawless skin.

"I've never had plastic surgery," she says. "I have wrinkles, but wrinkles are not what makes you old. People overlook them."

Ask about fillers. Plumping up the skin beneath a wrinkle is an alternative to peeling off wrinkles from the surface, says Dr. Monheit. Dermatologists use several substances as wrinkle fillers, but the best known is cattle-derived collagen. Collagen is a fibrous tissue that forms a supporting network just under the surface of the skin. The doctor injects the collagen into your wrinkle, and a lump appears above the skin surface. When the lump fades (in as little as 6 hours), the wrinkle will have been smoothed away.

The problems with collagen? It's temporary—results last from 4 to 15 months, Dr. Monheit says. And some people may be allergic to this form of collagen, so the doctor must first perform an allergy test.

If you do prove allergic to cattle collagen, ask about a newer method called autogenous tissue implant, says Dr. Elson. A patch of skin harvested from another part of your body is sent out to a company that processes your own collagen from the skin. The processor then returns to your doctor a syringe filled with the collagen for an injection.

A wrinkle filler called Fibrel may last up to 5 years, says Dr. Monheit. Fibrel is a gelatin-based material that is mixed with your own blood serum and injected beneath a wrinkle. Your body responds by making its own collagen, which, in turn, fills out the wrinkle. Drawbacks? Fibrel injections hurt more than collagen shots, and the procedure is more time-consuming, Dr. Monheit says.

"The best filler would be something natural from your own body," says Michael Sachs, M.D., a plastic surgeon in private practice in New York City. A technique for wrinkle filling that's still in the experimental stage is called fat transfer, or microlipoinjection. The doctor extracts a tiny amount of fat from another part of your body, such as your belly or buttock, and injects it beneath the wrinkle. There's no danger of an allergic reaction since this is you being injected into you. However, results are short-lived. Researchers aren't sure why, but the fat cells just don't seem to last long in their new location.

Surgical thread can plump up a wrinkle, too, says Dr. Sachs. "The surgeon places a protein-based thread directly under the wrinkle line, where it stimulates local cells to produce their own collagen. In about 6 months or so, the thread dissolves, and the remaining collagen will fill out the wrinkle for 2 to 5 years." Dr. Sachs developed this procedure. Check with your doctor about its availability.

Scrape them away. A procedure called dermabrasion, which is often used to remove acne scars, can also be very effective on wrinkles around the mouth but not on areas where the skin is very thin, such as around the eyes, Dr. Sachs says. A special instrument called a dermabrader literally sands away the top layer of skin, leaving a scab that will heal within about 10 days, he says. A drawback is that dermabrasion often removes pigment from the skin, adds Dr. Resnik. So if you choose this method of wrinkle removal, you'll need to always wear makeup on the treated areas.

When You're Thinking of Surgery

There's a wide range of surgical options for wrinkle removal, says Dr. Tobias. Some surgeries will lift and tighten facial skin, smoothing wrinkles in the process. Other procedures remove wrinkly bags and pouches or fill out wrinkle folds in the skin. Here are two options.

Smooth the eye area. Over the years, eyelids may crease into heavy folds that make you look tired all the time. With a traditional blepharoplasty, or eye-lift operation, a surgeon trims and removes this excess skin for a firmer, younger-looking eye area. Or you may have wrinkly bags above or beneath the eyes that are composed primarily of fat. A new procedure invented by Dr. Sachs, called fat-melting blepharoplasty, can help. A surgeon inserts a heated probe through a tiny incision at the corner of the eye and vaporizes the water content of the fat, which literally melts away the pouches. Recovery times can vary from a few days to a week or more, depending on the procedure used, Dr. Sachs says.

Get rid of gaunt. One of the natural processes of aging is the gradual loss of bone along the jaw and of soft tissue beneath the cheeks. Solid silicone implants can fill out the aging hollows and wrinkle folds that result, says Dr. Tobias. Solid silicone implants have not been associated with the difficulties that have been seen with liquid silicone implants, he adds. Working from incisions within the mouth, a surgeon can insert these forms under cheeks and along the jowl line.

INDEX

Underscored references indicate boxed text.

A

Abdominal fat
  exercise for, <u>208</u>
  stress and, 255
Accidents. *See also* Injuries
  falls, 169–70
  gender differences in, <u>6</u>
  reducing risk of, 167–68
  traffic-related, 170
  workplace, 169–70
Acetaminophen, 78, 226
Acetone, 307
Achilles tendon, shortening of, 117, 119
Achromycin, sun sensitivity from, 37
Acidity, 12, 18
Additives, chemical, 12, 18
Adhesions, in bursitis and tendinitis, 78
Adrenal glands, 11
Advil, 168, 274. *See also* Ibuprofen
Aerobic exercise
  benefits of, 22–25
    abdominal fat loss, <u>208</u>
    arthritis prevention, 25, 49
    back pain prevention, 53
    cancer prevention, 24
    cellulite loss, 80
    depression prevention, 25
    depression relief, 94–95
    diabetes control, 99
    diabetes prevention, 24–25
    energy boost, 23
    HDL cholesterol elevation, 85–86
    heart disease prevention, 24
    injury prevention, 168
    lung health, 225
    memory boost, 177
    menstrual cramp relief, 24
    metabolism boost, 22–23, 189–90
    osteoporosis prevention, 25
    sex drive, 23–24
    sleep improvement, 23
    stress relief, 257–58, 271
    stroke prevention, 25
    weight loss, 212
  bursitis and tendinitis from, 75, <u>76</u>
  endorphins release with, 53
Afrin, 240, 251
Age spots, 37
  melanoma distinguished from, <u>38</u>
  preventing, 38–39
  treatment, 39–41
Aging, 3–5, 6–7
  diet effect on, 42–46
  gender differences, <u>6</u>
Alcohol consumption
  effects of, on
    beer belly, <u>208</u>
    bladder irritation, 218
    breast cancer, 84
    cholesterol level, 84, 153–54
    depression, 94
    fatigue, 115
    gout, 125
    HDL cholesterol level, 153–54
    high blood pressure, 158, 161
    memory problems, 180
    metabolic rate, 192
    osteoporosis, 199, 201
    reaction time, 221
    respiratory system, 225
    sleep apnea, 240
    snoring, 251
    stress, 258
    stroke, 267
    ulcers, 275
  for heart disease prevention, 153–54
  motor vehicle accidents and, 170
Allergy. *See* Asthma
Allicin, 84
Allopurinol, for gout, 128
Alpha-hydroxy acids, 3, 80, 307
Alpha-linolenic acid, 267

use for
    bladder infection prevention, 31–32
    cancer prevention, 31
    constipation prevention, 31, 102
    gout, 125
    heartburn prevention, 103
    incontinence prevention, 61
    respiratory diseases, 226
    skin health, 30–31
    urinary tract infection prevention, 58
    varicose vein prevention, 282, 283
    weight loss, 31, 210
Waxing, 280
Weight, healthy, 206
Weight-bearing exercise, 8
Weight lifting
  blood pressure surges from, 100
  effects of, on
    arthritis, 48–49
    bone health, 203
    breast sag, 68–69
    cellulite, 80
    constipation, 102
    diabetes control, 100
    injury prevention, 168
    metabolism boost, 189–90
    upper arms, 213
    for weight loss, 212–13
  varicose veins and, 282, 283
Weight loss, and
  arthritis, 48
  back pain prevention, 53
  cholesterol reduction, 86
  diabetes control, 98
  double chin, 108
  exercise, 212–13
  gout, 126
  heart disease prevention, 152
  impotence prevention, 163
  incontinence, 61

lowering high blood pressure, 158
nutrition, 209–12
prostate problems, 216
sleep apnea, 239–40
varicose vein prevention, 282, 283
Weight-loss strategy, 207–9
Weight-loss supplements, 213–14
White noise machine, 250
Wine, for heart disease prevention, 153
Workplace
  accidents and injuries, 169–70
  stress and, 255
Worry, 298–301
Wrinkles, 4, 10, 302–10
  prevention, 303–5
  from smoking, 242
  treatment, 305–10, 306
Wrists, bursitis and tendinitis in, 75–77, 76

Y

Yoga, 99, 115
Yogurt, 104–5
Yohimbine, 164

Z

Zeaxanthin, for cataract prevention, 297
Zinc, 45, 179
  deficiency and
    hair loss, 134
    heart disease, 155
  use for
    colds, 226
    eye health, 297
    impotence, 165
    memory boost, 179
    prostate problems, 216
Zyloprim, for gout, 128